HYGIENE PROMOTION
A practical manual for relief and development

SUZANNE FERRON, JOY MORGAN and MARION O'REILLY

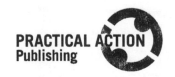

Practical Action Publishing Ltd
Schumacher Centre for Technology and Development
Bourton on Dunsmore, Rugby
Warwickshire, CV23 9QZ, UK
www.practicalactionpublishing.org

ISBN 978-1-85339-641-0
© CARE International, 2007

First published in 2000
Reprinted in 2002
This edition published in 2007
Reprinted 2010

A catalogue record for this book is available from the British Library.

CARE International's mission is to serve individuals and families in the poorest communities
in the world. Drawing strength from its global diversity, resources and experience,
CARE promotes innovative solutions and advocates for global responsibility.
CARE facilitates lasting change by:

o   Strengthening capacity for self-help;
o   Providing economic opportunity;
o   Delivering relief in emergencies;
o   Influencing policy decisions at all levels;
o   Addressing discrimination in all its forms.

Guided by the aspirations of local communities, CARE pursues its mission with both excellence and
compassion because the people whom CARE serves deserve nothing less.

Spanish and Portuguese versions of this books are available at:
www.careusa.org/careswork/whatwedo/health/water.asp

Since 1974, Practical Action Publishing (formerly Intermediate Technology Publications and ITDG
Publishing) has published and disseminated books and information in support of international
development work throughout the world. Practical Action Publishing is a trading name of Practical
Action Publishing Ltd (Company Reg. No. 1159018), the wholly owned publishing company of
Practical Action. Practical Action Publishing trades only in support of its parent charity objectives and
any profits are covenanted back to Practical Action
(Charity Reg. No. 247257, Group VAT Registration No. 880 9924 76).

Cover design by Meena Arnold Design & Distribution
Index preparation: Indexing Specialists (UK) Ltd
Typeset by S.J.I. Services
Printed by Replika Press Pvt. Ltd.

Contents

Acknowledgements

WE ARE PARTICULARLY grateful to Susanne Niedrum for realising the need for this manual, for contacting us, for organizing the funding and for seeing this manual through to completion. We hope you like the final product Susanne!

We thank those who read, used and commented on the draft manual, particularly John Adams, Vicky Blagborough, Ben Elers. Without your efforts this manual would have been half what it is now.

We thank Peter Lochery for receiving and collating the reviewers comments on this manual, and for organizing the final pre-print version and the Spanish, Portuguese translations and CD versions.

We thank those of you whose work has inspired the thoughts and examples incorporated into the text, particularly Simon Ameny, Andy Bastable, David Charles Edwards, Jeff Crisp, Adrian Cullis, Andrew Cunningham, Rennee De La Haye, Sue Emmott, Helena Evans, Manan Ganguli, Gill Gordon, Maurice Herson, Jamila Kerimova, Ann Kiely, Veronica Kloster, Rose Lilonde, Annie Lloyd, Richard Luff, Woldu Mahari, Othman Mahmoud, Shona McKenzie, Cathy Mears, Tim Norwood, Mathew Onduru, Martin Oudman, Bob Reed, Stephen Rusk, George Schroeder, Vivien Walden and the people they were working with in those emergency situations. We would also like to thank those who gave us permission to insert parts of their work and writings into this text.

We thank the artists for their illustrations, drawings and ideas, particularly Ham Kakembo for selecting pictures and organizing the pictures and the layout of the first draft, Joseph Kariuki for the cartoons in the text, Petra Röhr-Rouendaal for the flexiflans and WASH Motivator, Fred Omusula for the unserialized posters, Tony Okuku for the story-with-a-gap pictures, Henry Koské for the three-pile sorting pictures, and Nduhiu Change for organizing them.

We thank CARE International (UK), CARE International (USA), the Dulverton Trust and Oxfam (GB) for funding the writing and production of this manual.

We thank those individuals and organizations that have provided administrative support especially CARE International (Kenya, Uganda, UK) and Lizzie Bell. We would also like to thank Oxfam for their assistance and for many of the field examples.

We also thank John Alexander, Terry Andrews, Andy Bastable, Richard Beedell, Deborah Betts, Dan Bishop, Jill Butler, Paul Eunson, Mary Healey, Ann Henderson, Denise Hurlburt, Caroline Hunt, Tine Jaeger, Bobby Lambert, Cathie Loden, Jean Long, Alma McGhee, Moira Noble, Patricia McPhillips, Helen Pankhurst, Peter Poore, Patta Scott-Villiers, David Smith, Gill Volpe and Gillian Wells for their encouragement and assistance in producing this manual.

Many individuals and organizations not named here have also been instrumental in the development of this manual and we are grateful for their support too.

Finally, we want to thank you for reading this manual and we hope that you will find it both interesting and useful.

Joy Morgan, Suzanne Ferron and
Marion O'Reilly
July 2007

The second edition

THIS SECOND EDITION is an updated version of the original edition. The three authors have between them spent a further 20 years working on hygiene promotion in humanitarian relief and 10 years working in development contexts. This manual has been revised with this additional experience in mind. The second edition contains updated information about the internationally agreed (Sphere) standards for humanitarian response and a greater emphasis on rights-based programming. The planning chapter has been strengthened with problem tree and risk analysis. The chapters on assessment and monitoring and evaluation have been made more practical. The manual also contains more recent field examples in each of the chapters. The flexi-flan pictures have been replaced with those of Petra Röhr-Rouendaal from *Where There Is No Artist* (1997).

About this hygiene promotion manual

WHILE SEVERAL TEXTS on refugee health care explicitly state that health promotion in emergency settings is important, they do not detail how it could be done. The conditions facing those affected by crises and those working with them warrant the development of more specific guidelines, taking into account the variable nature of emergencies and current issues in the provision of emergency relief. This manual attempts to fill a gap in the current literature on health and hygiene education in relief and rehabilitation settings but is also applicable to development settings.

The manual is written mainly for fieldworkers on projects or programmes aiming to reduce the incidence of water- and sanitation- related diseases. It may also be useful to programme managers or ministry officials struggling to integrate water, sanitation and hygiene education/community management into their projects, and for health care workers attempting to address the high incidence of diarrhoeal diseases in either development or emergency programmes.

The manual draws together the experiences of hygiene promotion fieldworkers in humanitarian settings over the last 15 years, experiences from development programmes and the insights of current hygiene promotion theory. The approaches that we have described are flexible enough to be used in a variety of settings. The illustrations and materials have been designed and pre-tested for use in the Great Lakes region of Africa, but could be adapted and used almost anywhere. Working in collaboration with people and allowing them to take more control in the design, implementation and management of water and sanitation systems is central to the aims of hygiene promotion and this concept is also central to this manual. Such action for change cannot be achieved by using didactic approaches to

education that do not encourage the development of problem-solving skills. This manual stresses the need for education that fosters capacity building by not relying on the simple provision of information alone.

It is often assumed that there is little scope for participatory learning outside the development field, but we have tried to look beyond this limited perspective. Wherever there are people there will be opportunities to build on their knowledge and skills through a more interactive type of learning. When we talk about people in communes or settlements, or refugees in camps, it is not to highlight the distinction between them, but rather to explore the learning potential common to both. We hope that the flexibility of approach will maximize the opportunities for promoting hygiene in such challenging environments.

Encouraging participation

Trainers and facilitators who are unfamiliar with participatory methods may initially find it difficult to adapt their style of teaching towards a more learner-centred approach. Participants may also find it difficult to express their opinions if they have been used to a different style of teaching. They will often expect a more formal approach to workshops and training sessions, and they may be surprised at the extent to which they are required to participate. Some may not think that they are learning unless they have taken reams of notes from a lecturer. However, with practice, both participants and facilitators will become more comfortable with the methods used.

There may be other reasons why people feel uncomfortable with the style of participatory sessions. They may lack confidence in themselves and their own opinions. Women, especially, may defer to traditional decision makers in the family and community, and may therefore be reluctant to contradict their husbands or elders. People may not feel that they can bring about change and may therefore feel that it is not worth participating. They may also be afraid of the consequences of participating in group discussions if the issues being discussed are seen to be contentious. These fears, however, are not insurmountable. A participatory approach can generate greater enthusiasm and involvement the more it is used and the better the facilitators become at allowing the participants to direct and shape their own learning and exploration.

Recent commentators on the use of participatory learning have had misgivings that the techniques might be employed simply as a 'bag of tricks' for use *on* the community instead of *with* the community. There is indeed a danger that the activities will be used as an end in themselves rather than as the means to an end. The main purpose for using such techniques should be to stimulate open and creative discussion about a particular situation from the perspective of participants. If the facilitator fails to 'hand over the stick' and relinquish control of the discussion, this will not happen.

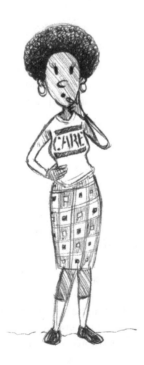

Preventing helplessness

The avoidance of helplessness and dependency may be critical in promoting mental, physical and social health, as well as in saving lives. Men, women, boys and girls affected by a crisis are less likely to feel like helpless victims if they are involved in making decisions about how aid is provided. Participatory hygiene promotion seeks to do this and it is therefore as vital to emergency relief as it is to development work. In recent years the new rights-based approach has sought to recognize people's right to humanitarian assistance and the importance of meeting standards in the provision of aid. The Sphere project and its associated manual sets out these standards and champions the importance of both participation and hygiene promotion in aid interventions. However, many technical and medical programmes still assign low priority to hygiene and health promotion and many aid workers have little experience of using participatory methods. This manual tries to provide practical information and ideas on how to approach hygiene promotion in different emergency and rehabilitation settings.

Mixing hygiene promotion approaches during different emergency phases

Throughout the manual we emphasize the use of empowering approaches but do not exclude the necessity of using other strategies. It is possible in fact to move in and out of these approaches, depending on the situation. A directive approach is probably necessary in the early stages of an emergency when people are overwhelmed by the ordeal of their flight to safety. For example, at the height of a cholera outbreak, it may be necessary to enforce the use of latrines or areas specially designated for defecation while operating a campaign providing messages on what to do in order to prevent sickness. This may be effective during the acute stage of an emergency, as people may be more willing to listen and respond to messages. In the long term, message-based health education is unlikely to have a sustained impact on people's lives. A more empowering approach to hygiene promotion becomes easier to undertake in the intermediate, recovery and resettlement phases of the emergency. At this point the blanket message-based health education could be refined into a strategic social marketing campaign to create a market demand for improved water supplies or sanitation facilities. At the same time, more empowering participatory approaches to hygiene promotion could be focused on specific vulnerable or 'at risk' groups.

Using the manual

The manual has been divided into six chapters. A detailed list of the headings and sub-headings of each section is contained in the Contents at the front of the manual. The comprehensive Index is intended to assist you to find your way around and to identify the sections that interest you most.

The introduction chapter contains the theory and principles of promoting hygiene in emergencies and in development contexts. It is written in a more formal style than the rest of the manual. The project cycle has been used to structure the next four chapters, with separate chapters on assessment, planning, implementation, and monitoring and evaluation. For each phase of the cycle we have tried to provide suggestions for working with communities to promote health and hygiene in a variety of contexts. The final section is the Appendices, which contain details of how to do the various activities mentioned in the main chapters and contain pictures to be used and adapted for these activities. It also contains some examples of job descriptions, training schedules, a menu of excreta disposal technologies with their advantages and disadvantages, information about common water and sanitation-related diseases and community management, a glossary and an annotated bibliography.

We intend the manual to be used as a resource for both relief and development workers. It is difficult to direct you to specific parts of the text for ideas about either emergency or development contexts. There are very few sections that can be identified as purely relief oriented. We feel that part of the richness of the text comes from contrasting and comparing a range of situations. All situations are different and even the same situation differs over time and with various people's perspectives. Each community will be different and some activities may work well with some groups and others may not. This is regardless of the stage in an emergency relief or development process. The material provided is not meant to stifle creativity nor prevent the invention of new activities and approaches. The example activities and resource materials may need to be adapted to suit specific local conditions.

Go ahead and experiment!

List of boxes

List of figures

List of tables

Abbreviations and acronyms

CMC — community management committee
DRC — Democratic Republic of Congo
HAPI — Humanitarian Accountability Partnership International
IDP — internally displaced person
LFA — logical framework analysis
LLIN — long lasting insecticide treated net
LQAS — lot quality assurance sampling
MDG — Milliennium Development Goal
NFI — non-food item
O&M — operation and maintenance
ORS — oral rehydration solution
PLA — participatory learning and action
PRA — participatory rural appraisal
PTSD — post-traumatic stress disorder
RRA — rapid rural appraisal
VIP — ventilated improved pit

Introduction

Emergency contexts

EMERGENCIES ARISE WHEN communities have difficulty in adapting to and coping with the changes brought about by a disaster. This can occur as a result of disasters such as floods, droughts and earthquakes. It can also occur because of changes in social conditions such as those caused by wars or political expulsion. People's ability to survive these catastrophic events is related to their socio-economic status and their degree of preparedness.

In 1994, the Great Lakes region in Africa saw some of the largest population movements in history. Regional conflict left many thousands of people displaced from their homes or living in exile. Those who returned to their homes continued to live in uncertainty and relative instability as they attempted to rebuild their lives. The lack of tolerance for cultural and ethnic differences combined with political, social, economic and environmental factors underpin conflicts such as these, which have become known as 'complex emergencies'. Rather than resulting in a return to normality, such emergencies often leave populations struggling with chronic crises. In the mid-1990s, the majority of emergency relief assistance was related to complex emergencies.

In 1998, devastating floods swept Asian and Latin American countries including China, India, Bangladesh, Nicaragua and Honduras, causing among the worst 'natural' disasters in history and claiming many thousands of lives. Over-exploitation of resources, massive deforestation in the uplands, giant dams and river control systems are blamed for the flooding. In 1998, almost a third of all emergencies were weather related and since then the proportion of 'natural' disasters has continued to rise, in part due to global environmental degradation.

In parts of Africa, HIV/AIDS constitutes a chronic emergency that is undermining the fabric of society while conflict and its aftermath has left thousands of people struggling to survive or rebuild their lives. Political instability and insecurity continue to undermine the health and well-being of much of the population of the Democratic Republic of Congo (DRC) and the Darfur region of North Sudan, while drought and food insecurity threaten populations in several African regions. As well as the annual floods to which they are prone, South and East Asia have been the victims of the 2005 tsunami and a major earthquake.

Phases of emergencies

Disasters or emergencies are sometimes described as following a four-phased linear progression as detailed below:

Acute phase, which may last for days or weeks and is usually characterized by people in transition or newly arrived at a location, camp or settlement. Their focus is on acquiring the basic necessities: food, water and shelter. Their physical safety may be uncertain. Depending on the conditions that prevailed before and during their flight, there may be high levels of illness, malnutrition and physical injury. High rates of sickness and mortality may be evident (the crude death rate may be out of control at over 2.0 deaths per 10,000 population per day[1]). A high incidence of water- and sanitation-related diseases is likely

---

[1] The Sphere manual gives mortality rates disaggregated for different geographical regions.

because of the lack of sanitation, water and the most basic requirements for personal and family hygiene. Families may also have become separated and communities fragmented.

Intermediate phase may endure for weeks or months and is characterized by increasing stability in the camp or settlement. Basic provision of food, water, sanitation and medical care is in place, though it may be inadequate. Mortality and morbidity rates should be decreasing (crude death rates between 1.0 and 2.0 deaths per 10,000 population per day). If communities have managed to stay together, social structures and hierarchies may have been re-established or new ones built.

Establishment phase may follow the intermediate phase when it becomes apparent that a prolonged stay in the camp or settlement is likely. The infrastructure for long-term habitation will be either established or developing, and new or previous systems of community organization will be operating. Schools may be functioning, religious groups mobilized and government structures may be involved in the delivery of services. Morbidity and mortality rates are unlikely to be higher than the normal rates expected for the population of the local area (normal crude mortality rate in developing countries is 0.5 deaths per 10,000 population per day). People may be able to engage in routine daily activities such as cultivation and attending the market.

Resettlement phase involves the migration of people back to their communities of origin where, to a greater or lesser extent, they will try to re-establish their former existence. They may build new settlements, or return to situations where the previous infrastructure has been damaged, for example, ransacked housing, damaged water and sanitation systems. Social structures may need to be revived in the absence of those formerly responsible for their management and organization.

Conceptualizing emergencies in this way is over-simplistic and may not apply to every situation but nonetheless may be useful, as particular interventions may be required during different phases. The decisions made by relief workers about these emergency interventions will have consequences for months, perhaps years, following their implementation (e.g. development).

Effect on health and hygiene patterns

In the course of an emergency, and particularly following displacement to large camp settings, normal patterns of water use and hygiene behaviour are often disrupted and individuals rendered more susceptible than usual to water- and sanitation-related diseases. Normal social structures and support networks may also be disrupted or reorganized so that some individuals become more vulnerable to exploitation and insecurity as well as to shortages of the basic essentials for survival.

The mental health of refugees, displaced people and returnees is often a cause for concern as trauma and displacement can result in depression and despair. Little is known about the effects of collective or prolonged trauma on communities in developing countries as research has concentrated on the impact of war on individuals from industrialized countries. However, post-traumatic stress disorder (PTSD) is known to be associated with recurrent painful and intrusive recollections of painful events, irritability, restlessness, explosive anger, and feelings of guilt, anxiety, and depression. Approaches to relief and rehabilitation that treat people as passive and dependent victims may further serve to undermine the mental health of people struggling to recover from trauma and displacement.

Hygiene promotion needs to be integrated into the relief or rehabilitation programme as part of a holistic strategy that encourages greater participation and more accountability of the programme towards those who have been affected. It is often thought that children are not as traumatized as adults in complex emergencies. However they often notice more than is recognized. They too have a right to participate in decisions about the provision of support. Encouraging participation may then be seen as a way of harnessing resourceful responses and saving time in both the short and the long term. The problem remains of how participation can be made possible. While

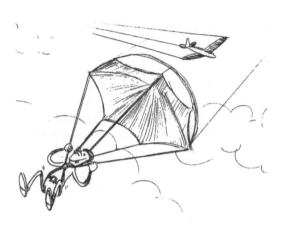

influenced by the need for publicity for their activities in order to ensure further funding. They may be perceived as being 'short-term, short-lived, top-heavy, centralized, standardized, resource-intensive, donor-dependent and neglecting of local administrative structures and social norms' (Duffield, 1994). Once involved with relief for those affected by complex emergencies, organizations may become part of the dynamic of the conflict and may even help to perpetuate it. Interventions may become self-justifying and undermine the need for disaster mitigation (Duffield, 1994).

development organizations struggle to reorient their practice towards working in partnership with the poor, many emergency programmes still fail to recognize this as an important objective. Participation requires commitment at all levels and also some risk-taking by those individuals and agencies who are courageous enough to dare to be different and who can act as a catalyst for change.

Preventing loss of life during an emergency must take precedence, but the interplay between mental and physical health should not be underestimated.

Developmental approach to relief

Development programmes are characterized by a long-term perspective that develops and builds on local structures and maximizes opportunities for community participation. Interventions try to be sensitive to local power structures, but also try to avoid marginalizing less powerful individuals or groups. They seek to discourage dependence on aid and aim to create systems and structures that are sustainable by the population in the long term.

Do relief. . . think development!

Relief programmes are often criticized by those who work in longer term development programmes. They are seen as being driven by their own priorities rather than those of the affected population. To this end, they are significantly

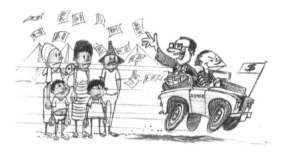

Over time both aid workers and affected populations find security in their roles: the former as active, authoritative problem solvers, and the latter as passive, dependent recipients of aid. It may be difficult to move towards a more collaborative and participative way of working. The pressures exerted on agency staff to take immediate action to save lives mean that often their work is hastily planned and implemented, and mechanisms for evaluation are not put in place early enough. Aid workers are often expatriates who may have a very limited knowledge of the cultural and social traditions of the refugees or displaced people they are working with. The often rapid turnover of staff on short-term contracts can prevent adequate institutional learning from the situation, and may mean that the same mistakes are repeated time and time again.

> *No relief programme can be neutral in its effect on development, they either support it or they undermine it.*
> Williams, 1995

> *Relief aid can distort local markets and create a degree of dependence amongst the people it is designed to benefit. It can be used by the parties in a conflict to feed their soldiers and supporters, thereby prolonging or intensifying the war.*
>
> Crisp, 1997

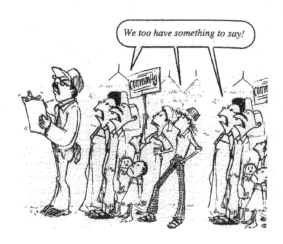

The way agencies intervene in emergencies may adversely influence affected populations, creating a disincentive to self-help and hindering appropriate social and political adjustments.

Relief needs to be informed by development theory and practice that emphasizes the need to facilitate cooperative actions, participation in decision making and political reform. The provision of relief should support people to cope with change, and promote positive change where appropriate. Recent emphasis on a rights-based approach to interventions forces aid workers to recognize the obligation that they and governments have to provide an acceptable level of assistance in an acceptable way. The Sphere manual of minimum standards outlines this approach and is underpinned by a variety of legal instruments such as human rights law, humanitarian law and the Geneva conventions. The emphasis is no longer on simply saving lives but also on promoting 'life with dignity'.

Participation and accountability

The term 'participation' is open to many interpretations, and its meaning is frequently obscure. The key is to analyse the interests represented in the catch-all term 'participation'. Different people will perceive the advantages of participation differently. For example, a nominal form of involvement might be getting refugees to dig drainage soak-pits as a contribution to a water supply scheme. However, people's enthusiasm for a project depends much more on whether they have a genuine interest in it, rather than whether they merely participated in its construction. A representative form of participation would encourage refugees to express their views on how interventions should be carried out, including their roles in them. An empowering form of participation allows people (including those from marginalized groups) to decide on their own priorities for action, and how agencies might facilitate them to take action. If participation means that the voiceless gain a voice, then power relations within that society will often be challenged and conflict should be expected. Participation may thus become the focus for struggle.

> *It is important to recognize that people who have been affected by the emergency are a resource, not a crowd of helpless victims.*
>
> Gosling and Edwards, 1995

A World Bank (1991) discussion paper on participation formulated a taxonomy of participation ranging from information provision to control and decision making. The paper stressed that there is no correct level of participation, and that the optimum level will depend on circumstances. While this may undermine the political and radical nature of participation, it appears to give a clearer representation of the reality that relief and development workers struggle with.

There is a tendency to assume that it is always good for people to take an active part in all community projects, but participation is more complicated than that. There are always tensions regarding who is involved, how, and on whose terms. While participation has the potential to challenge patterns of dominance, it can reinforce existing power relations.

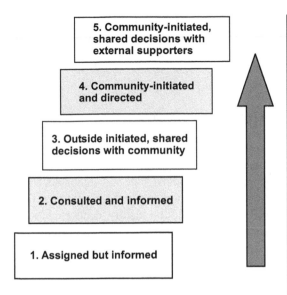

5. Community-initiated, shared decisions with external supporters

4. Community-initiated and directed

3. Outside initiated, shared decisions with community

2. Consulted and informed

1. Assigned but informed

Figure 0.1 Participation steps
Source: UNICEF, 1999.

People have always participated on the most favourable terms they can obtain. They find out what each agency is offering and what it will want in return, judge its suitability to their interests and opt in or out of projects accordingly. Sometimes they resort to manipulation, sabotage and covert resistance to express their interests. Participation may also happen for negative reasons. For instance, people may not be confident that their interests will be represented unless they are physically present. For some, choosing to participate may not be a feasible option, for example, women with heavy domestic responsibilities may find that they cannot sustain the expenditure of large amounts of time away from the household and some may grow tired of being 'active citizens'. Participation therefore may not always be in the interests of the poor. The value of participation depends on the type of participation and the terms on which it is offered. In some cases, opting out may be the most empowering option (White, 1996).

Ways must be found to increase people's participation in keeping with the call for a developmental approach to relief. In its response to emergencies, the international community and those involved in humanitarian assistance must become

Box 0.1 Reasons why women don't participate

A study conducted by the CARE water and sanitation project in Byumba, Rwanda, found that a mixture of socio-cultural and organizational issues contributed towards women's failure to participate in the project:

○ The community had traditional views of women's roles as mothers that did not encourage their involvement in broader community activities;
○ Men's permission was usually needed for women to move outside the home;
○ Decision making and economic control within the family was usually the responsibility of the male head of household;
○ Information about the project was directed towards men, and low levels of literacy and the lack of training among the women presented a barrier to their involvement;
○ Those in charge of the project did not take sufficient measures to interest the women in the project, and women in turn did not feel that they needed to be involved.

Source: CARE, 1993, personal communication.

Box 0.2 Promoting accountability

In camps in Aceh and Sri Lanka that were formed following the Asian Tsunami in 2004, some NGOs provided information boards where they described programme activities and lists of the costs of the non-food items that they planned to distribute. In other contexts, suggestion boxes have been placed in communities or settlements so that individuals can feed back comments to the agencies involved.

more accountable to beneficiaries or claimants (as the new rights-based language dictates). Humanitarian Accountability Partnership International

(HAPI) suggests accountability involves two sets of principles and mechanisms:

1. those by which individuals, organizations and states account for their actions and are held responsible for them;
2. those by which emergency affected communities may safely and legitimately report concerns, complaints and get redress where appropriate.

Hygiene promotion activities usually involve programme staff in frequent and regular face to face contact with people affected by emergencies and hygiene promoters are often responsible for collecting monitoring data. They are therefore well placed to ensure a good two way flow of information and feedback between the programme and the community and can play an important role in helping to make sure that the programme responds to changing needs, including the need for protection, as the humanitarian situation evolves.

Protection

In recent years the aid community has become more aware of the limits of responding only to people's physical needs, especially in complex emergencies where people's greatest fear may be that they will be the object of violence or coercion. Young men may be forced to fight or young girls kidnapped to provide for armies on the move. Protection policies and interventions have mainly been applied in programmes where conflict is a feature but even following natural disasters people may become more vulnerable to violence or coercion, for example, when women feel forced to provide sexual favours in return for food or cash when crops have been destroyed, or when domestic violence becomes more commonplace because of feelings of inadequacy amongst male breadwinners after their means of livelihood has been destroyed. Protection policies are informed by legal frameworks and interventions try to raise awareness about legal requirements and responsibilities. Most countries are signatories to human rights laws and conventions but where this is not the case or they neglect their duty to enforce them, lobbying and advocacy on an international scale may help to bring them into line. At a local level, pressure may be brought to bear by discussing the practical implications of these laws.

Affected communities

Any community is usually made up of people from a variety of backgrounds, rich and poor, non-literate and professional, élite and oppressed. Great variations in experience and perspective reflect differences in cultural history, gender relations, socio-economic status, age and education.

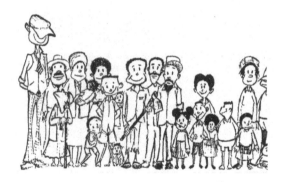

In this respect, communities affected by disasters are no different. However, the social structures that contribute to cohesion in most stable communities have often been fragmented. Families may have parted. During times of conflict, men will often stay on to fight while women flee with their children, the elderly and the disabled in search of safety. The trauma of uprooting and increased vulnerability to physical and sexual attack is compounded by the loss of normal family ties, property and possessions, and by forced changes in roles and status. People who are rendered particularly vulnerable by displacement include women (especially female heads of household), unaccompanied children, the elderly, the sick and the disabled.

Women's experience

Although the experience of displacement is harrowing for all displaced people, women are often the most seriously affected. The harassment of women and girls may be the cause of flight, and is a continuing threat from the day they leave their homes to find safety. They may lack physical protection, they may also be in constant threat of being captured or killed. The continuous danger of rape and sexual harassment mark their journeys world wide. Once arriving in the new situation, women continue to be vulnerable to physical and sexual violence even from their own men, who themselves may be suffering from acute stress and breakdown. Fear of physical and sexual harassment within and outside displaced settlements can keep women and girls confined to their homes (Wallace, 1990). The mental and physical suffering experienced by those women and girls who have been, or fear being, molested or raped is to date unsatisfactorily dealt with and may even be ignored by officials.

> *Many women in Darfur sought refuge in camps after their villages were burned by militia and they were subjected to physical and sexual abuse and sometimes to rape. Even after their arrival in the camps they were not safe as they had to venture outside regularly to collect firewood and were often attacked as they went about this essential chore.*
> Oxfam, 2004, personal communication

The traditional gender roles of a woman include that of water carrier, caretaker of family health, teacher of hygiene practices and user of water for production. In emergencies, women may have to take on a wide range of additional roles and responsibilities within the family and community, and at the same time they have to adjust to living in an alien situation. As refugees, many women and children become heads of household for the first time in their lives. In addition, women often take responsibility for social education and trying to maintain cultural cohesion; two of the most critical factors for coping, especially in the early days of flight and disruption. Yet programmes for refugees are not always targeted at women or children as household heads, and it is often the case that the allocation of land, food, tools, jobs and legal identity papers are made directly to adult male household heads, leaving these women and children in even more vulner-

able positions. Training and employment programmes are often targeted at men, again leaving women and children – who usually have less education and fewer employment skills than men – in a very weak position to care for themselves or their families. In many situations, even where a woman or child is not officially the household head, male heads of household may neglect their responsibilities because of family breakdown and stress. Divorce and serial marriage are common in communities living under stress, leaving women with the sole responsibility for the children (Wallace, 1990).

> *In some tsunami affected communities, more men than women survived, leaving a skewed gender balance of up to three men to one woman. The effects of the imbalance are being investigated. There are concerns that young women will be pressured into early marriage with negative consequences for their health, fertility and education.*
> UNFPA et al, 2005

Women's health and food needs are frequently poorly met in emergency situations. Food rations are often distributed through men and adult male household heads, giving men control over supplies and consequently greater power. This is inevitably open to misuse. It is certainly still the case that women and children may get less than their allocation, or be asked for favours in order to receive their ration. Sexual violence and coercion are often associated with displacement due to conflict but can arise in any context where resources are scarce. With the overburdening or breakdown of health care services, which is frequently a feature of emergencies, there is the potential for an increase in sexually transmitted infections including HIV transmission.

While women are often responsible for family welfare, their access to employment is limited. When seeking formal employment they, like most displaced people, often suffer discrimination. But, in addition, they may lack the skills to get anything more than the lowest paid jobs and even then they are often paid lower wages than men. Aid agencies tend to employ more displaced men on their projects and often target their employ-ment work to male heads of households, mainly for reasons of speed, ease of communication and the belief that the men are responsible for all the women and children. The fact that a women or a child may often be responsible for feeding the family forces many women into illegal activities such as brewing and prostitution for their sur-vival.

Living in a hostile environment, with little im-mediate hope of a return home, many refugees see education as vital. It is often seen as the only way to create a better future for the next genera-tion and many women request that education serv-ices for their children be set up immediately dur-ing the acute emergency phase. There is also a real need for basic education courses such as literacy classes and language training to equip them with the new skills required in the host country.

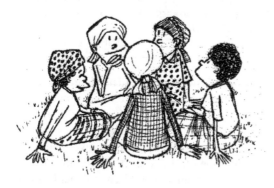

HIV/AIDS in emergencies

Emergencies make people more susceptible to becoming infected with HIV, while AIDS suffer-ers and their carers are often more vulnerable than others to the impact of emergencies.

Evidence is emerging to suggest that HIV transmission increases with displacement due to conflict for many reasons (see box). For those already HIV positive or suffering from AIDS, dis-ruption to health care and public health services may cause a deterioration in health status or may hasten the progression of the disease, thereby increasing the stress on families and carers. An emergency response programme may uninten-tionally increase transmission rates by creating opportunities for sexual transactions between

> *Factors fuelling the HIV pandemic include: massive population displacement, disruption of family and social structures, disruption of social networks, sexual interaction of emergency affected people with military or paramilitary personnel, the economic vulnerability of women and unaccompanied minors, the frequency of commercial sex work, the frequency of sexual violence and coercive sex, psychological trauma, the disruption of preventative and curative health services, unsafe blood transfusions at a time of increased blood transfusion requirements, the increased use of illicit drugs, and the high prevalence of sexually transmitted infections...host refugee/IDP [internally displaced person] interaction, especially rural people with lower HIV prevalence and less HIV knowledge interacting with urban population with higher both.*
>
> Khaw et al, 2000

vulnerable individuals. HIV/AIDS, like gender, can be considered as a cross-cutting issue in water, sanitation and hygiene promotion programmes. As a minimum there should be a rapid analysis of the HIV context and awareness raising with staff to ensure that response activities do not exacer-bate the situation and that they are designed to prevent increased transmission if possible. The specific needs of infected and affected individu-als and families should be considered along with those of other vulnerable people. Some initial considerations on how to do this are listed in the assessment and planning chapters on pages 25–27 and 40. More detailed background information on HIV/AIDS and on mainstreaming can be found in documents listed in the Bibliography section.

Working with communities

People who are affected positively or negatively by a project may be referred to as 'stakeholders'. This term will include the target population, project staff, donors, government departments, local organizations, other populations affected by the project, and the private sector.

Stakeholders can be identified through data collection and effective liaising and communication

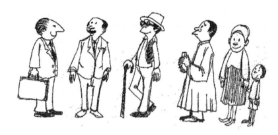

with other organizations and structures at all levels. Venn and flow diagrams can be useful to promote discussion on stakeholder relationships with community members (see page 111 in the Appendices). The importance, influence and needs of key stakeholders should be identified.

Influence is the power that stakeholders have to control decisions, facilitate implementation or exert influence over the project. It is the extent to which stakeholders are able to persuade or coerce others into making decisions and following certain courses of action. *Importance* indicates the priority given by the project to satisfying those stakeholders' needs and interests through the project. In general, their needs and interests can be determined by examining the goal, purpose and outputs of the project. The levels of importance and influence of each stakeholder determines the extent to which their needs should be considered by the project.

Key stakeholders are those with significant influence or importance for the success of the project. Good relationships with key stakeholders are essential for the project's success and their needs will have to be addressed by the project. Those stakeholders with high importance and low influence require special initiatives by the project to protect their interests. Where a group of stakeholders have high influence and low importance they could pose a significant risk to the project if their needs are not met, and should be closely monitored. Those with low influence and low importance are unlikely to be the subject of the project's activities and their views can be ignored. Details of how to do a stakeholder analysis and an example can be found in the appendices on pages 224–26.

The views of key informant and influential stakeholders should be sought regarding the potential strengths, weaknesses, opportunities and threats posed by the project. Some examples of points to consider are listed below:

○ A project's *strength* may also be a *weakness*. Providing employment opportunities for local people may entice them away from jobs within local structures, whose capacity is thus undermined.

○ *Opportunities* to extend the influence of the project locally may involve supporting local structures, for example, by collaborating with them on training or by sharing materials and resources. Extending the impact further, opportunities for sharing information and pursuing joint advocacy strategies with other organizations may contribute to national or international policy decisions.

○ *Threats* to the success of the project may be posed when its interests potentially conflict with those of others, for example, when a scarce resource such as water or health care has to be shared with the host community.

Analysing the potential of the project in this way can help to identify areas where discussion, negotiation, and compromise will be required in order to avoid conflict or the marginalisation of particular groups.

Life-saving interventions should not be insensitive to the skills and capacities of the affected population. Agencies must set in place mechanisms for collaboration, taking into account the knowledge, opinions and priorities of different groups. The leaders of affected populations often do not expect to be involved in decision making. However, if they have access to the information gained during agencies' assessments, the involvement of local leaders and community representatives in planning and decision making could become a reality. Monitoring and evaluating participation in planning, decision making and implementation is also vital if agencies are to become more accountable to the men, women and children affected by emergencies. Indicators that reflect levels of participation should be measured alongside the more familiar mortality and morbidity data.

The host community will often be another important stakeholder. They may require special attention to make sure that they are included in the

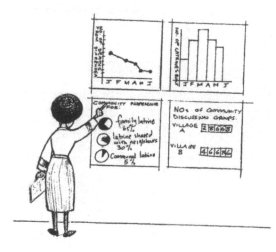

project activities. Often they are left out of project decisions and become marginalized. Even when the host community welcomes the displaced people in the short term, in the longer term they often come to resent the impact of the displaced on their environment, health and services. They often consider that displaced people are given favoured treatment, for example, free food, free medical treatment, ample supplies of water. It may be necessary to lobby for basic service provision for host communities in some circumstances in order to avoid conflict.

Sudanese refugees in Eastern Chad brought herds of camels, goats and donkeys with them when they crossed the border. Conditions in the host villages were very basic. While the refugees had access to clean piped water, the host community used water collected from shallow wells dug into the dry river bed. The visitors' animals shared their sparse grazing pasture causing some resentment while a local school serving several host villages had to close because the teachers left to take up jobs with international NGOs.

Oxfam, 2005, personal communication

Community management
Experience has shown that the long-term maintenance of water and sanitation installations should always be taken into account, even in emergency situations. This is especially important where

permanent water supplies are being constructed or renovated. People will not automatically assume responsibility for keeping the system functional in the longer term, and may think that this will be taken care of by the agency concerned. The community may well have 'participated' in construction work but (as we have said before) this does not automatically mean that they will feel a sense of ownership for the completed project. Recent research (Schouten and Moriarty, 2003) has shown that ongoing institutional support is necessary to ensure sustainability and it cannot be assumed that training water and sanitation committees and pump attendants will be sufficient to ensure effective community management.

Benako and Lumasi were two camps in Ngara, Tanzania established for Rwandan refugees in 1994. Benako camp was set up very rapidly and in an unplanned manner with refugee participation limited to paid manual labour. Agencies provided tools, construction materials and expatriate labour to establish and run the camp. Lumasi was set up more slowly and in a planned manner. Refugees were involved in the planning, implementation, operation and maintenance of all camp facilities from the beginning. Minimal material inputs were provided by relief agencies to encourage refugees to use local materials under their own initiative. By 1996, when external funding was dwindling, both camps had almost become permanent settlements. Benako needed to cut services dramatically, while Lumasi was able to maintain its more modest services because of its low reliance on external funds. Interestingly, morbidity and mortality rates were consistently lower in Lumasi than in Benako.

Schroeder, 1997

It is important to consider the following points:

○ Do people in the community consider that the project responds to a priority felt need?
○ Have women and children as well as men been involved as far as possible in the initial discussions on the proposed project?

o Does the project have the support of local government and community leaders? (If respected community leaders are available they should be leading the discussions rather than the agency involved.)

o If people do not attend meetings, try to find out why not and whether alternative arrangements can be made.

o Ensure that the issue of long-term maintenance is raised as soon as possible with community groups. Ask them how they intend to repair the system if it breaks down or what provision they have made for this in the past. Ensure that issues of financial accountability are also discussed.

o Try to ensure open and ongoing dialogue about the project. It is important to remain flexible and to encourage suggestions from community members on how the project should proceed.

o Formal agreements and contracts should be drafted when discussions have been finalized.

An overview of community management is included in the appendices.

Hygiene promotion

Health effects of water, sanitation and hygiene practices

Improvements in water supply, sanitation and hygiene are important barriers to many infectious diseases. Research carried out by Esrey and Habicht (1986) and Esrey et al (1991) in a range of development contexts, showed that safer excreta disposal led to a reduction of childhood diarrhoea of up to 36 per cent. Handwashing, food protection and improvements in domestic hygiene brought a reduction in infant diarrhoea of 33 per cent. In contrast, improving water quality alone produced limited reductions in childhood diarrhoea by 15 to 20 per cent. Reductions in other diseases, such as schistosomiasis (77 per cent), ascariasis (29 per cent) and trachoma (27–50 per cent) are also related to better sanitation and hygiene practices. Only the reduction in guinea worm can be totally ascribed to the quality of water (Van Wijk and Murre, 1995). Studies of the joint effect of water, sanitation and hygiene interventions show that the greatest health improvements are found when interventions occurred together (68 per cent). Besides reductions in diarrhoea, improvements in nutritional status, including the reduction in the prevalence of stunting and wasting of children by 38 per cent, as well as savings in time and energy expenditure have been reported (Esrey, 1995). A recent meta analysis of 17 hand washing studies (Curtis and Cairncross, 2003) showed a mean reduction in diarrhoea incidence of 43 per cent. Another recent meta analysis by Fewtrell et al (2005) suggests that hygiene (mainly hand washing) is the most significant factor (42 per cent), then excreta disposal (32 per cent). The impact of water quality (30 per cent) suggests that point of use treatment may be effective in reducing diarrhoea. Hand washing also appears to reduce the incidence of colds and flu (Ryan et al, 2001).

The two most important practices for hygiene promotion programmes to target are:

o Safe excreta disposal;
o Hand washing with soap after contact with excreta (adult, child or infant).

The contribution of water- and sanitation-related diseases to morbidity and mortality is exacerbated by population displacements. Studies of displaced people in various countries have shown that diarrhoeal diseases contribute to between 25 and 50 per cent of all deaths. Lack of water for bathing (leading to skin and eye diseases) is a major cause of morbidity, especially among those under five years of age (Toole and Waldman, 1990). Following the influx of Rwandan refugees to Goma in 1994, 50,000 deaths were attributed to an 'explosive epidemic' of diarrhoeal diseases including cholera and dysentery (Goma Epidemiology Group, 1995). Deaths from cholera are usually far fewer in number than those from other types of diarrhoea, but in this case they made up approximately 25 per cent of all deaths. The disease was spread by rapid contamination of drinking water sources, inadequate sanitation, poor hygiene and overcrowding. Providing improved water and sanitation facilities is vital for improving health in refugee camps. However, the provision of facilities alone does not necessarily ensure that people will use them effectively. Many emergency and development water and sanitation projects have failed in the long term because pumps or other facilities have not been maintained. Hygiene promotion tries to ensure that the potential benefits of such facilities are optimized and sustained both through improved use and maintenance of facilities, and through improved hygiene practices.

Approaches to promoting health and hygiene

The terms 'hygiene education' and 'hygiene promotion' and their relationship to health education and health promotion need to be explained. In this context, hygiene promotion is an umbrella term used to cover a range of strategies that aim to prevent water- and sanitation-related diseases, and optimize the short- and long-term effects of water and sanitation interventions. It includes the use of education, learning and social marketing strategies, and also encompasses the community management of engineering installations, which is vital if facilities are to have a lasting impact.

Hygiene promotion has traditionally been seen as the provision of information to induce behaviour change (hygiene education). This kind of didactic approach to hygiene promotion does not attempt to empower people to make decisions, or take account of the context or culture of the target population. Message-focused didactic approaches were founded on the belief that giving people information about the causal link between their behaviour and ill health would automatically change their attitudes towards damaging practices and would ultimately cause them to change their behaviour. Such approaches assume that when people understand how water and sanitation diseases are transmitted, unhygienic practices will be dropped and improved ones adopted. However, message-based approaches to disease avoidance often have very disappointing results.

Social marketing has shown that positive messages reinforcing status and personal dignity are often more likely to influence behaviour. It has been shown to work well where the intervention is first developed in a small-scale participatory manner and then applied on a larger scale across camps, urban centres, counties or regions. This

---

Box 0.3 Hygiene promotion

Hygiene promotion:

- ○ is the planned and systematic attempt to enable people to take action to prevent water- and sanitation-related illness, and to maximize the benefits of improved water and sanitation facilities;
- ○ combines insider/affected population knowledge (what do people know, do and want) with outsider knowledge (e.g. the causes of diarrhoeal diseases, communications and learning strategies);
- ○ includes (but is not exclusively) the provision of information and learning opportunities regarding aspects of personal and environmental hygiene, including water provision, excreta disposal, drainage, solid waste disposal and vector control (more commonly known as hygiene education);
- ○ makes better hygiene possible in an emergency by providing essential items that may be in short supply, such as water and food storage containers, soap, and menstrual protection materials;
- ○ provides the crucial link between people in the community and the technical interventions during all stages of a project cycle.

Hygiene promotion has a narrower focus than health promotion, but both attempt to enable people to take action to prevent illness.

Source: Curtis and Kanki, 1998; Ferron, 2003.

---

approach is not without its contradictions and has been criticized for being manipulative. It is centred on the user's perspective yet it has a firm agenda. It uses participatory methods to develop the marketing strategies but it is not necessarily intended to be empowering.

While changes in behaviour often require access to knowledge, and frequently a change in attitudes, this is not always the case. It is also important to realize that individuals are not solely responsible for their own health. Many factors such as poverty, housing, food supply and cultural norms and values may compromise their capacity to accept and act upon health or social marketing messages.

People also have widely differing ideas about health and disease that are socially and culturally determined (Kleinmann et al, 1978). These are not necessarily consistent within any one culture. The risk of aid workers imposing their own interpretations on the needs of a displaced community is therefore very great. Aid programmes must learn to be more sensitive to claimants' different perceptions and interpretations of need by according them more control in the planning and implementation of programmes.

Health and hygiene promotion are being redefined to stress a more facilitative and enabling approach to promoting health, with the realization that control over one's life and the capacity and confidence to make one's own decisions are crucial to promoting and maintaining health. Hygiene education cannot just be a matter of providing information and persuading people to change their behaviour; it must be part of a broader health promotion framework. Such a framework attempts to address the structural determinants of health, such as the provision of adequate quantities of safe water, the provision of sanitation facilities, adequate and appropriate food rations and access to health care. At the same time, health promotion should facilitate individual action within the existing constraints by supporting people's capacity to control the factors that determine their own health and the health of others.

Naidoo and Wills (1994) outline a schema of descriptive approaches to health promotion that can be readily adapted to hygiene promotion, as follows:

○ *Medical/preventive* – identifies and makes provision for those at risk, for example by the distribution of soap and the chlorination of water;
○ *Behavioural change* – encourages individuals to make lifestyle changes through, for example, one-to-one counselling during home visits or social marketing campaigns to promote latrine use or improved hygiene practices;
○ *Educational* – increases knowledge and skills, for example by implementing training for hygiene educators;
○ *Empowerment* – involves working with the community to meet perceived needs through advocacy, negotiation and networking;
○ *Social change* – addresses inequalities such as women being expected to work voluntarily as educators while their male counterparts are paid as labourers.

An eclectic approach is needed that suits the population, and the time and place, and is aimed at the individual and the structures that influence individuals and groups. People themselves should be at the centre of any approach to health and hygiene promotion, even in the emergency setting. By building on people's existing capacities they can be empowered to make decisions about their lives and to take action for change. The health promoter becomes a facilitator of change, stressing the need for not just two-way

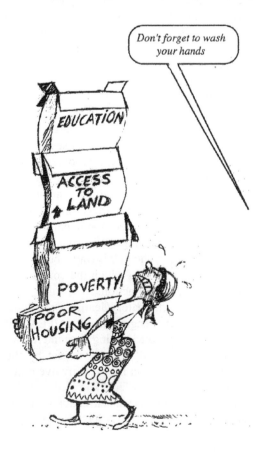

communication but also multi-way communication (Narayan and Srinivasan, 1994; Linney, 1995).

Within cultures there are sub-cultures, and differences in interpretations of the world abound. Education itself influences how we perceive the world and may create barriers between the educated and those with no formal education. Working with counterparts from a culture similar to those affected does not automatically ensure a 'cultural fit' for health promotion. While the health promotion provided by people from the same national culture may be more appropriate than that provided by someone from a different culture, appropriateness also depends on the type of training that is provided, the attitude of the promoters and facilitators and the techniques and tools that they use. Participatory learning and action (PLA) provides an accessible method of ensuring multichannel and cross-cultural communication that can overcome some of these difficulties.

Participatory methodologies

One of the principles of adult learning is that adults need to be seen by others as being capable of self-direction (Knowles, 1990). In addition:

o Adults have substantial life experience that they bring to the analysis of a new situation. They can help each other or learn by sharing their experiences, hence learning should start with what they already know and seek to build on it.

o People move through stages when learning: they are unlikely to be ready to accept new information on a subject unless they have identified it as an issue that is relevant to them. Learning will be more effective when the content is related to people's real lives.

o Communities contain individuals with a wealth of experience, skills, talents and ideas. Telling

people what to do encourages dependency. Building on their own capacities can foster creative approaches to problem-solving.

Paulo Freire has been the inspiration behind many literacy and health education programmes by stressing the idea that feeding students knowledge so that they can regurgitate it later is counterproductive. With experiential learning, the learners become the subject of the inquiry, and enthusiasm for future learning is generated by the rewards of present learning. This philosophy underpins the participatory research and PLA approaches to health promotion (Chambers, 1992; Pretty et al, 1995; De Koning and Martin, 1996). PLA, which has evolved from participatory rural appraisal (PRA) and rapid rural appraisal (RRA), employs techniques derived from applied anthropology to facilitate learning. The use of PLA in health education recognizes that people have knowledge about their own situation, including the factors that affect their health. It also recognizes that education involves the exploration and analysis of a situation and this can lead to action to change it. PLA emphasizes the importance of indigenous knowledge but allows the space to challenge that knowledge with new ideas and explanations.

The rationale for employing participatory methods of learning and/or PLA is to encourage dialogue and discussion. However, these two approaches are not synonymous. PLA seeks to explore people's different perceptions of reality, and uses dialogue to tease out consensus and promote mutual understanding with the intention of empowering communities to act. During this process they may arrive at a decision to confront the forces that are preventing them from changing things for the better, and in this way it becomes a social change process in which the community sets its own agenda for action.

The use of participatory learning methods, however, is less challenging than PRA/PLA as it simply involves people learning in an interactive way. The agenda will usually be set by the facilitator of the session but will involve much more than the simple transfer of knowledge, which is known to be of limited value in enabling people to put into practice what they have learnt.

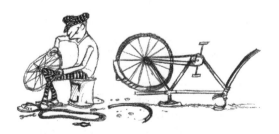

The use of 'pure' PRA/PLA may not be possible at the height of an emergency, but we advocate its use in principle whilst recognizing that time constraints may initially preclude a community-set agenda. PLA techniques can still be usefully employed in the emergency setting to give people a voice in planning the intervention, and to ensure that any learning or education is culturally sensitive and begins with what people already know. It will also help to establish an appropriate approach for the long-term benefit of the community. Learning the PLA approach will take time. If its potential is to be maximized, a reorientation of practice at all levels is required.

Facilitators and participants will gradually learn to appreciate the significance of PLA through continually evaluating their own efforts. The techniques employed (some of which have been adapted for inclusion in this manual) are not meant to be a 'bag of tricks' providing instant solutions, but as a means of allowing people to learn through dialogue. They also provide a practical way of enabling those involved in the provision of relief to listen more to the people who have been affected.

The understanding of the term 'participation' has evolved over time as ways to involve people more centrally in the development process have been sought. Along with participatory learning, participatory planning and evaluation methodologies are recommended by this manual, though they may represent a range of interpretations of the concept of participation. For instance, participatory evaluation initially used conventional methods of data collection, such as questionnaire surveys, but emphasized the need to provide feedback to the community. In recent years, participatory evaluation has come to be seen as a process in which community members actually help to carry out the evaluation regardless of their literacy levels, through the use of different methods of data collection and feedback. Both these approaches to participation are valid and may be useful to meet the needs of different stakeholders. This manual stresses the need to involve people as much as possible in relief and development efforts, and to foster an environment that allows them to assume greater control. To achieve this in reality is not always easy and may be less so in an emergency context, where the interests of donors and agencies often take precedence. We therefore suggest a range of approaches that emphasize people's involvement, but that vary in the degree to which control is shared.

Understanding behaviour change

Understanding the complex interaction of relationships that influence the way people behave is a vital prerequisite for planning hygiene promotion interventions. There are numerous models that try to explain the nature of behaviour change. A simple model is provided by Hubley (1993), which draws on Green and Kreuter's (1991) description of the factors necessary for behaviour change:

1. *Predisposing factors* affect the likelihood of people considering a need to change. These include demographic factors unlikely to be affected by the hygiene promotion programme, such as age, sex and socio-economic status. They also include other factors likely to be affected by a project, such as knowledge, beliefs, values and attitudes. A *belief* is what a person holds to be true, and a strongly held belief based on tradition or religion is less likely to be open to change. In some communities where diarrhoea is commonplace among young children it is believed to be a normal part of growing up. In this case, challenging this belief would be part of the hygiene promotion process. *Values* are what people consider to be important to them, and are often shared at the community level. The value placed on

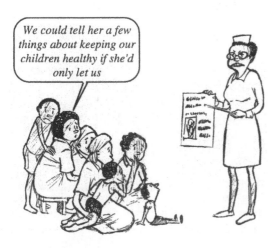

We could tell her a few things about keeping our children healthy if she'd only let us

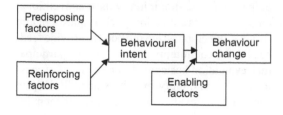

Figure 0.2 Behaviour change model

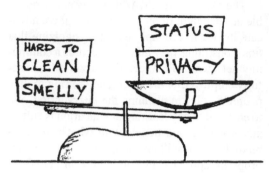

privacy, for example, may determine the kinds of latrines found to be acceptable. People are more inclined to change if they understand and value the benefits that the change might bring. An *attitude* refers to an outlook on something and may be regarded positively or negatively. Many different beliefs may combine to create an attitude. For example, attitudes to latrine use may be influenced by a variety of beliefs: they may be considered smelly and hard to clean and at the same time useful for privacy and contributing positively to the status of the owner.

2. *Reinforcing factors* are those things that support changes and that encourage them to be sustained. These include the attitudes and behaviour of respected and influential individuals in the community, and those of family and peers. They may also include the use of incentives or sanctions and regulations to encourage compliance with changes in practice.

3. Each belief will impact to a greater or lesser extent on the overall positive or negative judgement of its value. Changing attitudes does not always bring about a change in behaviour. Sometimes exposure to a previously untried behaviour is required to change people's attitude toward it. This is where intent to change behaviour (*behavioural intent*) becomes an important step towards behaviour change.

4. *Enabling factors* refer to the material preconditions necessary for carrying out a behaviour. How realistic a proposed new behaviour is will determine the ease with which the change can be made. Enabling factors may include access to acceptable facilities and the time, skills or resources necessary to use them or develop alternatives. It may mean addressing the absence of basic domestic requirements that make good hygiene practices possible, for example water

containers and soap. Promoting changes that make life more difficult or less comfortable are unlikely to be viewed positively in the long term, especially if people have an alternative. Some changes, once tried, may act as a disincentive to future change because they take up too much time, are not practical or have other perceived negative effects.

The combination of all these factors will affect an individual's or community's disposition to try the new behaviour and then to adopt it. The complexity of the situation and the numerous structural, cultural, social and behavioural determinants of health must all be taken into consideration if a health promotion strategy that saves lives by promoting the affected population's own adaptive capacities is to be achieved.

Planning hygiene promotion activities

Planning models usually consider two options: the top down, directive and project-based model; or the bottom up, participative and community-based model. The former is easier to control, manage and evaluate but usually imposes a set agenda on the community. Programme plans are formulated in advance, often using a systematic planning blueprint such as the logical framework analysis (LFA) that details, prior to the initiation of the project, what is to be achieved and how. A detailed guide to the 'log frame' is shown below.

In the alternative model, control and decision making lies with the community, so independence is promoted. It encourages skills development, long-term commitment and sustainability, but requires skilled facilitators and a flexible timescale. In this situation, the community would determine

Table 0.1 Logical framework guide

PLAN DOWN

Narrative summary	Measurement indicators	Means of verification	Assumptions
FINAL GOAL The impact to which the project is expected to contribute. What are the wider problems that the project will help to resolve?	**MEASURE** (direct or indirect) to determine the extent to which the FINAL GOAL is fulfilled. What are the quantitative ways of measuring, or qualitative ways of judging, whether the FINAL GOAL has been achieved (quantity, quality, time)?	**TESTING** the accuracy of the indicators chosen to measure the FINAL GOAL. What sources of information exist and does other information need to be generated?	Important **EXTERNAL EVENTS**, conditions or decisions necessary for achieving the SUPER-GOAL and sustaining the FINAL GOAL in the long run. What needs to happen outside the project to make sure the project is successful?
INTERMEDIATE GOALS The effects that are expected to be achieved as a result of the project. What are the intended immediate effects on the project area or target group? What are the expected benefits or disbenefits and changes, and to whom will they go?	**MEASURES** (direct or indirect) to determine the extent to which the INTERMEDIATE GOALS are fulfilled. What are the quantitative measures or qualitative evidence by which achievement and distribution of effects and benefits can be judged (quantity, quality, time)?	**TESTING** the accuracy of the indicators chosen to measure the INTERMEDIATE GOALS. What sources of information exist and does other information need to be generated? Does provision for collection need to be made under inputs–outputs?	Important **EXTERNAL CONDITIONS**, events or decisions outside the control of the project necessary for the FINAL GOAL to be attained. What conditions external to the project are necessary if achievement of the INTERMEDIATE GOALS is to contribute to reaching the FINAL GOAL?
OUTPUTS that the project management should be able to guarantee. What outputs are to be produced by the project in order to achieve the project purpose?	**MEASURES** (direct or indirect) that determine to what extent the outputs are produced. What kind and quality of outputs, and by when will they be produced (quantity, quality, time)?	**TESTING** the accuracy of the indicators chosen to measure the outputs. What sources of information exist and does other information need to be generated?	Important **EXTERNAL CONDITIONS**, events or decisions outside the control of the project necessary for the INTERMEDIATE GOALS to be attained. What are the factors not within the control of the project that are required to facilitate progress from outputs to the project?
INPUTS of goods and services necessary to undertake the ACTIVITIES that will produce the outputs required. What time-frame?	**MEASURES** to determine the extent to which inputs have been provided and activities carried out. What personnel, materials and equipment have been provided, and what information collection, training, campaigns, etc. have been carried out, over what time period?	**INFORMATION** available about these inputs and activities. What are the sources of information and does more information need to be generated?	**EXTERNAL FACTORS**, events or conditions or decisions outside the control of the project necessary to realize the outputs. What external factors must be realized to obtain planned outputs on schedule? What and whose decisions and actions are needed for project inception?

THINK UP
The arrows show the flow of logic on the guide. Logical thoughts flow from the lower left corner, moving first horizontally to the end of the bottom line and then diagonally from the end of that line to the start of the line above it, and so on until reaching the final box at the top right hand corner. You think that making these inputs, performing these activities, and with these external factors holding true, you will achieve the intermediate goals – and so on

Adapted from Srinivasan, 1990, DIID, 1997b and WEDC, 1998)

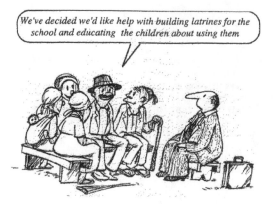

their own health priorities and decide how they would tackle them.

In reality, a mixture of the two approaches is often used in development programmes. Systematic planning may be viewed simply as a first step to initiating a community-oriented agenda. It is often thought that a bottom-up approach is not appropriate in emergency programmes and that in such a situation people are unable to make decisions or assume control. In fact, both approaches are still possible and may run concurrently. For example, it may be necessary in the acute phase of an emergency to use a directive approach to promote the use of demarcated areas for defecation or to convey specific messages about preventing illness. It may also be possible to research the positive beliefs, values and attitudes that different groups in the community associate with the key hygiene practices and so develop positive social marketing messages for a campaign. At the same time, it may also be possible to engage people in small group discussions, enabling them to take community-defined actions to address some of the sanitation problems in the camp or settlement. Given that the directive approach may have only a limited impact, it is important to maximize the opportunities for working in a more facilitative way and to work towards a community-defined agenda for action.

Overview of manual

The pictures below provide an overview of the project cycle and form the basis for the four main chapters of this book.

Stage 1 – Assessment and analysis: Where are we now?

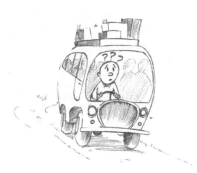

Collection of information to enable identification of the problems to be tackled and the resources available for resolving them. Problems should be prioritized in order of their impact on the project community. This comprises the baseline on which the project cycle is based. These issues are covered in detail in Chapter 1 of this manual.

Stage 2 – Planning: Where are we going?

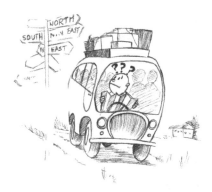

Prioritize the information and decide which are the most important areas to address. It may be possible to deal with several issues simultaneously, but the sequence of activities may be important. Define aims and objectives, remembering to consider how you will measure project success. Draw up an action plan that includes activities, resource requirements and a time frame. This will involve considering who you will work with, who will be the target group, what you aim to achieve with them and how long it is likely to take. These issues are covered in Chapter 2.

Stage 3 – Implementation: How do we get there?

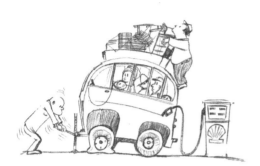

Once the plans have been drawn up and agreed, they can be implemented. The activities carried out in the implementation phase will depend on what was found in the assessment and could be limited to hygiene education or could include wider hygiene promotion activities of social mobilization and community capacity building. Chapter 3 discusses these issues in detail.

Stage 4 – Monitoring and evaluation: How shall we know when we've got there and how can we do it better next time?

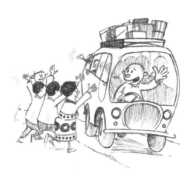

Maintain records of activities undertaken, training or education sessions held, and participants' evaluation of them. Use this information and compare with baseline data from the assessment stage to compare subsequent changes in the situation. This information must then feed back into the project cycle in order to determine how we can do it better next time. These issues are explored in Chapter 4.

1
Assessment and analysis: Where are we now?

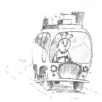

ASSESSMENT INVOLVES THE collection of data to guide decision making. In an emergency, a rapid assessment should provide information as to whether to intervene and if so the type and scale of activities and the priorities for the allocation of resources. In the aftermath of a disaster there will always be a tension between starting implementation quickly with inadequate information and taking valuable time to formulate a more effective response. A balance must be struck. Rapid assessment information can be complemented with more detailed baseline data once essential interventions have begun. This section deals with the process of collecting and analysing information. Specific assessment techniques are referred to and details of how to use these can be found in the data collection tools section in the Appendices. More detailed information about planning and implementing priority interventions, monitoring and evaluating their effects and changing the interventions to suit evolving contexts are subjects covered in subsequent sections of this manual.

Collecting information

Data are usually described as qualitative or quantitative. *Qualitative data* examine the nature of a problem or issue, whereas *quantitative data* are based on numbers and can indicate the extent of a problem or issue. Certain data collected using qualitative techniques, for example, the mapping and scoring exercises described in the Appendices, may also contribute towards a quantitative analysis of a situation. Often a combination of approaches is used to provide the opportunity to cross-check and clarify data gathered from different sources. When three or more methods are used as a means of cross checking, this is referred to as *triangulation*.

Rapid assessment

At the height of an emergency you will probably have to content yourself with essential information. A rapid assessment will involve the collection of the most relevant data as quickly as possible. This will allow for an informed, if not perfectly planned, response. A few days should be adequate to find out enough information to plan subsequent action. More information should then be gathered as the project proceeds. Rapid assessments rely mainly on qualitative information gained from discussions with various people and from general observations of the situation and any quantitative information is usually an estimate of numbers affected. Key informant interviews and group discussions may be used to obtain views and opinions from individuals or groups. It is important to make sure that women are represented and enabled to speak. Try also to identify other potentially marginalized people

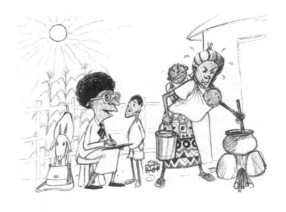

Box 1.1 General criteria for good assessment practice

The criteria for good assessment practice are:

○ *Timeliness*: providing information and analysis to inform key decisions about response;

○ *Relevance*: providing the information and analysis most relevant to those decisions;

○ *Coverage*: adequate for the scale of the problems;

○ *Continuity*: providing relevant information throughout the course of a crisis;

○ *Validity*: using methods that can be expected to lead to sound conclusions;

○ *Transparency*: being explicit about the methods used, information relied on to reach conclusions and about the limits of the accuracy of the data relied on.

Source: Darcy and Hofmann, 2003.

---

such as ethnic minorities, widows, elderly people or those with disabilities. An exploratory walk, a mapping exercise and two or three focus group discussions (as described on pages 32–35 and 105–9) may be enough to provide essential information initially for a particular location.

Baseline information requirements

In an acute emergency the initial, rapidly collected essential data will not be sufficient for detailed programme planning or for judging the success of the programme when compared later during evaluation. The use of a range of baseline data collection tools enables a more comprehensive picture to be drawn of affected communities as the emergency evolves. As well as providing information against which changes can be measured, baseline data can highlight the most vulnerable and thus help to target assistance. It can reveal skills and capacities within affected com-

munities and highlight continuing risks to health that may need to be addressed through health promotion initiatives. Collecting data is a dynamic process and you will be constantly learning and revising what you already know. Assessments do not just take place at the beginning of the project cycle but need to be updated as work progresses, especially in rapidly changing situations. All too often they are regarded as a one-off start-up activity, whereas reviewing the scope, scale and nature of emergency interventions on an ongoing basis is important to ensure that programmes remain responsive to needs.

In the emergency context it is frequently the case that not enough information is collected because there is enormous pressure to be seen to act immediately and to save lives. Remember that without baseline data you may not be sure whether your interventions have had the desired impact and you will be unable to measure whether they are effective or not!

It is beyond the scope of this manual to consider other key factors that affect the well-being of populations affected by an emergency, but a comprehensive analysis of threats to their life, health and dignity is important for a detailed understanding of the context in which water, sanitation and hygiene promotion activities will be implemented. High rates of malnutrition may be aggravating the rates of diarrhoeal disease or an outbreak of measles may be causing more deaths than those due to inadequate water and sanitation. Emergency teams will need to remain flexible and work closely with the local and national authorities and other agencies to ensure an effective response. Communities may be unwilling or unable to invest time and interest in sanitation initiatives when their basic food needs are not being met as their priorities will lie elsewhere. Their security may be a more urgent need than trying to prevent diarrhoeal disease. For example, in Darfur in Western Sudan in 2004 some beneficiaries declined the distribution of certain non-food items that they were afraid would make them vulnerable to attack and robbery, even though these items would have been extremely useful.

Table 1.1 provides a list of questions that will need to be addressed for planning and implementing

Box 1.2 Ten questions to ask when making an assessment for a hygiene promotion project

1. What were 'normal' practices before the emergency?
2. What are the widespread 'risky' practices in the community?
3. Who and how many employ the 'risky' practices in the community?
4. Which 'risky' practices can be altered?
5. Who uses 'safe' practices and who and what motivates and influences them to use these?
6. What communication channels are available and which are trusted for promoting hygiene?
7. What facilities or materials do people need in order to carry out the 'safe' practices?
8. How much time, money or effort are people willing to contribute for those facilities/materials?
9. Where will those facilities/materials be available?
10. How will people know that the facilities/materials exist and where they can be obtained?

Souce: Adapted from Curtis, and Kanki, 1998.

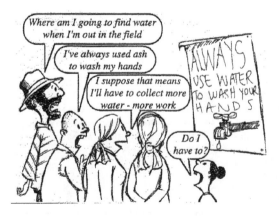

hygiene promotion activities in an acute emergency situation. When assessing these factors consider who is involved, what they do and what they do it with. *Later on*, it might be possible to gather information about a wider range of hygiene practices. Table 1.2 lists all hygiene practices considered important in development contexts. Information about water- and sanitation-related diseases that are common in emergencies, including their transmission patterns and ways in which they can be prevented can be found on pages 233–42 of the Appendices. While it is useful to gather at least the essential baseline information before acting, there may be activities that can take place concurrently. For example, if a particular water source is found to be a risk for cholera infection in the initial assessment, there may be simple activities that can be undertaken straight away to try to prevent people from using that water source. One of the camp leaders could be asked to hold a meeting to explain the dangers of using that particular source and to enlist people's help in identifying ways of tackling this. It might be appropriate to ban people from collecting water from the contaminated source. If community leaders' are involved they may be more willing to undertake to ensure that a ban is enforced.

Gender issues and different groups

As has been discussed, a 'community' is never an homogeneous entity. It will always contain different groups who have different priorities and whose interests may conflict. It is difficult and perhaps unrealistic to expect consensus on certain issues. However, every attempt should be made to try to identify these different groups, to seek their views and to involve them actively in the project. Some groups may find themselves frequently discriminated against and their views ignored. Women are often not adequately involved in the decision making and planning of aid programmes. This has undermined the success of many water and sanitation programmes as women are frequently the main water carriers and users. They are usually responsible for and influential over the health of their children and families, although they are not usually expected to perform the role of decision making at community level. Within communities women are also not an homogeneous group. For example, single women may have different priorities to women

Table 1.1 Essential information and ways to collect it

Data required	Example questions	Possible collection methods
Size of population and level of emergency	Size and density of population affected and over what area? What is the crude death rate in the population (per ten thousand per day)? What are the main causes of disease and death in the community? Are certain groups of people suffering more from these illnesses? Is there a history of particular epidemics in the area e.g. cholera or malaria or are people at risk of epidemic outbreak e.g. low coverage of measles immunisation, low immunity to malaria, overcrowded conditions, poor environmental conditions?	Discussion with government and NGO workers; clinic records; discussions with refugee leaders and community representatives, community health workers, and traditional healers; counting and mapping funerals and burials
Priority needs and vulnerable groups	What are the priority problems according to the refugees? Do people feel safe? Do they have adequate shelter, fuel and cooking utensils, food and items essential for personal hygiene and dignity? Does this vary with age, gender or social group? What are the needs of the disabled and elderly? Are there risk factors for HIV?	Mapping, discussion groups, matrix ranking, pocket chart, three-pile sorting
Social structures and communication channels	How is the settlement organized? Who makes and influences decisions within the community? What structures and groups exist within the community and what is their purpose? What outreach workers exist in the community? How do people get their information? Which communication channels are thought to be most effective? What proportion of the population are literate?	Mapping, key informant interviews and focus group discussions with refugees, government workers and other organizations, Venn diagrams, stakeholder analysis
Hand washing practices	Is hand washing at key times the usual practice and what do people use for hand washing? Do men, women, boys and girls wash hands after defecation, after cleaning a child's bottom? What is used for hand washing? If people use soap or ash for hand washing, what advantages do they associate with this practice?	Key informant interviews and focus group discussions with adults and children, exploratory walks, mapping, observation, three-pile sorting
Defecation practices	Where do people defecate? Has the current situation forced people to change their defecation practices? Is there evidence of faeces near to dwellings? If people use latrines, what advantages do they associate with those latrines? Do children use the latrines? Is infants' excreta disposed of in latrines? Will the latrines need emptying? If the facilities are shared, how will people clean their hands after using them?	Key informant interviews and focus group discussions with adults and children, mapping, three-pile sorting, time-line, exploratory walks, observation
Water sources	Which water sources do people use and what do they use this water for? Is the drinking water source likely to be contaminated? Do people distinguish between water used for drinking and water for other uses? Are communities involved in managing the water points?	Key informant interviews and focus group discussions with users at water sources and near dwellings, exploratory walks, observation, pocket chart, three-pile sorting

Table 1.1 (Contd)

Data required	Example questions	Possible collection methods
Water collection and storage practices	Which household members collect drinking water? Are drinking water containers clean and sufficient in number? Do they use balancers, such as leaves, to stop water splashing? If yes, are these balancers washed before use? What do people use to store drinking water in?	Focus group discussion, home visits, exploratory walks, observation, three-pile sorting, gender roles
Special needs for women	Are there special problems for women? What do women use to protect themselves during menstruation? Have breastfeeding or other child care practices been altered? Are women able to carry out their domestic tasks without fear of attack?	Key informant interviews and focus group discussions, observation, gender roles
Beliefs about the cause of disease	What is the understanding of the relationship between water, sanitation and disease? Is it the same for all groups? What do people think causes diarrhoea?	Key informant interviews, focus group discussions, story-with-a-gap, three-pile sorting
Vector control	Is there a problem with rats, mosquitoes, lice? Are there any other problems associated with vector control? Is solid waste or waste water accumulating near to dwellings?	Clinic records, focus group discussions, three-pile sorting, observation
HIV/AIDS	What background information is there on HIV in the affected and surrounding community? Who will be made more susceptible in the current emergency context and how? Which agencies/institutions are involved with HIV/AIDS initiatives? Is there an intermediary who could facilitate access to HIV-affected individuals/households?	UNAIDS website, clinic records, key informant interviews

with dependants or partners. The consideration of gender is not just about discrimination against women. It refers to the fact that men and women have different roles and responsibilities in society and that this frequently gives rise to different needs, priorities and perspectives. Without understanding the roles played by these different groups, or the barriers to their participation in certain activities, incorrect assumptions will be made by project planners.

The young and the old, the poorest members of the community, boys and girls of different ages and the disabled may all have varying needs and perspectives in terms of the provision of water and sanitation facilities. Any project must be sensitive to these differences. A good baseline survey will try to identify as many of these groups

Some Sudanese refugees in Chad began adapting blocks of communal latrines constructed by international NGOs to better suit their requirements. Two cubicles in blocks of ten were reserved only for urination and bathing and people collected local materials to build more of these simple cubicles closer to their shelters.

This was preferred by the women and was said to be the customary practice in their villages in Sudan. The plastic sheeting used in some of the communal facilities was not popular as it was easily damaged and transparent in the sunlight and so this was also modified.

O'Reilly, 2004, personal communication

Table 1.2 Key hygiene practices checklist

Hygiene Practice Categories	Key Variables
Sanitation	○ Location of defecation sites ○ Latrine structure and cleanliness ○ Disposal of children's faeces ○ Use of cleansing materials ○ Number of users ○ Sanitation preferences for different groups
Water	○ Placement of latrines in relation to water sources ○ Different water sources used, and daily and seasonal patterns ○ Average distance to water ○ Amount of water used per person per day ○ Water quality at source and home ○ Water storage practices ○ Methods of water treatment ○ Water handling in the home ○ Water use and reuse ○ Hand-washing (including religious rituals) ○ Bathing (children and adults) ○ Clothes washing ○ Previous experience of water source management
Food	○ Food handling and preparation ○ Food storage practices ○ Food reuse practices ○ Breastfeeding, weaning practices and beliefs ○ Washing and drying of utensils
Environment	○ Household refuse disposal ○ Management of domestic animals ○ Evidence of stagnant water around dwelling or water point ○ Vector control problems ○ Slaughtering facilities ○ Burial of the dead

Souce: Adapted from Almedom et al, 1997.

as possible and involve them in the data collection process. If facilities are being designed it is very important to try to ascertain people's preferences:

Box 1.3 Check list for considering the views of different groups during assessments

Do you have information from female and male groups? How many of each?

Were key informants drawn from different sections of the community (rich, poor, leaders, women, elderly, disabled, adolescents)?

Which vulnerable groups have you consulted?

What special provision has been made to include women, children and vulnerable groups?

Were women available to interview women?

Were the different results compared and discussed with women and men separately?

○ Are men and women used to sharing latrines?
○ How will they feel about sharing bathing facilities?
○ What might be the particular problems that women face if the water points are situated outside the camp, for example, might there be problems with security?

It is important to identify and talk with as many groups of beneficiaries as possible to make sure that the fullest picture is obtained. However, the need for detailed information from all groups has to be balanced with the amount of time available to gather this information.

HIV/AIDS

Given the nature of the HIV/AIDS global pandemic, it is important to understand the nature of the potential risks of HIV and design the programme to mitigate these risks. Obtain background information of the HIV profile in the location of your programme. The UNAIDS website is useful for this. Consider who will be made more susceptible to transmission in the current emergency context and how the welfare of those already infected and affected by the virus may be made

Box 1.4 Planning and implementation for HIV/AIDS

o Carry out HIV awareness raising activities for project staff: they should know basic facts about transmission and understand susceptibility and vulnerability issues in relation to the current programme context.

o Ensure men, women and children access water and sanitation facilities safely.

o Consult with communities to ensure the distribution of aid, for example, non-food items, or the location of facilities does not put them at increased risk of attack.

o Ensure that all water and sanitation facilities are accessible by the chronically sick or disabled – the type of technology used should not be a barrier to access.

o Talk with affected families about the specific needs associated with caring for people suffering from AIDS, for example, increased water requirements for hygiene and hydration.

o Find other ways of consulting with people whose caring responsibilities prevent them from attending meetings.

o Where gaps in knowledge of HIV are identified within the community consider how these can be addressed in a culturally sensitive way and by whom.

o Be sensitive to ways in which programme activities may increase the susceptibility of groups or individuals, for example, separating rural men from their families to carry out paid work in towns where payment for sex is more likely to occur.

worse by the emergency. Identify the agencies/ institutions involved with HIV/AIDS initiatives. Try to find out if there is an intermediary who could facilitate access to HIV-affected individuals/households. Box 1.4 has further details of considerations that are needed in areas affected with HIV/AIDS.

Tools or methods of data collection

Separation of information
In order to differentiate the level of needs between different groups within a sampled population, information must be separated into different groups. This is referred to as *disaggregation* of data. Only by disaggregating data can the differences in health, service levels and needs be clearly identified in different socio-economic groups, particularly when those groups are in the minority. For example, a latrine use study may show that most people in a settlement have access to latrines. Disaggregation of information may show that female household heads have less access to household latrines than their male counterparts, or that children under five years of age are discouraged from using latrines. Disaggregating the information reveals these differences and allows project planners to address the actual needs of all sections of the community.

Choice of data collection tools
The choice of methodologies to be used will depend on the local situation and on the project objectives. A mixture of qualitative and quantitative data will be needed. Important considerations will include:

o *Who is the information for?* Community members and field workers may find that information provided by participatory learning at the local level, using less extractive qualitative methodologies, is useful. Donors, aid agencies and government departments may value quantitative data that meet particular statistical criteria. However, increased recognition of the need for aid programmes to be accountable to affected populations requires that their views on programme design and delivery are considered and qualitative methods best capture this kind of information.

o *What resources are available to collect the data?* The numbers and skills of personnel and the time they have available will affect the choice of data collection. Logistical requirements for the collection of different types of data and training implications will also affect what can be done in the time available. In keeping with the participatory focus of this manual, we touch briefly on the more extractive process of classical, quantitative data collection such as the use of questionnaire surveys, but emphasize the use of PLA methods for their community learning potential. Opportunities to provide feedback to the community should always be sought even when less interactive methods of data collection are employed.

o *Who will collect the assessment and baseline data?* It is unlikely that you will have the luxury of time when you start to work on data collection. You will need help from other people but who should you approach? There may be other project staff who can assist with data collection, perhaps other project staff from different organizations such as local government workers and local community health workers linked to nearby clinics and health centres. There may be other agency staff who would be interested to find out more about the situation in the community. There may also be members of the community who are willing and interested to learn and share their experience with you and with others – these might include health workers, teachers, community representatives or extension workers. It is likely that for initial data collection you may consider working in small teams covering different affected areas. These teams should already have experience of data collection and ideally require a minimum of orientation. At later stages, you can invest more time in training and facilitating other groups of people to monitor and use information for the project.

Working through interpreters

In some cases it will be necessary for fieldworkers to use interpreters to talk with the community. This can make the natural flow of discussion between the fieldworker and the community extremely difficult. Interpreters should be native speakers, preferably from the same social group as the target community.

In societies where it is not appropriate for men to talk to women, both female and male interpreters are needed. When the ideal interpreter is not available, it is important to be aware of the dangers of using interpreters from a different group, class or gender; these include misinterpretation, misunderstandings, suspicion and guarded responses. Where interpretation cannot be avoided, the following suggestions may help to reduce problems:

o First explain to the interpreter what you are intending to do. Explain that on this occasion, you want to understand exactly what the interviewees or discussion group are saying rather than a summary of their responses or the interpreter's own views.
o It is sometimes useful to have a trial run with someone else in the team to expose the interpreter to some of the vocabulary that she/he may need to translate.
o Ask her/him to translate what you say and the response of the other person(s) as closely as possible.
o Talk naturally, maintain your natural eye contact with the person you are talking to.
o Allow the interpreter to translate what you have said after a sentence or two.
o Keep your conversation simple and clear. Be aware that the interpreter may elaborate on what you say and may sometimes have difficulty in translating some terms or phrases.

Surveys

Fieldworkers often embark on surveys as the primary choice for data collection, particularly if they have had little exposure to participatory methods. Some strengths and weaknesses of the use of surveys are considered in Box 1.5

Using questionnaires

Questionnaire surveys are not always used in the first phase of an emergency as the situation may be evolving very quickly and any information gathered may soon be out of date. However, if they are used, they need to be: *well designed* in order to produce the same answers when repeated, *measure* what they set out to measure, and be *sensitive* to change. Careful structuring of the questions is necessary to avoid biasing the

Box 1.5 Strengths and weaknesses of surveys

Strengths:

○ A lot of statistical information can be gathered systematically in a relatively short time over a wide area;

○ If the survey methodology is sound, the results from a sample can be extracted to a bigger population and the results compared with similar surveys carried out at different points in time or in other communities;

○ Different types of information can be collected at the same time and compared against each other e.g. nutrition surveys can include basic hygiene questions or level of education can be compared with health seeking behaviour;

○ Some stakeholders may feel more confident in the validity of data collected through surveys.

Weaknesses:

○ Responses may be superficial if questions focus on 'what' and 'how' rather than 'why' and it may be easy for the respondent to say what she/he thinks the interviewer is expecting to hear;

○ Specialist advice and close supervision is required to ensure statistically valid methodologies;

○ Significant time and resources are necessary to design the questionnaire, recruit and train the survey team, carry out the survey and analyse the data and both time and resources might be stretched in the early stages of an emergency;

○ In an emergency, the situation may be changing so fast that a survey will rapidly become out of date;

○ The methodology is extractive rather than interactive so cannot easily be used as a learning tool by the participants.

Source: Adapted from Feuerstein, 1986.

responses and the questionnaire will need to be pre-tested in the field and then modified if necessary before use. It is also preferable to keep the questionnaire as short as possible as the longer it is, the more time it will take to analyse. Do not try to ask all the questions that are possible and consider which questions may be better answered by using other means such as a focus group discussion. In the field, a cross-checking mechanism is needed to ensure consistency, for example, a small number of questionnaires should be reviewed each day to ensure they have been properly completed and that the interviewers are using a similar approach. Work out how much time it takes to administer the questionnaire during the pre-test and remember to allow time and resources for training the interviewers, producing and translating the questionnaires and analysing and reporting on the data. The amount of time needed to plan and implement a survey is often underestimated, so if questionnaires are to be used they should be brief and easy to administer.

Work out how the data will be analysed and reported on *before* you start the survey as this will influence the design of the questionnaire. Cross-check the data for reliability by comparing it with information collected using other tools. For example, you could complement questionnaire *data* with observation of practices at the household or water point and with information gained from more in depth qualitative discussions with people. A sample questionnaire used in the 1997/8 cholera outbreak in Uganda is included on pages 118–20 in the Appendices. It includes some observations, some closed questions with answers limited to 'yes' or 'no', and some open-ended questions requiring the opinions of the person being interviewed.

Interviewers will require training to make sure that they are able: to make the person being interviewed feel at ease; to ask the questions and fill in forms correctly; to observe the things required; to be non-directive so as to minimize the effect of observer bias. The following points on the next page, on training interviewers are important.

Tips on training interviewers

Interviewers:

o will need to know the exact purpose of the interview and be able to explain this simply;
o must dress appropriately;
o should know how to introduce themselves and respect the fact that someone is giving up their time to answer the questionnaire;
o should explain how long the questionnaire will take;
o must accept that some people may not want to answer the questionnaire;
o should wait for a response to each question; be silent then probe;
o should remember to thank the respondents once they have finished;
o should explain to the respondents whether the results will be made available through village or camp meetings;
o should ensure confidentiality and ensure that individual comments will remain anonymous;
o may need to carry an official document with them to identify themselves;
o should know exactly how to mark the responses on the questionnaire;
o should keep records of how many men, women, boys and girls were interviewed;
o should clearly mark each questionnaire with the name of the interviewer and the household name, number or code;
o should meet other interviewers at the end of each working day to discuss the progress of the survey and confirm plans for the next working day.

Role plays can be used when training interviewers providing good and bad examples of interviewing techniques. In this way, questionnaires can be pre-tested as part of the interviewer training.

Sampling

If the population you are working with is very large, you will not be able to interview everybody. A smaller 'sample' of people can be selected to represent and give information on the population as a whole. In many refugee situations precise population figures are unavailable. It is also of-

ten the case that where figures are given they are exaggerated. Unless grossly exaggerated, however, this will probably not make a difference to the sampling number. There are two main types of sampling. The first type of sampling involves a non-random process of selection and is highly suited to small-scale projects and participatory methods of data collection. The participants may select themselves, for example, those willing to participate in a public mapping activity, or a group may be identified by the project organizer and invited to attend a focus group discussion. This type of sampling is also known as *purposive sampling*. There is no rule of thumb for the number of different discussions, interviews or observations for the size of population as this will depend on the differences within the community. Investigations are complete when sessions are no longer providing any new information. For example, in one focus group you may find that some women dispose of children's excreta in the latrine and others throw it in the bushes. In the next focus group discussion some women say that they throw it in the bushes and others that they use potties. In the next, the women may give the full range of answers given previously. If, in a final focus group, all the answers are again the same, you can probably assume that you have exhausted the possibilities and you can stop sampling. This is sometimes called *sampling to redundancy*.

The second type of sampling aims to collect objective information from a minimum number of people, while still making sure that they represent

---

Box 1.6 Random sample sizes

For populations under 100 use 30–50 units.

For populations between 100–300 use 50–70 units.

For populations between 300–1,000 use 70–90 units.

For populations over 1000 use 90–100 units.

Note: Unit here means households, groups or individuals.

Source: Dale, 1998.

the full range of people in the population. This is the usual method employed when carrying out questionnaire surveys when you have a large population to study and want to carry out a statistical analysis on the findings (for example, health outcomes). This type of sampling is known as *random sampling*. With random sampling it is important to know how to choose the sample and how big it should be. Specific statistical power calculations are used to determine the sample size needed but Box 1.6 gives a rough idea of how many people (or households) could be selected.

Sample selection should be made from the whole community in a way that is likely to sample all types of people in the community. One way is to use a list of names of male and female household heads to generate a map showing all the households in the area to be surveyed. Where the number of households ranges from 200 to 500, one name in every three to seven would be selected for sampling. Where the number of households is 10,000, one name in every 100 would be selected for sampling. Sample sizes can be reduced when you already know the population well but if the different community groups or villages are of varying sizes, you need to 'weight' the sample size. That is, you need to make sure the number of people interviewed in each community or village is proportional to the size of that community. You do this using the following formula:

Number of people in the community × number of the sample required

———————————————

Total number of population being studied

An example using this formula is given in Box 1.7.

There are also several computer programmes that calculate sample sizes. The following website is free and allows you to calculate the sample size on screen. However, you need to understand the concepts of confidence intervals and confidence levels: www.surveysystem.com. EpiInfo is a computer programme that allows you to analyse survey data. It can be downloaded from www.cdc.gov and it also allows you to calculate sample size. Again, a certain degree of familiarity with statistical terms is required.

Box 1.7 An example of a weighted sample size

The catchment area for the Fatumasi clinic has six villages with a total population of 3,620 people. You need 100 people for questionnaire interviews. Add another 10–15 questionnaires in case you find that some are not answered properly and have to be discarded, making your sample size 115.

In village A, there are 345 people so you use the above formula:

$$\frac{345 \times 115}{3620} = 11$$

Village B has 1072 people so again you calculate:

$$\frac{1072 \times 115}{3620} = 34$$

Then you do the same for all the other villages.

Another approach to *random sampling* is known as *cluster sampling*. The sampling takes place in two stages. First, the whole population is divided, on paper, into smaller discrete geographical areas or clusters, such as villages. For each village, the population size is known or can be estimated. Clusters are then randomly selected from these villages with the chance of any village being selected being proportional to the population size of the village. This means that each person in the whole area has an equal chance of

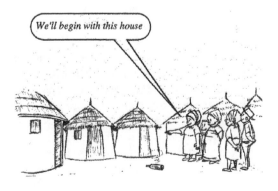

We'll begin with this house

being selected. In the second stage, the individuals are chosen at random from within each cluster area or village, as described previously. If communities are far apart or very big, cluster sampling is a good approach, as logistically it is easier.

The lot quality assurance sampling method (LQAS) is a method of sampling that uses a sampling size of just 19 to give statistically 'reliable enough' data to show differences between different project areas and to indicate intervention priorities. By combining the data from several project areas, known as 'supervision areas' an overall coverage rate can be obtained. A minimum of five 'supervision areas' is suggested, giving a total sample size of 95 individuals or households. Training materials for the LQAS method can be found on the CORE website: www.coregroup.org.

Another type of data collection methodology often used to determine the factors associated with disease outbreaks is an epidemiological tool known as the case-control study. It allows comparisons of health or health-related practices to be drawn between individuals within a community. People contracting a disease (*cases*) can be compared with those who have not contracted the same disease (*controls*) for a range of possible risk factors such as sources of drinking water, hand-washing practices or food hygiene. Those practices that are most common among 'cases' but rare among 'controls' are likely to be the practices most associated with the outbreak. Ideally, cases should be as similar to controls as possible, so that the only difference between them is their health status and the factors associated with it. Cases and controls can be selected randomly and information collected from them using questionnaires or the participatory tools mentioned in the data collection tools section of the Appendices. Where out-patient clinics are available and widely used, randomization will be automatic as cases and controls randomly select themselves by attending the clinic on that particular day. For example, the controls could be those attending the clinic without diarrhoea, while the cases could be those attending with diarrhoea. This type of survey is referred to as a clinic-based case-control method.

Participatory data collection

Getting started

It is essential to start the data collection process by approaching the community leaders in order to explain what your organization is able to offer and obtain their permission to work in the camp, village or settlement. You will need to find out if there is a perceived need for the project that you hope to initiate. Discussions about what is expected of the project and what can be provided will also be necessary. Roles, responsibilities and contributions should be detailed in a written document to make a formal community contract agreement (see pages 254–56 in the Appendices). Village or camp leaders will be able to give you other vital information and details on the existence of formal groups in the community or useful key informants that you may want to speak to, but use your own judgement to identify vulnerable groups or individuals who might otherwise be omitted.

Participatory tools

Exploratory walks, mapping and discussions (group or one-to-one) are probably the best methods with which to begin an emergency assessment. A range of data collection tools appropriate for hygiene promotion projects in emergencies are outlined in the data collection tools section of the Appendices.

Some of these may be more useful later for the collection and clarification of detailed information and ideas. It is important to remember that some communities *or groups* within communities may not have time to contribute to participatory data collection. In refugee camps, for example, women often spend many hours queuing for food and water so data collection must be sensitive to their work loads.

Things to consider when conducting a participatory exercise are:

o Define the parameters of what you want to know and whom you need to work with.
o Select an appropriate tool and have an idea of possible resources.
o Ensure an appropriate location and time to do the exercise. Not everyone will have the time for participatory data collection.

○ Make sure invitations are accessible to people and that they can understand them easily.

○ Ensure that people know why you are there and what the aim of the exercise is.

○ Facilitate the session rather than direct it – allow the participants to take as much control as possible.

○ Probe more deeply if you can, or if you feel that the outcome is unclear. At appropriate moments try to clarify certain issues by feeding back your impressions of what has been learnt – encourage other participants to do the same if they want to.

○ Monitor the process – be aware of some people dominating the exercise – be aware of your own potential for directing the process and choosing the methods of representation.

○ Record the event giving date, location, who was involved, for example, single women from Giti commune, children from Murambi water point, and how many people were involved.

○ Suggest that the information is copied on to paper for preservation if done on the ground. Ask community members how they would like to preserve it and where.

○ Enjoy the exercise – it should be fun and stimulating. You will learn more than you expect.

Ideally, the methods used should encourage people to discuss their own situation and by exploring it, allow them to identify solutions to their problems. Even in the data collection phase of the project, the facilitator should be there only to initiate discussion and keep the activity on track. One of the hardest things about being a facilitator is to try to keep silent and let other people do the talking. If you can facilitate discussion rather than direct it, however, there is more chance that the learning will be culturally appropriate and you will also start from the level that the learners are at. In this way, data collection sessions also become an entry point into the hygiene promotion activities. They may also provide the opportunity for fieldwork training for some of the facilitators who will subsequently work with different sections of the community.

Exploratory walks

Exploratory walks are quick and easy to organize. They allow you to observe life in the community.

Choose sites that are representative of your target area and ask a group of local people to show you round, preferably at dawn or dusk so that you can see more hygiene activities. During the walk you can observe water sources, water collection and handling practices, excreta disposal, refuse and waste water disposal practices. You will have the opportunity to discuss your observations with those you are walking with and to talk to the people you meet along your way about their hygiene problems and how they manage with the facilities they have available. Details of how to do exploratory walks are contained in the Appendices on page 109.

Mapping

A mapping exercise may be a useful way to start the process of assessment. Information on different aspects of camp or village life can be represented by drawing on the ground with a stick and using other available materials such as leaves, sticks or stones as symbols of key structures. Different groups of people will produce different maps according to their priorities, so every attempt should be made to ensure that as many types of people as possible contribute to the map, such as old men, young men, married women, single women, children and poorer households. It may be necessary to hold separate mapping sessions for those individuals or groups who do not express their views openly or when examining sensitive subjects. If the group or groups desire, information can be shared and discussed between groups. Chambers (1992) lists the range of information that maps can convey (see Table 1.3). Among these are community facilities such as roads, water sources, markets and clinics, or demographic information on community organization, numbers of men and women, boys and girls, pregnant women (perhaps using one seed to represent each month of pregnancy), female-headed households and number of dependants or sick children or problems such as lack of drainage, open defecation sites or shelters without plastic sheeting. Mapping is open to ideas and reactive responses from participants depending on the priorities they identify. Having identified the location of vulnerable households, the map can also ensure that facilitators can locate these

Table 1.3 Some information that can be recorded on a map

Infrastructure	Health	Social Organization
○ Roads	○ Sick children	○ Leaders
○ Water sources	○ Sick adults	○ Elders
○ Latrine facilities	○ Malarial areas	○ Representatives
○ Solid waste management	○ Pregnant women	○ Markets
○ Areas of poor drainage	○ Disabled persons	○ Meeting places
○ Markets		○ Women's groups
○ Health centres/clinics		○ Female-headed households
○ Hospitals		
○ Schools		

groups. Maps should be transcribed on to paper in order to preserve them and so that they form part of the baseline information against which progress may be measured. The community may also like to identify somewhere to keep the maps and other information that is produced, for example, the school or other public location. Details of how to conduct a community mapping exercise can be found on page 105 in the Appendices.

Interviews

When information is needed rapidly at the onset of an emergency, interviews with key informants are useful for collecting data as well as for beginning to gather support for an activity or project. Select people who have a good overview of their community initially, for example, respected leaders, elders, women's representatives, health workers, teachers. As time allows, increase the range of stakeholders to get a wide range of views and perspectives on a subject. Information can be gathered by asking questions informally but systematically, for example, to find out which hygiene practices are considered ideal or acceptable and why. A discussion checklist or more formal interview schedule should be prepared for the interviewer to study beforehand. Decide on possible lines of questioning and the exact wording of any

translations that might be required. Try to avoid leading questions such as, 'when do you wash your hands with soap?'. Use open questions instead, such as, 'what do people do when they have used a latrine?' Interviewing may require some specific training to enable the interviewer to learn or improve their interviewing and discussion techniques. Details of how to undertake key informant interviews can be found on page 107 in the Appendices.

Focus group discussions

Group discussions should ideally involve a small, homogeneous group of people, for example, elders, young men, single women, married women, or female heads of household. This is to ensure that people can talk openly and freely about a particular issue. Often, discussing sensitive issues such as sanitation and hygiene practices may not be possible or appropriate in large or mixed groups. The facilitator's task is to keep the discussion in focus so that an issue is explored in depth while allowing and encouraging discussion between participants. Initially the facilitator will probably decide on the topic to be studied, but later on, as people become aware of how the process works, they may also decide on issues they would like to explore. Mulenga (1994) claims that the medium of discussion groups is particularly favoured in Africa. Details of how to conduct a focus group discussion can be found on pages 105–7 in the Appendices. Other discussion-based tools are also covered in the appendices. Many of these tools use the stimulus of pictures or dramas to encourage discussion around a particular topic, some of which are best drawn by the group (for example, pie charts and body mapping on pages 115–16). Others work better with pre-drawn pictures (for example, three-pile sorting on page 149). Sets of pictures designed for use with each of these exercises are also included in the Appendices. However, the facial features, clothing and scenery may need to be adapted to suit the community you are working with.

Structured observation

Structured observation is a systematic technique of observing and recording particular practices to find out which hygiene practices are common or rare. Structured observation should be carried out by a team of trained observers, who visit households, often very early in the morning as people get up. They then sit as quietly as possible in a space where they can see and take note of what is happening. Child defecation is likely to be one of the practices of interest, in which case households with young children (under three years of age) should be selected for the observation. Structured observations may not be acceptable to some people so it is important to ensure that fieldworkers do not impose themselves when families are unsure or unwilling. Permission should be sought prior to visiting. Details of how to carry out structured observations can be found on pages 108–9 of the Appendices.

Using the information

Once data have been collected, they must be analysed and presented before they can be of real use.

Analysing information

An important aspect of participatory data collection is that the participants are also directly involved in the analysis of the data. Participatory data collection techniques should provide the opportunity for participants to analyse the problems and suggest solutions during the sessions. During some of the initial focus groups it may be possible to tape the proceedings, with the participants' permission, in order to study the responses in greater depth afterwards. This can also be a way for the facilitators to assess their facilitation skills.

It is important to give feedback on the findings of the session to the group members at a later date. In any event, notes should be taken during the discussion session and used to confirm certain points or clarify the group feeling about particular issues while the discussion is in progress or once the discussion has finished.

An important limitation to quantitative data collection is that the participants are not usually involved directly in the analysis of the survey information. Ways must be sought to involve both interviewers and the community. At the very least,

those who collected the data should also be involved in collating them and ideally, community members should be included. Fieldworkers may require translators for transcribing questionnaires and checklists into local languages and for transcribing findings into the reporting language. It may be possible to use other members of the team who are fluent in the reporting language to translate for them when reviewing and documenting their information, although this is often a very time consuming job.

Quantitative data

A system of collating the information will need to be devised, such as the use of tally sheets, where a line is used to record answers to each question and then grouped together in fives for easy counting. Once the responses have been counted they may be turned into percentages by dividing the number of responses by the total number in the survey and multiplying by 100, for example:

$51 \div 173 = 0.2947976$

$0.2947976 \times 100 = 29.47976$ per cent

These percentage figures should then be rounded to the nearest whole number – in this case 29 per cent.

The LQAS training package, which can be found on the internet, contains example data collation forms. Computer programmes such as SPSS are available but can be expensive and, as with EpiInfo, require some familiarity with statistics and statistical terms.

Qualitative data

Whilst the responses from focus groups or other qualitative data methodologies can sometimes be tallied, the results cannot be translated into

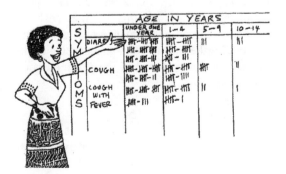

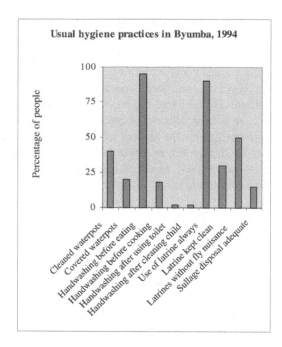

Usual hygiene practices in Byumba, 1994

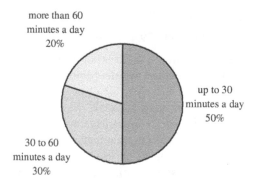

more than 60 minutes a day 20%

30 to 60 minutes a day 30%

up to 30 minutes a day 50%

Figure 1.1 Data obtained from a quantitative survey carried out in Rwanda in 1994

percentages as above. Qualitative data is what people actually say and this has to be analysed by categorizing the information and identifying themes. Further information on analysing qualitative data can be found in the Appendices on pages 116–18.

Presenting information
A way must then be found to present these results in a way that will be understood by the community and other stakeholders. Obviously, if

people are numerate they may understand percentages easily. It will still be a good idea to give a graphic representation of the results in the form of a bar or pie chart. These charts will need to be explained to people who have not learnt skills with numbers.

Figure 1.1 has been drawn from information obtained with the community using questionnaires and group discussions, this time from a development programme in Byumba, Rwanda. They give you an example of how some of your information could be presented. If you do not have a computer and printer to help with all the data analysis and compilation of tables and charts, hand drawn charts, diagrams and tables can be more attractive and just as effective. They can also be enlarged more easily, which may be useful for discussing with larger groups or pinning on noticeboards. The pie chart shows that most of the people in Byumba spend less than one hour collecting water each day, and half of them spend less than 30 minutes collecting water each day. Column graphs (or bar charts) can be used to present and compare data obtained on hygiene practices. The actual numbers are of less importance than the general trends, for example, whether a practice is common, very common or rare. However it is important to clarify in the diagrams what the numbers represent. When talking about percentages, indicate the size of the sample from which the percentages have been drawn. When reporting on focus group discussions, say how many people were involved. Do not present the results as percentages as this may mislead people to think that the numbers represent the whole population rather than those interviewed in the focus group discussion. For example, 'Many of the 80 participants interviewed in four focus group discussions walked for more than 30 minutes to the nearest water point...', is preferable to saying 70% of the participants interviewed, etc.

This data can be triangulated with information from exploratory walks, mapping exercises or short questionnaires to find out how well it represents the situation of the wider community. In the example provided of a bar chart, the bars represent the proportions of various practices reported in focus group discussions and mapping exercises. Bar charts could also be produced from practices

reported through pie charts, voting exercises and questionnaire surveys. With more time, this could be done separately for particular groups found within that community. It is likely that practices will vary in different social groups, for example, for different income-level groups and for people with different education levels. Other differences might be notable, such as cleansing and hand-washing practices of Muslims and Christians. Differences might also be noticed between woman-headed households and male-headed households. Later in the project, a repeat data collection exercise would enable you to prepare new charts. If the project has been successful in enabling people to take action, then the proportion of people practising better hygiene will have increased. In the bar chart in Figure 1.1, the two least common hygiene practices were hand washing after using the toilet and washing hands after cleaning a child. These are proven high risk behaviours and ought to be the focus of the initial hygiene promotion activities. Also, covering of water pots, hand washing before preparation of food, and safe sullage (wastewater) disposal are practices that are seldom carried out and may pose health risks to most people. 'Hand washing before eating' and 'consistent use of latrines' are practices performed by most people and therefore would be the lowest priority for emergency hygiene promotion interventions with this community. The use of pictograms may make the presentation of information easier for beneficiaries to relate to, understand or comment on. The example above illustrates that out of every ten children, six are healthy, three have malaria and one has diarrhoea.

Pictures from this manual can be used and adapted or you may prefer to work with local people to develop ideas yourself.

Sharing information

Sharing these findings and discussing them with the community (or key representatives of the community) will help you identify priorities for hy-

giene promotion interventions. The community may provide you with useful insights into the causes and traditional beliefs around those risky hygiene practices. Together you will be able to identify who is responsible for those practices within the household and how they can best be reached. Figure 1.2 represents a community where covering water pots was found to be a common practice but hand washing with soap after cleaning a child or using a latrine was rare. In this example, promoting hand washing, especially with soap, after defecation and after handling infants' excreta could be chosen. Raising awareness with mothers and child carers about the dangers of infants' excreta might be required. Other issues around the availability and convenience of access to soap and water for hand washing at these times may also need to be addressed. This sort of information could be revealed in focus group discussions.

When decisions are being taken about where to begin implementation, comparing the hygiene practices of different communities may help to

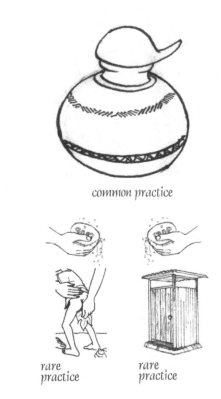

common practice

rare practice   *rare practice*

Figure 1.2 Common and rare practices

In villages affected by the protracted conflict in DRC, an observation walk and focus group discussions were carried out by project staff examining hygiene practices. The results were then fed back to a community meeting using a chart with symbols to represent the frequency of the high risk practices observed in each community. A lively discussion followed. 'Now we are naked and we must make changes' was the comment from one participant at the meeting.

Oxfam, 2002, personal communication

highlight those groups of people with the greatest health risks and therefore the most urgent needs.

If the community feels that it is appropriate, a meeting can be arranged to present and discuss the results. The discussion can be used to cross check the findings and to generate action to change the situation. You may find it useful to produce a table showing the information you have collected. For the purpose of programme records and donor reports, baseline data reports should consolidate the information collected. An example of a situation report is provided in the Appendices on page 226. Another way to give feedback on the results to the community or even to other stakeholders is to present the findings in the form of a drama. Details of how to organize a drama can be found on pages 77–8 and 207.

Preparing for evaluation

Most manuals leave evaluation to the last chapter but it is important to plan how to evaluate from the start, especially in emergencies, as there is a tendency to assume that monitoring and evaluation are less important than the practical task of saving lives. Keeping accurate progress records of a project is vital if those who work in emergencies are to be accountable for what they do.

Indicators derived from the information collected during the assessment and baseline data collection will need to be monitored at different stages of the programme cycle to ensure that the interventions are actually making a difference to people's lives. This is dealt with in more detail in Chapter 2 and 4.

Moving on

This chapter has covered the process of collecting information as part of an emergency assessment. It has detailed types of information that may be necessary for different purposes and the tools or methods that can be used to collect that information. Different ways of using the information have been discussed, including the importance of sharing information with the affected population. Having obtained sufficient information to know where you are now, you can move on and decide where you are going. Planning is the subject of the next section of this hygiene promotion manual.

2
Planning: Where are we going?

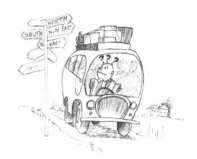

In the last chapter we discussed how you can learn about and understand the situation. This chapter discusses planning. Planning is the process that helps you to decide what can be done, how it can be done, by whom and when. There are many different ways to plan; some are less formal than others. As many donors and organizations (including CARE and Oxfam) are using the 'logical framework approach' to project planning, this is the one that we have chosen to focus on.

Planning framework

Just as obtaining baseline information is crucial to a hygiene promotion project, so is the setting of realistic goals. This section outlines what final and intermediate goals are and shows you how to define them, in order to get your own project where you want it to be. Setting aims and objectives for a project is not easy, nor is creating a 'logical framework'. You will need time and energy to concentrate on 'where you are going'. However, unless you take the time and make the effort to plan, you are likely to waste more time, energy and resources in the long run, and less likely to achieve what you set out to do.

What are aims, goals and objectives?
The terms 'aims', 'goals' and 'objectives' are frequently used interchangeably. There is no universal consensus on their precise meaning. However, aim or goal is often used as a general statement of intent while objectives refer to the precise steps necessary to achieve that aim or goal. The internationally agreed Millennium Development Goal (MDG) for water is: by 2015, to reduce

by half the proportion of people without access to safe drinking water measured by the proportion of the population with sustainable access to an improved water source. The World Summit on Sustainable Development of 2002 added: halve by 2015 the proportion of people without access to basic sanitation. The other MDGs that link to hygiene, sanitation and water supply improvements are included in Table 2.1.

CARE uses the terms 'final goal', 'intermediate goals' and 'output objectives' within a project hierarchy that has five different levels:

1. *Final goal* refers to the impact of this project and other interventions, the sustainable improvements in human conditions or well-being (it may be an MDG);
2. *Intermediate goal* refers to the effects of the project, the changes in behaviour or improvements in access to or quality of resources;
3. *Output* objectives are the specific products of project activities necessary to achieve the intermediate goals;
4. *Activities* are the interventions/processes implemented by the project;
5. *Inputs* are the resources needed by the project, for example, funds, personnel, materials and equipment.

This hierarchy is one that is used by many donor and aid organizations (although the terminology may vary; for example, *intermediate goals* are sometimes referred to as *purpose* objectives or *specific* objectives and *outputs* may be referred to as *results*). The hierarchy forms part of the logical framework, so-called because there is a logical connection between each level. A water, sanitation and health education project could be viewed as depicted on page 41 in Figure 2.1.

Table 2.1 Millennium Development Goals linked to hygiene, sanitation and water supply

MDG	Link to Hygiene, Sanitation and Water Supply
Eradication of poverty and hunger	A lack of water resource management, poor hygiene, unsafe drinking water and lack of sanitation are key links in the cycle of food insecurity, poor growth, disease, malnutrition and poverty. Irrigated agriculture provides a large proportion of the world's food and irrigation comprises over 70 per cent of overall water use
Universal primary education	Diarrhoeal diseases and parasites reduce attendance and attention. Girls often stay away from school unless there are female-only latrines. Time spent collecting water takes precedence over school attendance and this burden often falls on girls. Teachers are unwilling to live in areas without adequate water and sanitation
Promotion of gender equality	Women bear the brunt of poor health and the security risks from lack of private sanitation or washing facilities, and the burden of carrying water. Increasing women's roles in decision making to match their responsibilities, and bring about a more equitable division of labour, are known to help improve water supply, sanitation and hygiene. Demonstrating this can help to improve women's status in other ways
Reduce child mortality	Diarrhoea causes 2 million deaths per year mostly amongst children
Improved maternal health	A healthy pregnancy and hygienic labour practices reduce the risk of maternal illness. Hand washing is a simple yet effective method of improving maternal health
Combating disease: *(HIV, malaria and others)*	Of the global burden of disease, 23 per cent is a result of poor environmental health, 75 per cent of which is attributable to diarrhoea. HIV treatment is more effective where clean water and food are available and HIV-infected people get sick less often if they have good hygiene practices and use improved sanitation and water supply facilities. HIV-infected mothers require clean water to make formula milk. Water management reduces opportunities for malaria mosquito breeding sites. Clean water and hygiene are important in reducing a range of parasites including trachoma and guinea worm
Environmental sustainability	Water resource management is key to environmental sustainability. Water resources are under stress. Public health improvements can address the environmental degradation resulting from urbanization
Global partnerships for development	Public, private and civil society partnerships help deliver water and sanitation services to the poor

Source: DFID, 2004.

Hierarchy of goals, outputs and activities

When setting objectives (intermediate goals and outputs) remember to define how they will be measured and how you will know if they have been achieved. If they are too vague, difficult to measure, impossible to achieve, unrealistic or without a time frame, you will not be able to measure whether or not you have achieved them.

The acronym *SMART* is often used to define the criteria for useful objectives (intermediate goals and outputs):

Specific
Measurable
Achievable
Realistic
Time bound

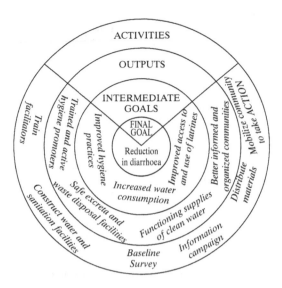

Figure 2.1 Hierarchy of Goals, Outputs and Activities
Source: Adapted from Davis and Lambert, 1995

Oxfam has more recently added the use of the acronym *SPICED* to help refine objectives and make them more people centred:

Subjective
Participatory
Interactive
Consultative
Empowering
Diverse

We have tried to include all these elements in the example logical framework for an emergency hygiene promotion project on pages 130–34 of the Appendices.

How many objectives are necessary?

The project framework should have only one final goal. It is also useful to limit the number of intermediate goals to one and the number of outputs to about three or four, and not more than six. The specific conditions encountered will determine the intermediate goal and outputs chosen. As the project develops, so will the intermediate goal and associated outputs. Refining the intermediate goal, or modifying or dispensing with output objectives and activities, may be indicated by monitoring and evaluation. However, usually

it will be necessary to consult with the donor organization before such changes can be made.

Who sets the objectives?

Joint decision making over the setting of project objectives is very important. If the project objectives are not seen by the community to be worthwhile, there is little chance that they will actively participate in achieving those objectives. In the acute phase of an emergency it may be necessary for project staff to define project goals and objectives. If this is the case, try to ensure that field staff, at least, are able to input into project planning at this stage as they can reflect field reality in the planning framework. When funding deadlines are tight, the logical framework is sometimes constructed by head office but the lack of consultation with field staff may mean that the implementers are unlikely to 'own' it or use it as a tool for planning and monitoring.

It is important that project communities define their own objectives as far as possible and as early as possible in the project. Where the baseline information collection is done in a participatory manner it will provide the beneficiaries with the opportunity to identify their own objectives and indicators as a response to the problems and needs discussed. These objectives will not be static but will develop and change as the project proceeds, and as greater insight is gained into the prevailing problems.

This may seem to run contrary to many planning models (including the logical framework) that attempt to ascertain all the necessary information from the outset of the project in order to provide a predictable blueprint for action. However, the logical framework should be viewed as a tool for

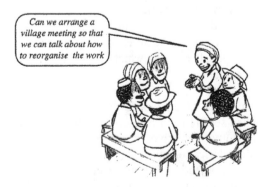

planning rather than as an inflexible procedure that must be followed to the last detail. As Narayan (1993) suggests, participatory planning and management provides a new challenge for managers:

> Because no two communities are alike, joint decision-making implies a certain element of unpredictability. Since no government agency, external sponsor or non-governmental organization can tolerate total uncertainty, the challenge for managers then becomes managing unpredictability by reducing the unknown to acceptable levels without prematurely imposing inappropriate structures.

Factors influencing objectives

There have been discussions over the past few years about standards of service provision in emergencies. Under the Sphere Project, aid agencies agreed minimum standards for disaster response including hygiene promotion, sanitation and water supply. The central standard relating to hygiene promotion is contained in Box 2.1. Hygiene promotion is integral to the other standards set for water supply, excreta disposal, vector control, solid waste management and drainage and the complete set of standards and indicators can be found in the Appendices.

The setting of project hygiene promotion objectives will be influenced by:

o The general project objectives, for example, if these include a plan to protect water sources, then promoting the management of the sources and safe handling and use of the water for drinking purposes would be a hygiene promotion objective.
o The results of initial community surveys or discussion groups highlighting target groups and problem issues and how they are perceived by the local community.
o A review of structures and organizations in the local area with which the project can collaborate.

Project goal and objectives

When setting the final goal, intermediate goals and output objectives, it is important not to sacrifice clarity for quantity. It might be useful to think of objectives in terms of clusters so that the cluster as a whole with its relevant intermediate

---

Box 2.1 Sphere hygiene promotion standards: Programme design and implementation

The Humanitarian Charter (developed under the Sphere Project of the Steering Committee for Humanitarian Response) is concerned with the most basic requirements for sustaining the lives and dignity of those affected by calamity or conflict, based on international human rights, humanitarian and refugee law. Water, sanitation and hygiene promotion are defined under one technical sector with hygiene promotion as the umbrella for both water and sanitation. The three key elements in hygiene promotion in emergencies are:

o *mutual sharing of information and knowledge;*
o *mobilization of communities;*
o *provision of essential materials – facilities.*

Hygiene Promotion Standard 1

Programme design and implementation
All facilities and resources provided should reflect the vulnerabilities, needs and preferences of the affected population. Users should be involved in the management and maintenance of hygiene facilities where appropriate.

Key Indicators are:

o *Key hygiene related public health risks are identified;*
o *Programmes include an effective mechanism for representative and participatory input from all users, including in the initial design of facilities;*
o *All groups within the population have equitable access to resources or facilities needed to continue or achieve the hygiene practices that are promoted;*
o *Hygiene promotion messages and activities address key behaviours and misconceptions and are targeted for all user groups. Representatives from these groups participate in planning, training, implementation, monitoring and evaluation;*
o *Users take responsibility for the management and maintenance of facilities as appropriate, and different groups contribute equitably.*

Source: Sphere Project, 2004.

Box 2.2 The SAFE project in Bangladesh

SAFE was a household sanitation and hygiene pilot project undertaken by CARE Bangladesh with technical assistance from the International Centre for Diarrhoeal Disease Research. SAFE followed CARE's 1991 cyclone relief project around Chittagong and covered about 9,100 households. Behaviour change interventions were focused on the potential benefits of improved water, sanitation and hygiene that were most valued by community members.

Latrine use and faeces disposal

○ *All family members >5 years of age usually defecate in a hygienic latrine;*
○ *Young children (3–5 years) defecate in latrine or fixed place;*
○ *Children's faeces are disposed of hygienically;*
○ *Latrine is maintained clean (inside and out) – especially shared latrines;*
○ *Yard is kept clean and free of human faeces (and garbage).*

Hand washing

○ *Hands are washed with ash/soap before eating, feeding children, food serving/ handling;*
○ *Hands are washed with ash/soap/mud after defecation, faeces disposal or contact with any human faeces, including washing the child's bottom after defecation;*
○ *Hand washing technique includes all of the five following – uses water, washes both hands, uses ash/soap or mud, rubs hands at least three times, hands are dried hygienically – by air-drying or using a clean rag;*
○ *Mud/ash/soap is kept near the kitchen (or other convenient place) for hand washing;*
○ *The rag used for hand drying is kept exclusively for hand drying and washed daily.*

SAFE achieved dramatic improvements for all targeted behaviours and a 66 per cent reduction in diarrhoea prevalence. The project demonstrated that hygiene behaviour change programmes can be successful within nine months.

Source: Bateman et al, 1995;
Zia and Lochery, personal communication.

goal, output, and activity indicators will fulfil all the criteria of SMART and SPICED, even if the component objectives do not. There is no blue-print for setting objectives and many different styles of objective setting may be encountered. The crucial thing is to be aware of what will be measured and how when monitoring and evaluating the project. The LFA approach to project planning provides a logical step-by-step description of objectives and how they relate to each other. The LFA planning matrix is frequently used in longer term development projects and also in many emergency situations. A detailed guide to the logframe is shown in Chapter 1 and an example of a logframe is given on pages 130–34 in the Appendices. It is a complex but comprehensive model, and is useful for outlining all the steps that should be considered when planning a project. The strengths of the logframe approach is the focus on achieving results[2] and ensuring that planners are explicit about the resources, assumptions and critical factors for success. It also requires checks on internal linkages and that attention be given to monitoring and evaluation indicators from the start. The major weaknesses are that it is time consuming and complicated, and may focus on targets and quantitative assessment rather than qualitative assessment.

One way of working out activities and outputs necessary to reach the goal is to develop a problem tree, applying the information you collected during the assessment. A problem tree can be done quite quickly on your own, in a small group or even in a large plenary. For information on how to develop a problem tree and turn it into a logframe, see pages 126–28 in the Appendices. Below are the goals and objectives from our example logframe for you to consider.

The final goal of the example project is: to contribute to the reduction of preventable, communicable diseases and to restore coping mechanisms of the affected community.

As the project is only a small part of what affects the final goal, we must focus on a more

---

[2] Results-based planning is a variation on the logframe terminology where objectives are renamed 'results' and written as if they had already been achieved. This gives the framework an even stronger results focus.

specific intermediate goal: (i.e. the contribution our project is supposed to make towards the final goal) to enable men, women and children in the target population to manage and use water and sanitation facilities optimally, and take preventive action to protect themselves against threats to public health.

In our example, to achieve our intermediate goal, four clusters of output objectives are necessary:

1. X men, women and children have access to and use safe sanitary facilities within six months;
2. X men women and children have safe, equitable access to water in compliance with Sphere standards within X months;
3. X men, women and children are enabled to practice safer hygiene in a dignified and culturally appropriate manner;
4. Community Management Committees (CMCs) are involved in planning and implementing all water and sanitation related activities in X camps/communities.

To achieve these, a total of thirty activities contained within the four clusters are necessary. Each cluster corresponds to one of the outputs.

Activities relating to first output:

1.1 Preparation of design options for discussion with communities;
1.2 Consultation with women to identify suitable sites and designs for sanitary facilities during X community meetings;
1.3 Setting up of X temporary defecation areas;
1.4 Construction of X gender-segregated latrine in line with international standards;
1.5 Training and equipping of X latrine attendants;
1.6 Construction of X gender-segregated washing facilities;
1.7 Construction of X community washing facilities (laundry);
1.8 Provision of potties for under five year olds.

Activities relating to the second output:

2.1 Trucking of water (first phase only);
2.2 Preparation of design options for water facilities;
2.3 Consultation with communities on siting of water facilities;
2.4 Installation of X water points in camps/villages;
2.5 Training of X water point attendants in camp/village;
2.6 Construction of X hand pumps;
2.7 Training of X hand pump technicians in camp/village;
2.8 Establishment of a stock of community spares for water pumps in camp/ village.

Activities relating to third output:

3.1 Collection and reporting of baseline data;
3.2 Identification of partners and counterparts for implementation of hygiene activities;
3.3 Training of X community hygiene facilitators and children's facilitators in camps/villages;
3.4 Development of IEC strategy and materials;
3.5 Provision of X non-food items (NFIs);
3.6 Provision of X community hygiene packs, monthly for six months (soap, disinfectant, laundry soap, for one family for one month).

Activities relating to fourth output:

4.1 Carry out stakeholder analysis to identify key collaborators and vulnerable groups and individuals;
4.2 Organize community selection of management committee;
4.3 Agree roles and responsibilities of all stakeholders in water/sanitation activities;
4.4 Arrange training for CMCs;
4.5 Set up monitoring system for water/sanitation facilities with CMCs;
4.6 Order NFI's, for example, water containers, soap etc.;
4.7 Support CMCs to arrange clean up campaigns;
4.8 Agree mechanisms and support for drainage and solid waste disposal.

We have inserted these activities in the example project framework in the Appendices on pages 131–34 in the column entitled 'narrative summary'.

Measurable indicators

It is now important to determine a way to measure the extent to which goals and objectives are being reached. To do this we need to define indicators to show us if the goals and objectives are being fulfilled. At first glance it would seem to make sense in a hygiene promotion project to measure changes in those indicators by measuring health. In fact, measuring health is not so easy, and we tend to measure the numbers of sick or dead people instead! Morbidity and mortality, however, turn out to be imprecise measures of the success of health or hygiene promotion interventions. This is mainly because they are affected by many different variables, and it is extremely difficult to obtain accurate figures that isolate the effects. For example, it is difficult to measure the effect of providing latrines on the incidence of diarrhoea because the incidence of diarrhoea might also be affected by factors like wealth, education, rainfall, food hygiene, breastfeeding, personal hygiene, individual immunity, uptake of immunizations, availability of clean water and access to health facilities.

It is not necessary to prove that improved water supply, sanitation and hygiene education have an effect on health because researchers have already proved that they do. Thus it has become acceptable to use surrogate or proxy indicators of health impact, such as the use of latrines, the use of soap for hand washing, the use of covers for water containers, and other indicators of hygiene practice. In this way the preconditions for good health are measured and related to the intervention rather than trying to infer the effectiveness of the intervention from increases or decreases in the incidence of diarrhoea.

Indicators that can be used to measure the output objective of community involvement in all project activities (design, siting, construction, operation and maintenance of technical and promotional activities) include community attendance at meetings, the number of hygiene promotion sessions held, self-rating by participants of the

degree of participation and involvement, the setting of objectives by various groups in the community, and actions taken to fulfil those objectives. In this instance one indicator is usually insufficient and sets of indicators will need to be used. In assessing the degree of participation it will also be important for the project to keep records of who participated, who did not, and the reasons for their participation or non-participation in order to identify ways to improve people's involvement. In our example project logical framework, some of the indicators are written as specific targets, for example, 'More than 80 per cent of men, women and children are using and maintaining latrines after X months'. To calculate the extent to which this has been achieved we can compare the percentage of people using temporary defaecation sites/latrines/children's potties at the start of the project (baseline) with the percentage of people using them after three months or even six months. Ideally this and associated indicators will also be monitored as soon as each facility is made available, to ensure that women, men and children find them acceptable and that there is some system in place to ensure they are kept clean. A standard way of measuring these indicators will have to be agreed on so that when they are assessed at different times by different people, they provide a reliable comparison.

Means of verification

The means of verification are the ways or methods by which the indicators are measured. These methods are the same as those used to obtain the baseline data and therefore may be interactive or extractive or a combination of both. Interactive methods might include focus group discussions, the use of pocket charts, mapping and other techniques of applied anthropology and participatory research. It is vital that information collected in this way is included in monitoring forms and project records. More extractive methods are surveys, questionnaires and direct observation. These methods may all be made more participatory by the involvement of the affected community in collecting the data and by ensuring appropriate feedback in a form that can be readily understood by different groups in the community. These methods have been explored in more depth

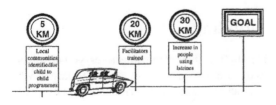

in Chapter 1 and in the 'tools for data collection' section of the Appendices.

Assumptions

There is never absolute certainty that project outputs will result in the achievement of the intermediate goals or that the intermediate goals will lead to the final goal. In working with projects we make assumptions about the achievement of the desired result from the project activities. The lower the uncertainty of the result, the stronger the project design. Unclear or wrong assumptions have probably caused more projects to fail than poorly carried out activities. In order to make sure that assumptions are considered, a column is included for them in the LFA matrix. These 'assumptions' relate to important events, conditions or decisions that are outside the control of the project but are necessary conditions to achieve the output, purpose or goal. By defining these assumptions and risks, their importance can be analysed and ways to actively manage their effects can be incorporated into the project design and implementation. Assumptions need to be re-examined during different stages of the project in order to safeguard the longer term future of the project.

In our example, we assume that peace and stability continue in the settlement area and that strong support will be provided by community leaders. Without stability and political support, the intermediate goal will not result in the final goal as planned. However, if the project takes place as planned and stability and support are in place, then we are confident that there will be some effect on the health of the target population within three months. We can be more certain of the result if we do more to manage the assumption. There are limits, however. For example, the project may not be able to greatly influence the security situation. When the limits are reached, the project should monitor those risk factors closely. However, assumptions such as whether the displaced community will be granted permission to build semi-permanent structures is an assumption that can be influenced by the project. Where possible, the project should include activities that reduce the risks that threaten the project's success. See the activity on risk assessment on pages 128–29 in the Appendices. Each objective does not need to have an assumption. Some assumptions will cover more than one objective. Well thought through plans will leave less to chance and make fewer assumptions. The assumptions box in the top right-hand corner of the logframe matrix is always left blank.

Project framework

Throughout this manual we have referred to the LFA model of project planning. The basic principle of the LFA approach is to formulate highly specific project objectives based on the analysis of all the factors involved, by all the stakeholders. Appropriate indicators can then be selected on the basis of the defined objectives. Regular monitoring of the chosen indicators provides the raw data for project evaluations, and enables the objectives and inputs to be adjusted as experience is gained. When using participatory evaluation techniques, adjustments to interventions can be made rapidly at all levels, with many simple corrections being directly implemented by the communities involved. A logical framework guide for this planning model can be found in Table 0.1 in the Introduction section. At first glance, it may seem complicated; however, once you concentrate on working out goals, objectives and measurements for your own project, the process will become easier. We have designed our example logframe for a hygiene promotion project in a refugee camp during the acute stages of an emergency, spanning into the intermediate stage. The example logframe can be found in the Appendices on pages 130–34. In a more stable setting, such as that afforded by the rehabilitation phase, different goals and objectives might apply. For example, there would probably be no need to distribute monthly hygiene kits to help bring the mortality rate under control and latrine construction might focus on family-level latrines rather than on communal facilities with caretakers, as at the start of the project.

Targeting

Having formulated the objectives, you now have to decide who are the key people to target, who will act as the intermediaries, who you can work with and how to go about it. Many aid agencies restrict their activities to specific sectors on the assumption that this allows for the most efficient use of scarce resources by developing expertise in a chosen sector. The potential limitation of this approach, however, may mean that the resulting interventions do not fit with the priority needs as defined by the affected communities. 'Targeting may not be a sufficient basis on which to understand or intervene in the complexities of people's lives' (Williams, 1995). People are part of a dynamic social process; they lead interdependent lives and focussing on only one aspect of their life will not ensure that rights are achieved. An attempt must always be made to carry out a broad-based needs analysis so that the wider context within which the targeted intervention will take place can be understood and other humanitarian actors lobbied to respond to the communities expressed needs where necessary (see Chapter 1). There are numerous vulnerable groups and vulnerability must always be assessed as it will be specific to a particular situation. However, from past experience we know that often women, older people, disabled people and minority groups will be disadvantaged, especially in a crisis situation. Pregnant women and children under five also form a group that are physiologically more vulnerable to ill health.

Whom to target

Projects are more effective if a small number of key messages are focused to specific target audiences. This concentrates the resources and increases the chances that behaviour change and action will result. Mothers are often designated as the *primary target audience* for hygiene education as they are often very influential in matters of hygiene and are usually the main carers of young children. While targeting mothers is useful for influencing change at the household level, there is also a need to involve their immediate family and other people around them who influence their practices (either positively or negatively). Women do not always have control over household expenditure so obtaining the support of the male head of household will often be important. This is sometimes referred to as engaging the *secondary target audience*.

It is important to work with stakeholders who need to endorse and support the project, such as community leaders, agencies and host government officers. These are sometimes referred to as the *tertiary target audience*.

How to target

It is important to consider how you will access each target audience. The questions in Box 2.3 may be useful to decide who the target audiences are and how to reach them. In conducting community group sessions it is important to appreciate that women may not always feel comfortable expressing their opinions in mixed company. Opportunities should be made to communicate with different types of women in settings in which they can feel at ease. Organizing sessions in places easily accessible to the women you want to reach and at suitable times in their busy work schedules will increase the likelihood of their participation. It may be necessary to get the support of influential men in the community for this to happen. Therefore they will need to have a good understanding of the project objectives if they are to help overcome any local resistance to women's participation.

Targeting children as a separate group is considered important for a number of reasons. Children often represent up to half of the community's population and the under five years age group is a highly vulnerable group in terms of

---

Box 2.3 Points to consider about target audiences

o Who are the members of each audience group?
o Where are they?
o How many of them are there?
o What languages do they speak?
o Who listens to the radio or watches TV regularly?
o What proportion can read?
o Do they read newspapers?
o What organizations and groups do they belong to?
o Which channels of communication do they like and trust?

Source: Curtis and Kanki, 1998

susceptibility to diarrhoeal diseases. In addition, older children are often heavily involved in domestic routines and in caring for younger brothers and sisters. They have opportunities to influence the behaviour of other family members, and will also form the next generation of parents. Learning made fun, practical and appropriate for their developmental stage will usually encourage them to be willing participants and will ultimately increase their potential to be better minders and later, better parents. Suggested activities are outlined in Chapter 4.

You may decide on a social marketing plan to reach the secondary and tertiary target audiences in order to raise the social status of improved hygiene in the community at large. This might include evening radio broadcasts to reach families and public meetings with a drama or video show to reach the tertiary target audience. Additional resources may need to be focused on the target audience in more participatory and intensive activities. This may include child-to-child activities in schools, home visits and women's participatory hygiene learning activities. Facilitator and supervisor training, support and supervision will be necessary. There may also be a need to involve latrine and water source artisans in the active marketing of their services to the community. Each of these activities will require ongoing monitoring and revision to gauge the extent of changing practices towards the project's objectives.

What to target

Faeces are the main source of diarrhoeal pathogens. Practices that stop faecal material contaminating the domestic environment are vital, especially for children. The priorities for public health in hygiene promotion projects are likely to include hand washing with soap after contact with faeces and the safe disposal of faeces (especially young children's faeces) preferably in latrines. Potential 'risk' practices need to be documented and their frequencies assessed. Practices that occur often and that allow faecal matter into the domestic environment are likely to be the important practices to target for change. Identifying the 'safe' practices to replace the risk practices

should be a process developed in collaboration with the community. Where several high risk practices are identified, consider feasibility as well as priority in terms of public health impact. Starting an activity that can progress relatively quickly can be motivating for communities, as well as good for staff morale.

Action plans

Once the overall project goals and objectives have been prepared, the details of what has to be done, by whom and when, have to be planned in detail. Certain activities will need to be carried out first before others are possible. Identifying these is known as a *critical pathway analysis* (see Figure 2.1).

A simple way to create one of these is to draw thick black lines on a Gantt chart to indicate that other activities cannot start until those before the line have been carried out or are underway. In our example, it is essential to meet local leaders as part of the familiarization process before any of the other project work can start. Likewise, the baseline data must be collected before the data can be analysed and the objectives set. The

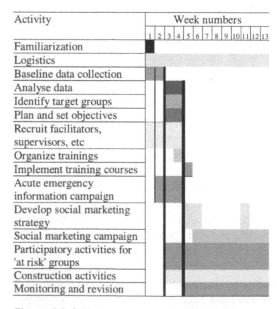

Figure 2.2 Critical pathway chart/Gantt chart

facilitators must be recruited before their training can be carried out. Identifying ways of working with the community can be done only after the recruitment and training of community facilitators, so that they direct the shape of the project activities after they have received their training. In an acute emergency, a two-week information campaign can be started before this, but without some assessment information the focus of the campaign may be inappropriate and much of the effort wasted.

Carrying out the plans

There is no easy route to setting goals and objectives. It requires time to work through them yourself, as well as together with the other project stakeholders – including project staff, government workers, host and displaced community representatives, and so on. Between you, there must be negotiation and compromise until you are all satisfied with the direction the project is going in. Chapter 3 deals with how to implement a hygiene promotion project in an emergency situation.

3

Implementation: How do we get there?

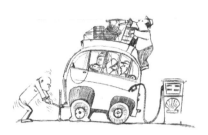

IN THE PREVIOUS CHAPTERS we have dealt with assessment of the situation and planning project activities. It is not possible to offer a blueprint for setting up a hygiene promotion project because situations, aims and objectives vary. This chapter recognizes the need for flexibility and offers you examples and ideas on implementation that can be adapted to suit your local circumstances. In this chapter we shall discuss the wide range of activities that are possible within a hygiene promotion project. A list of possible hygiene promotion activities in an emergency situation is contained in Box 3.1.

This extensive range of activities requires that the hygiene promotion team possesses a similarly extensive range of skills. This makes selection, training and management of hygiene promotion staff a critical component of the hygiene promotion activities.

Selection of fieldworkers

Whom to work with
Identifying key individuals and organizational structures to work with will be one of the first activities that the project needs to undertake and may include church, mosque and youth groups, women's associations, teachers, health care workers and extension workers, as well as groups concerned with health or water and sanitation facilities. In a refugee camp, this could also include attendants of public water points and defecation areas. Where communities have become fragmented, the hygiene promotion project may itself help to bring community members together to collaborate on activities they perceive to be important. It is preferable that, as far as possible,

> **Box 3.1** Possible hygiene promotion activities in emergency situations
>
> - Selection, training and management of field workers and volunteers.
> - Liaison and negotiation with community and other stakeholders.
> - Information collection and analysis.
> - Mass media campaigns and dissemination of information.
> - Stimulating social organization by supporting community leadership.
> - Distribution of tools and materials, for example, for environmental clean up campaigns.
> - Seeking views of different groups in the community on design and siting of facilities.
> - Organizing operation and maintenance systems for water supply and sanitation facilities.
> - Providing safe centres for women and children.

any work is undertaken in collaboration with existing structures but this may not always be feasible. The pros and cons of working with existing community health workers, for example, are listed in Table 3.1. Other development organizations that have been working locally or with the affected population may provide useful insights into the effectiveness of different approaches. Will the project provide a separate cadre of community facilitators who will work alongside existing organizations? Or will the project opt for a more integrated approach, for example, by training and supporting local health or extension workers to operate as community facilitators or hygiene promoters?

Table 3.1 Advantages and disadvantages of working with existing community health workers

Advantages	Disadvantages
Already trained and understand about disease transmission	May be unfamiliar with participatory approaches
Experience of community outreach work using a variety of communication methods	Hygiene promotion may not be their priority so potential impact on project objectives could be lost
Can incorporate hygiene into broader concept of health and explore other health issues such as infant feeding and nutrition	Burden of curative work may preclude them from dedicating time to hygiene promotion
More sustainable as they are already part of a structure expected to survive beyond the project	May require unlearning of didactic style in addition to learning a new style of facilitation

It is important not to duplicate services and to ensure that everybody is given the same accurate information. If it is not possible to work directly with other local structures, indirect ways of offering support and collaboration can be explored. For example, running a short workshop for local health and water and sanitation planners on establishing the project's objectives ensures their interest in the project from the start and may open up other areas of cooperation. Sharing course materials or providing posters for teachers or clinic staff may be another way of extending support for the project.

Children and learning

Children do not have the breadth of life experience and analytical skills of adults but their ideas and attitudes may be more flexible. They are often inquisitive and enjoy opportunities to find things out for themselves. The ways in which they learn will depend on their developmental stage. For example, infants like to imitate and learn by example, small children enjoy learning through play. As children grow older they are able to accommodate increasingly complex and abstract ideas. So how can children be engaged in the hygiene promotion process?

Children in school are a 'captive audience' and learning about hygiene can be integrated into the curriculum or incorporated in the form of specific projects reaching out to the community and forming an effective link between the school and home-learning environments. Where schools are not functioning or when many children do not attend school, they may be reached in other settings, for example, church or youth groups or perhaps simply in the places where they gather daily to play. Adolescents in particular are often very influenced by their peers and can be helped to become effective peer group educators.

The child-to-child approach recognizes the role that many children have in caring for siblings and the potential of children to learn from each other. It seeks to make learning enjoyable for children. They are encouraged to learn through experience and to apply what they learn in a practical way to improve the hygiene conditions within their own family and community. Through sharing and helping each other, they become more aware of their own ability to improve their situation. The child-to-child approach can be successfully implemented in schools and can reach out to non-attendees through activities carried out at home or in the community. A series of resource books, stories and activities is available from the Child-to-Child Trust and TALC in London.

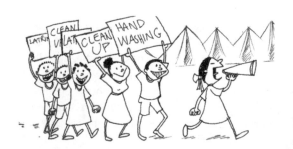

the skills and qualities of these people. The selection process for facilitators is therefore very important. The role of the community facilitator is

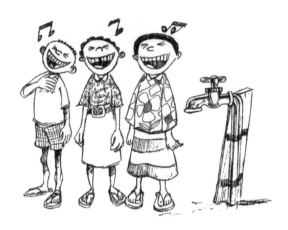

> *In the Occupied Palestinian Territories, an Oxfam programme worked with schools to help them make optimum use of their water supplies that were frequently disrupted. Additional water storage capacity was provided in the schools and water was recycled from drinking water fountains and hand washing facilities in the bathrooms for use in flushing the toilets. In one school there was initially some anxiety amongst the pupils about using the recycled water as they mistakenly thought it was being pumped into their drinking water tanks. Hygiene awareness activities were carried out through a school health club to encourage them to conserve water and to reassure them about the recycling system. As a result of this, the use of recycled water increased and pupils reported that they were much less likely to leave taps dripping than before. The school also made some savings on its water bills.*
>
> Oxfam, 2004, personal communication

> *In Azerbaijan, a series of story books and work books were developed jointly by the emergency project and the Ministry of Health to be used in refugees' schools and mainstream primary schools. The refugee project brought much needed funding for this endeavour. These books were accepted by the Ministry of Health and were used as part of the national health education programme supported by UNICEF. No other such programme existed in Azerbaijan.*
>
> Oxfam, 1994

> *A project in a refugee camp in Goma was working with thousands of unaccompanied Rwandan children of different ages. Clean water was available but not easily accessible to the children aged under five years, and the latrine building project was making slow progress. Many of the children were susceptible to illness because of poor nutrition. In August 1994 there was an outbreak of bacterial dysentery which was followed by an outbreak of non-bloody diarrhoea. A tent-to-tent treatment project combined with health education was commenced in the hope that it would limit the spread of the disease, but with little effect. It was decided to abandon this didactic approach to health education and to involve the children more actively in learning. They were encouraged to make up songs and rhymes about the spread of the disease and these were presented at a group concert which was broadcast on the UNHCR radio station to other camps. Within a week, the incidence of diarrhoeal disease had begun to fall and while the staff knew that they could not prove that this was a result of the dysentery song, they and the children were convinced that their innovative approach to health education had been effective.*
>
> Merlin, 1994, personal communication

Working with children

The tips in Box 3.2 have been prepared to help you work with children.

Who can be a community facilitator?

Community facilitators or promoters often play a central role in hygiene promotion programmes and the success of the project is often dependent on

Box 3.2 Tips for working with children

○ Begin by contacting parents, teachers and community leaders to discuss the project idea. Seek their permission and collaboration and find out from them what they think are the major issues of importance in the community. Some countries and organizations may have child protection policies in place that restrict who can work with children. Find out about these from the Ministry of Social Welfare or children's organizations such as Save the Children.

○ Work with groups of children of a similar age and include them when deciding the topics to be covered. Children of different ages will have different priorities and learning capacities. Find out about their experiences and ideas, for example on the subject of diarrhoea. Use games, stories, discussions and drawings to help them understand and encourage a sense of sharing and learning through cooperation.

○ Ask children to find out more about the topic by talking to their families and other community members. For example, they can find out what people believe about the causes of diarrhoea, how many are affected by it, and/or what they do to prevent or treat it.

○ Help children to share their discoveries with each other and to design activities to help tackle the problems identified. How can they overcome problems that may arise in sharing this information at home and apply it in a practical way when looking after their siblings? What ways can they use to communicate what they have learned to others? For example, inventing songs and games or producing posters and street theatre to put their message across.

○ Review the activities and encourage the children to think about what success they have had and how they might do things differently next time.

○ Decide how to involve teachers and parents in evaluating the success of the project. There will be many things to consider besides the health impact on children, such as the effect it had on their confidence as agents for change and the health of other family members.

○ The challenge posed by the child-to-child approach lies in seeking ways to make learning active and constructive for the child and his/her family. Encouraging children to think, observe, experiment and invent can make learning fun and can help them to apply what they learned into their daily lives.

to work with the community in small groups, ensuring that all participants have an opportunity to put their views forward. They will need to be able to identify and clarify key points in the discussion, challenge opinions and ideas on occasions, help resolve disagreements, and move the process on so that discussion leads to decision making and the planning and implementation of appropriate actions. They will need to have a positive attitude towards the people they will be working with and facilitating. The structure of the outreach work can be decided on following discussions with community members if time allows. The community may decide that a water and sanitation committee will suffice or they may also want to identify additional facilitators who will undertake group discussions and household visits. Whatever the community structure, it is wise to have some project facilitators who will support and supervise the community facilitators. The project facilitators will also be expected to carry out meetings and promotional work with the community. The skills and competencies required by the facilitator will depend on how the role is structured. Box 3.3 lists the criteria one emergency project considered to be essential for the selection of children's facilitators.

The number of facilitators or promoters required to work on the project will vary. WHO and Sphere suggest one community facilitator for every 1,000 people as a minimum, and if people are working as volunteers and if funds allow, then larger numbers will be more effective. It is often useful for facilitators to work in pairs and in some

Box 3.3 Selection criteria for children's facilitators in Azerbaijan

In a project for internally displaced persons in Azerbaijan, a children's health component was established. In each camp a group of three or four refugees was appointed to work as children's facilitators to implement the children's health work, one of which was the leader. The selection of the group was often difficult. These criteria helped to decide who should be included:

○ persons with creative potential (music, art, handicrafts),
○ ability to work with children, preferably with teaching background,
○ ability to organize activities,
○ ability to work with patience (calm temperament).

Source: Oxfam, 1994.

areas it may be better to have a man and a woman. One children's facilitator can probably not manage more than about 30 children and in the interests of safety it is wise not to exceed this. Supervisors of these facilitators can probably support and manage a maximum of 20 facilitators.

Literacy and numeracy requirements

Female community members who are respected by the community may carry considerable weight as opinion formers and role models in terms of their own hygiene practices. They have plenty of life experience and may be confident communicators, but may well be non-literate. This does not have to prevent them from making a valuable contribution; people who do not possess literacy skills often have considerable recall capacity and their lack of experience of formal education may make them more receptive to participatory educational methods. Methods of reporting that do not involve writing can also be explored (examples of these include pictograms, as shown on page 37). In some projects literate and non-literate women work together, each carrying out those functions that make the best use of their skills. A facilitator who is both literate and educated may be more

confident in coping with the organizational and liaison aspects of the role and more acceptable in this capacity to the community leaders and individuals in other sectors with whom she or he may need to collaborate. If quantitative evaluation is part of the job description then literacy and numeracy skills will be needed.

Male or female facilitators

Cultural norms may mean that mixed groups are unacceptable. Even if this is not the case, it is better to ensure that women are not inhibited from participating and it may be better to have women working with women and men working with men. This is not always possible in an emergency situation when it may be necessary for facilitators to be able to speak the local language(s), the host language and the international language. Frequently it is young men, with higher levels of education, who have more extensive language skills.

Age and marital status

Respect for age may mean that more mature individuals have greater credibility, especially when dealing with older people or those of higher status within the community. However, ability and education may compensate for lack of years in this respect. Similarly, marital status and motherhood

In Pakistan following the recent earthquake it was very difficult in some areas to recruit local female staff to work as health promoters or translators. Working in some of the more remote villages meant staff had to be able to stay away from home overnight and this was generally unacceptable. While men had more freedom of movement, they could not talk to women who were not members of their own family. Some agencies tried recruiting young unmarried women from the capital but they were not accepted in the villages. In the end Oxfam tried to increase access to women in the affected communities by recruiting married couples or brothers and sisters who could travel and work together.

Oxfam, 2005, personal communication

may be important for the credibility of women among their peers but may also be regarded as less important in the presence of other compensating skills or abilities. Children and young people often learn more readily from their peers.

Insiders or outsiders

In some situations it will be more appropriate for the facilitator to be drawn from within the local community where knowledge of culture and local language will be advantageous. In other situations, the detached perspective of an outsider would be more useful. A facilitator's ability to communicate with people in a language with which they are most at ease is important, but individuals may differ in their preference for working within communities they know very well. Some facilitators may focus their promotion activities on their family and close relatives. Some may demonstrate more confidence at a slight distance (perhaps in a neighbouring district), while others will feel more able to act as catalysts for change in very familiar surroundings. The project should be able to accommodate their preferences in this respect. If the facilitators are to come from within the community, should they be elected by the community members or accepted on the recommendation of community leaders? Who would do a good job? If the leaders appoint them, how acceptable will they be to the community and how motivated to work on their behalf? If the community has recently been disrupted, is it cohesive enough to be able to make democratic decisions about these matters? If facilitators are to come from outside the community, will they be able to speak the local languages or must they work initially through interpreters? Will they stay in the area after their contract is over? Will they use the skills they have developed in their own communities? It is helpful to establish some criteria for selection of facilitators and decide on the skills required to do a particular job. Suggestions for person specifications are contained in the sample job descriptions in the Appendices on pages 213–15.

Payment and remuneration

There are a number of issues to be considered in relation to the payment of salaries and whether or not people are paid will depend primarily on the urgency of the situation and the amount of time people are required to devote to the work. In the interest of long-term viability it is usually preferable that community facilitators work voluntarily. However, this may not always be feasible. Some communities are familiar with the concept of voluntary workers and individuals may be willing to offer some of their time on this basis. The degree of willingness may be influenced by the amount of time the role requires.

Women in particular are often busy with domestic routines and may not be able to find more than minimal amounts of time to fit around their daily tasks. Paying salaries to facilitators may enable them to devote their time entirely to the job. It can also increase the credibility and respect for the role among those who accord status to salaried positions. Gender inequities may be found here. It is often expected that women will offer their time voluntarily while men will receive payment for different types of work on the same project. Gaining support financially or in kind for the role from the community may not be easy since they may consider that there is nothing tangible to show for their investment. Paying salaries on a per diem basis for the number of days worked may be an option if the job is less than full time.

For some jobs such as the cleaning of public latrines, it may be necessary to employ people full time and to continue paying them for as long

> *In Saki camp in Afghanistan, a women's organization was formed to be, among other things, a channel for public health messages. The organization was not very effective. It lacked trained personnel, a supervisory system and resources. It was also dependent on women volunteers who were not paid, in a camp where payment by agencies was the rule rather than the exception. The value and weight given by the refugee community to work carried out by paid workers as opposed to volunteers was different. The work carried out by women on a voluntary basis was critical, but devalued by its voluntary nature.*
>
> Norwood and Mears, 1993

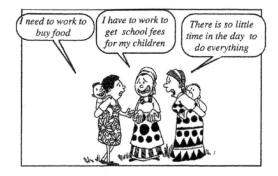

as such a system is used. In some areas of India where the caste system is still strong, certain castes are assigned the role of cleaning latrines or other tasks associated with waste disposal.

If salaries are to be paid, there may be implications for the long-term continuation of the role of facilitator. The crisis may be over, the project funds exhausted and yet the role of facilitator may still be required, but they are unlikely to continue to work for little or no remuneration. How long might the facilitators be required? How do their salary scales fit with the local and host levels? If their role is to continue beyond the lifetime of the project, what options are there for integrating the role into the structure of another organization or developing a community financing scheme for their salaries?

Where a community already has a strong culture of voluntary support for community initiatives it is particularly important not to undermine this completely by paying for all community-focused activities during an emergency. For example, some tsunami survivors in Aceh expressed reservations about the widespread implementation of cash for work projects, fearing that individuals would no longer offer their services for the benefit of the community without payment. Try to include some opportunities for voluntary work in the programme design where possible and ensure that the difference between paid and voluntary roles is easy to distinguish in order to avoid demoralizing the volunteers. If people agree to work voluntarily, come to an arrangement with them about the number of hours they are prepared to contribute and do not necessarily expect that they will make a long-term commitment of their time. Avoid overloading them with respon-

Animal and human faeces and solid waste were creating a health hazard in a Sudanese refugee camp in Eastern Chad. Poor sanitation and the onset of the rains gave rise to fears of an imminent cholera outbreak. The camp authorities suggested that the community should be mobilized to clean up and that payment should be provided to get the job done quickly. A health promoter lobbied for a different approach. Tools for cleaning were provided to community leaders who organised work groups within their sectors and an information campaign was mounted to raise awareness of the health risks. The health promoter visited the camp clinics every day to monitor diarrhoea rates as she had agreed with the authorities that an increase in the daily rates would signal the need to pay for the clean up operation. An outbreak was averted and community leaders continued to organize the environmental cleaning activities even after the end of the rains.

Oxfam, 2004, personal communication

sibilities so that the only way they can do the job is to gradually increase the amount of time they have to spend volunteering.

Payment of salaries at an elevated rate in order to get the job done quickly during an acute emergency has often led to problems in the long term. Host communities may leave their normal work to take higher paid relief work in refugee camps. Where refugees are employed, the host population may resent the lost opportunities to themselves. It also becomes increasingly difficult to get a job done for its real value. Salaries are not the only way that staff and volunteers can be remunerated and payment in kind may be a better option. Incentives might include daily allowances, provision of food or meals, provision of tools, soap or equipment to do a job, which could also be used by the person for non-project activities (for example, a bicycle). Other forms of motivation include:

○ visits to other places (perhaps with the purpose of generating new ideas for the project);

○ obtaining certificates for the training that allows people formal recognition of their achievements and possible access to future remuneration;

○ providing them with marketing and sales skills to be able to sell their products or services to the community.

Who manages the facilitators?

Facilitators and other hygiene promotion workers all require support and supervision. It is possible to manage effectively a maximum of 20 facilitators in an area where their work locations are close together and distances between work sites are short. Where distances are greater, fewer facilitators can be managed. The ratio of facilitators to staff is ideally 10 to 1 where they are working in one small camp or village and should not exceed 20 to 1 supervisor. However, where the project covers a large geographical area, the supervisor may only be able to manage four or five facilitators. In a large project, these supervisors will require managers – either a coordinator of the hygiene project or a coordinator of a broader programme. There are issues around selection and recruitment. What level of qualifications and experience should they have? Should the supervisors be male or female? How old should they be? Should they come from within the community or from outside it? What should be their remuneration? The key qualities of a supervisor will probably be organizational and administrative skills, commitment and a flexible, empowering approach to hygiene promotion. A possible person specification has been prepared for a hygiene promotion supervisor on page 213 of the Appendices.

Contracts and job descriptions

Having decided on the roles, responsibilities and rewards for the fieldworkers, these should be formalized in a clear job description, along with the terms and conditions considered necessary and appropriate for that job. A person specification should then be drawn up, stating those qualities that are essential (for example, able to make people feel at ease) and those that are desirable but not essential (for example, able to read and write in English; previous experience). Candidates who are likely to have the necessary skills can then be

selected. The selection process should be designed to test for these essential and desirable skills so that decisions are made on a candidate's ability to perform the job. For example, if it is essential that facilitators are able to communicate effectively with refugee mothers, part of the selection process might include observing the candidates as they discuss a relevant topic with a group of refugee mothers. Indicators with which to measure this ability should be set first to enable observers to measure the performance of candidates against relevant criteria. The criteria may include spoken language skills and appropriate body language. Selection can also be carried out during the training process. For example, two possible candidates can be trained for each post available and the better of each pair is then appointed to the post. However the selection process is designed, the process should be made clear to the candidates. Once selected, candidates need to be formally offered the job. This can be done on paper in a formal contract outlining the roles, responsibilities, time period, rewards associated with the job and the consequences of not performing the job. In this way, false expectations are minimized. Suggested items to include in an employment contract are listed in Box 3.4 and include signatures of agreement by both parties to the contract. Sample job descriptions for hygiene promotion supervisors, community facilitators, children's facilitators, campaign workers, waterpoint attendants, and community latrine attendants, including person specifications, are included in the job descriptions section of the Appendices on pages 213–16. Copies of the contract and the job description should be kept by the employee and the employer. All entitlements to be provided by the employer should be given at the agreed time. Failure to adhere to the agreed contract will demotivate the employee and may prevent them from performing their roles and responsibilities.

Before recruitment, it is worth considering how you will deal with staff or volunteers if they are unable to perform their roles. This is particularly relevant when the staff or volunteers are selected by the community. How will you deal with accountability and with whom? Box 3.5 contains an example from a refugee camp situation.

Box 3.4 Items to include in an employment contract

o Name of employer, name of employee.
o Date of commencement of contract (and completion, if fixed term).
o Rate of remuneration (salary and expenses).
o Frequency of payment (for example, weekly, monthly).
o Days and hours of work.
o Terms related to holidays, public holiday pay, religious days, time off in lieu, maternity and paternity leave etc.
o Terms related to sickness and injury benefits.
o Length of notice required for contract termination by both parties.
o Disciplinary rules applicable to employee.
o Grievance procedure.
o An attached job description.
o Dated signatures of employer and employee.

Source: Davis and Lambert, 1995.

Box 3.5 Selecting community health workers

The criteria for the selection of community health workers in Maza camp, Rwanda were set in consultation with groups of men and women from the Burundi refugee community. The criteria included:

o a high level of respect among the community;
o an ability to speak the local languages;
o a ratio of one male to one female worker.

At meetings set up with the wider community, health workers were selected and names cross checked with the crowd. Later the community substituted new health workers in place of those who were not suitable or who did not perform. Some health workers were seen to be too young and had been selected due to family ties with other important members of the community. It would have been useful to have selected from a wider group of people and then identified those most suitable for recruitment, with representatives from the wider community.

Source: Oxfam, 1994.

If your organization has a code of conduct, which may cover such issues as use of the agencies' funds and resources and guidance on staff behaviour, this should be made available in the language of the prospective employee with whom it should be discussed before they sign a contract of employment.

Training of fieldworkers

Training is an important aspect of hygiene promotion and should reflect the community learning processes. The course organizer will need to respect the knowledge and experience of the participants just as the participants will be expected to respect the knowledge of the community members they will work with. The use of participatory learning techniques should be encouraged and practised by the learners if they are to use them as part of their role as facilitators. Didactic teaching should be kept to a minimum. This may seem strange to the learners at first, especially if they are more familiar and perhaps more comfortable and confident with didactic approaches. Encouraging participants to discuss the methods and practise implementing them quickly increases their confidence. Trainees should be encouraged to review these exercises and materials so that they can use their own experience to determine which are the most effective tools to assist learning. The use of a variety of training methods and materials is recommended to maintain interest and provide a broader experience. Concentration will probably lapse after about 20 minutes if the participants are not actively involved in the session. Responses are likely to be slower in the afternoon following a meal. Training should not be confined to the classroom setting and fieldwork supervision and mentoring should form a major aspect of any training course.

> **Box 3.6** What adults remember
>
> Adults remember:
>
> 20 per cent of what they see;
>
> 40 per cent of what they see and hear;
>
> 80 per cent of what they **discover for themselves.**

Adult learning

As Brazilian educator Paulo Freire pointed out, the traditional approach to learning has often been to try to cram knowledge and information into people's heads. The problem-posing or learner-centred approach encourages people to think for themselves and stimulates action by setting real life examples of problems to be addressed. Adults learn better if their existing experience is valued and respected and if they are comfortable in the learning environment.

In many situations participants may be non literate and this may also mean that they are not visually literate and they will therefore find it difficult to 'read' pictures. However, the skills of visual literacy can be learnt quite quickly so it is useful to ensure that if pictures are used these are explained to others by a participant who is visually literate.

Training needs assessment

A training needs assessment is the first stage in carrying out any training activity but may need to be carried out rapidly in the initial stages of an emergency. There is no reason why the assessment process cannot continue as the project progresses. A training needs assessment should find out:

o The skills and knowledge that are required:
   – *what* people know and do already;
   – *what* they will be required to do.

o The target group:
   – *who* to train;
   – *how many* people to train.

o Practical issues such as:
   – *where* to carry out the training;
   – *when* to begin;

– *how long* the course should be;
– *which methods* to use;
– *what incentives* to provide.

These decisions will be influenced by the stage of the emergency. In some cases the participants may be required to unlearn some of the things that they already know, perhaps to rethink some of their attitudes about communicating and supervision. When the need for a rapid response and campaign-style information provision is no longer paramount, it will be possible to consider more people-centred ways of carrying out hygiene promotion.

Before a training course

Planning the course will entail the following steps:

1. Collect basic *background information* on issues that will be relevant to the training, for example, population estimates, risk factors for water- and sanitation-related diseases (see checklist on page 26). You do not need to have detailed information at this stage, as much of this will be collected during the participatory field sessions included in the training. Discuss this information with community leaders or representatives along with the role, recruitment, training and organization of facilitators. You should also try to make contact with potential trainees from a variety of different sectors of the community. Documents and reports relating to the area may also be useful.

2. Organize the *recruitment* of the people who will undertake the training. Arrange the selection procedure in the village or at a central location. Try to determine their training needs. This may take several days depending on the number to be selected and the urgency of the situation.

3. Clarify the *purpose* and *objectives* of the course. Plan the training programme and prepare materials. This requires planning each session and may involve the local production of materials. A one week course is likely to require at least two weeks planning. However, in an acute emergency, both may be condensed into a few days.

4. Organize the *logistics* for the duration of the course. This task will require several days and

should be done well in advance of the course, just in case anything takes longer than expected. Logistics includes the venue with suitable seating arrangements, storage space for any training materials to be used and possibly child-care arrangements. There should be scope for a variety of seating arrangements to allow a range of different training activities to be conducted. Participants will need to sit in a large circle for plenary sessions and in smaller circles for some group activities. Sitting in a large semi-circle may be helpful if a flip chart is being used for a presentation or summary.

5. *Accommodation* for the trainees will be needed if they are coming from outside the local area. Arrange regular breaks for food and drink if possible because low energy levels will not make learning easy. Some participants will be expecting payment for attending the course and careful consideration needs to be given to the levels of these payments to keep them sustainable or in line with host government policy. Arrangements for transport and carrying out community-based activities will need to be made.

6. Prepare the *timetable*. Arrange the topics in sequence, decide on the teaching methodology for each session and plan the approximate timing. Allow flexibility so that the learning needs of participants can shape the course.

7. Prepare the *learning materials* that will be needed. They may include teaching aids such as a flipchart, large sheets of paper and pens, blackboard and chalk, or cards, pens and a pin board. Slides, overhead transparencies, videos or multi-media projectors may also be required in addition to those other materials required for the participants to use in simulated

Keep the following adage in mind and concentrate on what is essential initially:
What is essential to know
What is useful to know
What is nice to know
Abbatt and McMahon, 1985

participatory sessions, such as case studies, picture cards, posters, pocket charts, flannelgraphs or flexi-flans and materials for mapping and modelling. Depending on time constraints, the participants may be able to produce some of their own visual aids such as props for community theatre or puppet shows and discussion pictures. While learning aids can greatly enhance a training session, they should not be allowed to dominate and distract from the purpose of the session. Effective learning is possible using no more than simple local materials such as twigs, leaves, seeds and stones.

8. Arrange for *follow-up* training, monitoring and supervision of activities after the course. Having worked all these things out, the activities can be detailed more clearly on a Gantt chart as part of the project plan. An example of a Gantt chart is given on page 48. Keep the above adage in mind and concentrate on what is essential initially.

Learning objectives and outcomes

For each training session it is useful to think about why you are doing this and what you hope to achieve from it. Setting learning objectives, for example: at the end of the session participants should be able to... demonstrate how to make up and give oral rehydration solution... list the causes of diarrhoea... demonstrate how to run a focus group discussion. These objectives will help to focus the session and provide a useful way in which the training can be evaluated.

During a training course

Training should focus on community processes and be community based as much as possible, using practical sessions held with the community in the field. This will enable the participants

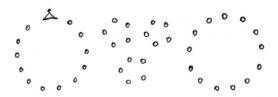

Possible seating arrangements

to learn in a real environment and help them to review and reflect regularly on the benefits to the community. This process can be enhanced with debriefing and evaluation.

Debriefing – is the process in which participants are asked to address such questions as:

○ How did the community find the activity?
○ What did you learn from the community about the activity?
○ What aspects of the activity contributed to/ inhibited communication?
○ Was it useful for encouraging discussion, analysis of problems, planning activities?
○ How would you go about organizing the activity in the community?

Ensure that you model the way participants are expected to interact with the community by the way you facilitate their learning. Make sessions as interactive and participative as possible, always trying to build on their existing knowledge and skills.

Evaluation is the process of reviewing the session, training day or training course. Evaluating previous activities is important, and feedback should be used to modify subsequent sessions. It can be done using the facilitation/evaluation wheel (see page 94), a simple questionnaire or with a flipchart placed in the training room for participants to record their positive and negative views – including style, content and pace of the sessions as well as satisfaction with the logistical arrangements. An overall evaluation of the training course should take place on the final day. This will involve the participants self-rating their satisfaction with the course, defining what they have learnt and what could be improved upon for next time. A visual evaluation sheet or mood metre showing different facial expressions that participants tick or circle to indicate how the course has left them feeling is shown on page 98. Evaluating learning is also important and can be done as the course proceeds using role plays, team quizzes or short written tests if the participants wish. Reviewing learning at subsequent follow-up training sessions is also a way to evaluate previous learning. The course organizer should

also reflect on his/her performance at each session, perhaps by keeping a course diary or by reviewing the day's activities with co-trainers or other colleagues.

After a training course
After the training course it will be important to help the participants plan how they can apply the training in the community. They can work with community leaders to organize activities or by initiating discussion groups wherever people normally gather. Review sessions can be arranged with the participants once they have started work so that they continue to evaluate their activities and develop their skills on the job.

Training methods
This section outlines various popular training tools.

Introductory exercises enable participants to make personal introductions in an informal atmosphere, while avoiding comparisons in terms of rank and experience that may inhibit some people from contributing. A number of introductory exercises are available. These include 'smiley Samuel', 'the name game' and 'favourite animals'. Details of how to carry out these exercises can be found in the Appendices on page 135–36.

Listening exercises are designed to improve listening and observation skills. They can help to shift people's views, allowing participants the chance to reflect on how they behaved in the exercise. It is crucial to follow listening and observing exercises with debriefing discussions. Some listening exercises include 'nodders and shakers', the 'folding paper game' and 'whacky whispers' and can be found on pages 136–37 of the appendices.

Lectures may be useful for introducing or summarizing a topic but they do not encourage reflection and should be used only if other methods are not possible. People quickly forget most of what they hear if they do not have the opportunity to relate it to their own experience through discussion and reflection. Attention tends to wane quickly, so lectures should be interspersed with

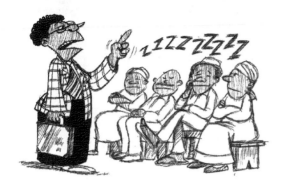

other methods to keep people interested. If you must lecture, focus on a few key points – the things you most want participants to remember – and repeat these points several times over. Avoid bombarding people with lots of information.

Brainstorming is a useful technique for generating ideas. Every individual in a group is encouraged to contribute ideas on a particular theme. The topics are not discussed during the brainstorm and the aim is to get as many contributions on a particular theme as possible, whatever the quality. They should be recorded and may be grouped together and discussed later. If brainstorming is new to the participants they can practise using a familiar topic such as the names of local fruits. Dividing the group into buzz groups of two people may give people more time to reflect on a topic prior to a brainstorm with the plenary group.

Discussion groups can be formed by splitting large groups into smaller groups of three or four people (or buzz groups of two people) to discuss issues in more depth than would be possible in a large group. The small groups can then be asked to give feedback on the main points of their discussion to the large group. This can be useful for collecting a range of ideas quickly. Feedback is important but it should not be allowed to become too repetitive; for example, each group could contribute only those ideas that are different from those already submitted. Discussion groups can also be used as a way to explore issues in depth and to develop problem-solving skills. The use of participatory techniques for training can be

simulated in the classroom by small groups of trainees. They can be used in this context to explore their beliefs and attitudes and to encourage their own learning through participation, as well as to help them become familiar with the learning strategies they will be using in the community. Some small group exercises involve the use of pictures and posters. Try to avoid discussing the detail of the pictures. Instead use the discussion to develop analytical/problem-solving skills. Small group exercises are included in the sample time-tables in the Appendices on pages 216–21 and described in more detail on pages 106–7, 109, 112–16, 167–200 and 211.

Case studies allow participants to work through a given real life situation and decide how they would tackle the problems as they are presented. Participants can be allocated roles and asked to consider their contribution from the perspective of that character. Significant preparation is needed for case studies but it can be useful for learning analytical and priority-setting skills. A shorter version involves presenting a group with a description of a situation and asking them to consider what went wrong or how they might have handled the situation differently. Details of how to use case-study material with examples of case studies is included in the Appendices on pages 148–50.

Drama is the process of acting out a situation and can be used in a number of ways as a means of communication. Drama can be used:

○ to communicate in an entertaining way with large audiences in the form of street theatre (pages 77– 8 and 208–9);
○ in a participatory way by community groups acting out a problem scenario of their choosing;
○ to involve children in thinking about health problems in their community and getting them to consider some of the solutions;
○ as a training activity for community facilitators.

Role-play is the use of drama in which people act out situations for themselves in order to acquire communication and problem-solving skills and

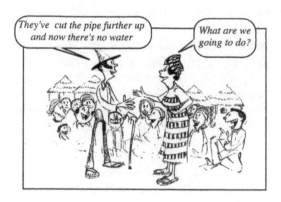

They've cut the pipe further up and now there's no water

What are we going to do?

Health promoters in DRC got local musicians to write a song about diarrhoea prevention following the volcano which caused widespread displacement in Goma in 2002. The already overcrowded, poorest area of the city was inundated with people whose houses were flattened by the lava. Poor sanitation and drainage and a lack of clean water led to fears of an outbreak of dysentery or cholera. It was difficult to evaluate the impact of the song, but it remained at the top of the local music charts for six weeks and many people in the town could be heard singing it!

Oxfam, 2002, personal communication

understand situations more fully. Role plays can help us learn more about people, their motivations and their behaviours. Role plays can vary in length from 10 minutes to a whole day. Participants try to imagine themselves in the roles of other people and respond to a situation as they think their character would do. This can help them to understand other people's views and to anticipate how they might respond in a similar situation. When performed in front of a group, role play can encourage discussion and can lead to working out solutions to a particular dilemma. The purpose of the role play should be carefully explained at the beginning of the session to help overcome possible reluctance or feelings of embarrassment. At the end of the session each of the participants should be debriefed and helped to disengage from their role characters. This can be done by asking each participant in turn to in-

troduce themselves again and to share their feelings about their roles and the role play. If this is not done, uncomfortable feelings brought out by the roles and between the actors may cause problems later. Examples of role plays can be found on pages 147–8.

Hot Seating is a type of role play with one participant taking the 'hot seat' and explaining an imaginary or real dilemma to the other participants who must then try to make suggestions as to how to solve the problem.

Songs can be a useful way of summarizing and memorizing information. Songs are particularly effective with children. Participants can be asked to invent songs about diarrhoea, or to adapt the words of a popular, easily remembered song with new hygiene-related words. The process of preparing new words and phrases, and singing them helps people to learn and remember the hygiene messages, and may influence later actions. Box 3.7 contains an example of a song used to encourage people to wash their hands.

Experiments and models can be used to demonstrate the concepts you are teaching. Experiments showing the effects of dehydration are very effective in the teaching of oral rehydration therapy. Some examples of experiments are included in the Appendices on page 210.

Box 3.7 The hand washing rap

You gotta wash your hands, you gotta wash them right. Don't give into germs without a fight.

Use water that's warm and lots of soapy bubbles, these are your weapons for preventing germ troubles.

Don't cut short your time, your fingers get between, it takes 20 seconds to make sure they're clean.

Gotta wash, gotta wash, gotta wash your hands

You gotta wash, gotta wash, gotta wash your hands...

The main hygiene promotion activity revolves around the hygiene education clubs in each of the 18 refugee schools. The children in the clubs produce poems, plays, songs and essays about the need for good hygiene and relate them to other children in the school, as well as taking the same messages to the residential blocks for the children who do not attend school.

Dadaab Refugee Programme, Kenya
CARE, 1997

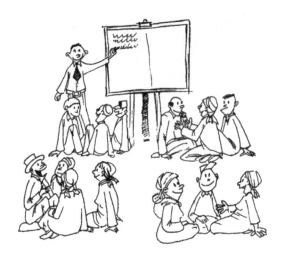

Stories can be spoken or read aloud, acted out or told using pictures. They can be used as teaching tools in several ways:

○ by incorporating a moral they can be applied to real life;
○ by incorporating local problem situations and identifying possible actions for their resolution;
○ by making it a creative activity to help children develop their understanding of hygiene-related activities;
○ by sensitively incorporating traditional practices and beliefs (in a way that avoids undermining confidence in local practices).

For an example of a story that could be used to stimulate people's imaginations and initiate a discussion on hygiene, see page 208 of the Appendices.

Length of training
Training sessions that aim simply to orientate people to the project may be as short as half a day to one full day. Those designed to impart basic communication skills to participants in an emergency campaign can be similarly brief. Training facilitators will take longer depending on their existing skills, background and availability. The project may have to take account of participants' other work and family commitments and, depending on the urgency of the situation, the course could be conducted part time over a longer period at times to suit the participants. Providing facilitators with regular opportunities to review their work and get feedback in the field is a way of continuing the training on the job.

Numbers of people to be trained
The number of people who can be trained at any one time will depend on the training methodologies used and the extent to which the participants are encouraged to participate in the training. Lectures and presentations lend themselves well to the transfer of information from one person to large numbers of people, whereas group discussions work best with smaller numbers. Working groups of six to eight people usually enable most of the participants to make a contribution, and three groups of this size, i.e. 24 people, could be effectively managed on one course provided sufficient time is allocated to allow each of the groups to give feedback to the whole group in plenary.

Sample training workshops
We have given five examples of training workshop timetables. The first is training for community facilitators who often play the key role in community hygiene promotion projects and are variously known as volunteers, animators, motivators, mobilisers or hygiene promoters. This workshop includes the use of simulated community group discussion exercises, role plays, case studies and dramas. The second is training for facilitators who work with children. The third training is for hygiene promotion supervisors, which emphasizes the need for a positive attitude towards staff and the community and negotiation skills in addition to an understanding of the principles of hygiene promotion. The fourth training

is to help those involved in information campaigns to communicate more effectively. The fifth training is for latrine and water-point attendants and includes raising their understanding of hygiene and their roles in promoting hygiene in the community. Each of the trainings emphasises active participation as a means of enabling participants to learn from one another. For instance, one learning objective is for participants to understand about disease transmission, but instead of a lecture on this subject, there is a series of exercises to explore and build upon the existing knowledge and experience of the participants and then enable them to relate this to a concrete situation. Learning in this way is more likely to increase knowledge and address the changes in attitude necessary to motivate changes in practice. The use of games, story telling, drama and puppets are emphasized in the children's facilitators course, as these are all techniques that can be used with children to collect information to enable them to learn more about the problems in their communities.

Training community facilitators

There are no hard and fast rules about the numbers of community facilitators to be trained. Large numbers of people may be required if they have very limited time to contribute. The number of full-time community facilitators required can be determined by population size or the number of water points. WHO and Sphere recommend a minimum of one community health worker (facilitator/ promoter) per 1,000 of the population. Other projects have employed a ratio of one facilitator to 500 people or even one facilitator per 10 households. While these figures can be used for approximate guidance, it is important to review them in the light of the level of community contact that the community health workers are able to achieve. We have prepared an example six day community facilitators' training course for about 20 participants, sometimes split into three small working groups for the training and community-based exercises. The training includes activities that take place in the community on most afternoons. The training objectives and timetable can be found on pages 216–21 of the Appendices. A facilitators' training course could take place in any building

or shelter with sufficient room to accommodate the participants, allowing them to work in small groups without distracting each other. This may be a school, hall or large tent. Training may even take place in the open under a shady tree, although the lack of privacy makes it a less than ideal venue. A training course for this level of participants should be built around a number of participatory learning exercises to be used by facilitators in the community to help people analyse the causes of ill health and plan activities to improve their situation. Exercises are simulated in the training to become both learning tools for the participants and course organizer and to start assessment work directly in their communities. A large number of exercises are included to illustrate the range of ways that people can be helped to learn. It must be emphasized, however, that the sample timetable is provided to stimulate ideas rather than to suggest a fixed model. The course could be made shorter or altered to include other methodologies as required to meet the project objectives. Box 3.8 suggests possible topics for inclusion in the community facilitators training courses.

Box 3.8 Topics that could be covered in community facilitators' training courses

o Beliefs about what makes people sick and how diseases are transmitted.
o Practices that lead to water- and sanitation-related diseases (see section A8 in the Appendices, pages 233–42).
o Preventing water- and sanitation-related illness.
o Barriers that prevent people from adopting preventive practices.
o Working with groups, individuals and the media.
o Working with children.
o Men's and women's issues in water and sanitation.
o Learning styles and adult learning.
o Participatory methods as an approach to learning.
o Methods of communication.
o Data collection, monitoring and evaluation.
o Planning a hygiene promotion project.

Training children's facilitators

Young people often communicate effectively with children, so this course is suggested for a group of 20 teenage girls and/or boys. An example of the objectives and timetable for a children's facilitators' training course can be found on pages 216 and 218. This course is based on the child-to-child approach outlined on pages 52–3. The course is intended to involve children actively in the education process and in helping the facilitators to draw on their own experience as learners and caretakers of small children. The training course is scheduled over five days, but the sessions could be organized over a longer period of time if necessary, to fit in with their school and family commitments. Some sessions could be removed or others added as appropriate according to the project's aims and objectives. The training venue should be selected to provide enough space for carrying out practical activities in small groups.

Training supervisors

The number of supervisors to be trained will vary with the project but on average one supervisor will be required for every 20 facilitators (community and children's). We have prepared an example six-day supervisors' course for about 20 participants, sometimes split into small group work and often using role-play simulations to practise important techniques for supervision. The training objectives and timetable can be found on pages 216 and 219 of the Appendices. A supervisors' course could take place in any building or shelter with sufficient space to accommodate the

The health promoter's role in the community is one of facilitation, not knowledge provision. Originally the training covered all aspects of sanitation and health but it became clear that the health promoters were instructing people. The training and approach were changed; now the focus is on problem solving and identifying existing good hygiene practices that can be built on and promoted to the rest of the community.

Slaya Health Education, Water and Sanitation Project, CARE, 1998

Box 3.9 Topics that could be covered in supervisors' training courses

o Practices that lead to water- and sanitation-related diseases.
o Preventing water- and sanitation-related diseases (see section A8 in the Appendices, pages 233–242).
o Barriers that prevent people from adopting preventive practices.
o Gender issues in relation to water and sanitation.
o Adult learning and behaviour change.
o PLA as an approach to learning communication skills.
o Role and attitudes of health workers and supervisors.
o Recruitment and selection.
o Training fieldworkers.
o Data collection and analysis.
o Needs assessment.
o Planning.
o Monitoring and evaluation.
o Report writing.
o Effective negotiations and meetings.
o Conflict resolution.
o Time management.

participants. However, one large room and one small room that are light, clean and quiet would be best.

A training course at this level should be built around the sort of work the supervisors will be expected to do, for example, aspects of assessment, planning, supervision, negotiation and report writing. They will require an understanding of what the staff they are responsible for are meant to do in the field. Box 3.9 suggests some possible topics for inclusion in the supervisors' training course.

Training communicators for information campaigns

Community leaders and representatives, and other experienced communicators, for example, teachers, extension workers, could all be trained to promote hygiene in a campaign. The maximum number of people to train at one time would be 40 people and the group would need to be split into smaller groups of no more than eight. A rapid training could be carried out in four hours to provide people with the basics for starting work but on the job support and further training will be necessary. A venue large enough to accommodate the participants and to allow space for group work is required to carry out the training.

A job description for campaign workers can be found on page 214 and an example training programme can be found on pages 216 and 220. The training comprises two sessions, one focusing on the priority messages to be communicated and the other on communication skills. It is a good idea to arrange follow-up sessions at the end of the first week of the campaign and again at the end of the second and final weeks to review the outcome of the campaign workers' efforts. Various methods of communication can be used, including dramas and radio messages broadcast over loudspeakers or megaphones (if available). Posters can be used to reinforce verbal messages and are most helpful as a backup to more interactive forms of communication. Time and effort devoted to the production of visual aids should not detract from vital person-to-person communication.

Training latrine and water-point attendants

Latrine and water-point attendants play a vital role in improving sanitation and hygiene conditions in camps and communities. Sample job descriptions can be found on pages 214–15. They can also be effective hygiene promoters among the users of the facilities they are responsible for and at home with family members. Latrine and water-point attendants should be selected from the users of those facilities. Again, the maximum number of people to train at one time would be 40 people, and the group would need to be split into smaller groups of no more than eight. They could be trained within one day. A venue large enough to accommodate the numbers is required to carry out the training without disturbance. This sample training course includes participatory methods for discovering their existing knowledge about hygiene and clarifying and correcting issues as required. The course also includes sessions on the importance of their role in the health and hygiene of the community and provides them with some experience of collecting data on the use of their facility and what they can use this

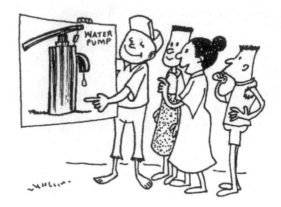

information for. The sample training course for both can be found on pages 220 and 221 of the Appendices.

Management of fieldworkers

Fieldworkers in emergencies require effective management in order to fulfil their roles and responsibilities. This applies when they are paid staff as well as when they are volunteers. During the initial phase of an emergency, basic management procedures that can be expanded at a later stage will be required. Management involves four key activities: planning, leading, organizing and controlling. The ability to convey clarity and understanding are two important skills of all good managers.

Teamwork

The team's effectiveness is determined by a shared goal, collaboration and coordination of activities and regular, frequent interactions.

Clarifying roles and responsibilities and selecting workers for their abilities to perform these functions is an important aspect of management and has been covered in the section on contracts and job descriptions above. It is useful for all members of a mixed discipline team to realize that working in these teams has a number of advantages and disadvantages. These are listed in the Box 3.10.

Jointly developing a shared goal and ways to achieve it (such as developing the logframe and action plans together) will increase the commitment of those team members to achieving that

Box 3.10 Advantages and disadvantages of working in a team

Advantages:

o Brings a variety of skills to tackle the task;
o Opportunities to learn from each other;
o Mutual support;
o Potential to motivate each other;
o Degree of independence from the organization.

Disadvantages:

o Goals can be out of tune with the project or organization;
o Team's views may go unchallenged;
o Competition leading to conflict.

Although each health educator worked with different groups of Rohinga refugees in Dumdumia camp, there were daily meetings between the health educators and the health education coordinator to discuss problems and share experiences and information. These meetings were very lively. Much communication with and feedback from the refugees came via the health educators. In addition to this informal monitoring system, special surveys were mounted if problems were suspected. The two-way flow of ideas and information from refugees to senior staff via the health educators was highly effective in identifying issues that needed to be rectified.

Herson and Mears, 1992

---

goal and make them less likely to put their own goals above those of the team. Goals and priorities for individual team members and task allocation can be done within the team after developing the shared goal. Jointly agreeing a set of ground rules or guiding principles that determine how the team works will provide members with an acceptable way of working together. Where the team includes people with responsibilities outside hygiene promotion, it is important that each team member understands how each of the roles will contribute to the project outcomes. These will greatly enhance the performance of the team. A technique for developing ground rules is included in the Appendices on pages 222–23.

Regular, frequent team meetings and encouraging open appraisal of problems and successes

Ground rules adopted by LWF's Karamoja Agro-pastoral Development Programme, Uganda, include:

o The programme aims to meet the needs of agro pastoralists in Karamoja;
o The programme is to be cost-effective and impact oriented;
o Deliver what you plan and say;
o All communication should be open and honest;
o Learn from your mistakes.

LWF, 1997

are ways that enable a team of people to learn from their experiences and to improve their effectiveness. Visits to other team members' work sites will help to promote understanding and integration. Further on the job training of staff and volunteers may be required in order to improve the abilities of individual team members to perform their roles and responsibilities more effectively.

Managing conflict within teams

Teams go through several stages when they work together. These are sometimes referred to as 'forming', 'storming', 'norming' and 'performing'. In the forming stage, team members get to know each other and understand their formal roles. In the storming stage, tensions and conflicts may arise that need to be resolved. If managed well, such conflict resolution can be positive. If left unresolved the team will not settle into the norming stage. The norming stage is where team members develop team spirit and an understanding of how they will work together. When the team is ready to focus on outputs, they enter the performing stage where they are functioning well, with mutual trust and respect and with a flexibility to deal effectively with difficult situations as they arise. Conflict can show itself in different behaviours, from disputes and fighting to unwillingness to communicate, putting someone down and polarizing opinions. Conflict is an inevitable part of working with other people who have different interests, backgrounds and experiences. Working through conflict can lead to improvements of plans and group dynamics. Conflict is complex and can stem from simple misunderstandings or differences in values and beliefs to differences in status, position or resources. Even minor conflicts need to be dealt with by the team leader or manager. In teams there are always trade-offs between individual and group objectives. Trust is particularly important and comes from respecting each other's views regardless of whether you agree with them. In conflict resolution (as with any negotiation) it is important to focus on a win-win outcome where both parties gain something from the settlement and neither loses anything they consider to be vital. Instead, the parties are encouraged to find a creative compromise which satisfies both parties. Some ways of handling potentially destructive conflicts are contained in Box 3.11.

Conflict can be resolved through a 'team review' process, where one member of the team is encouraged to openly review the positive and negative aspects of their performance in a non-judgemental team setting. Here the team member outlines the work they have been undertaking and encourages the team to discuss the issues raised. New ideas for solving problems and a greater understanding of each other's work will be generated. Team members can take it in turns to be reviewed or a team member can be reviewed when facing particularly difficult problems in his or her work.

Box 3.11 Some ways to resolve conflict in teams

- Active listening.
- Discussing agendas (personal).
- Sharing of mistakes and successes.
- Offering mutual support and constructive criticism.
- Socializing out of work.
- Monitoring of performance and feedback.

Meetings and negotiations

Meetings

Hygiene promotion projects in previous emergency programmes have included a range of meetings and negotiation activities. Meetings can seem like a waste of precious time, as suggested by the poster found on the wall of a Ugandan Ministry of Health official, see below.

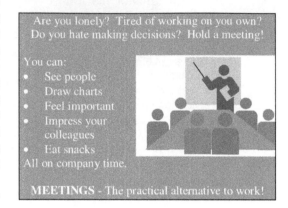

Are you lonely? Tired of working on you own? Do you hate making decisions? Hold a meeting!

You can:
- See people
- Draw charts
- Feel important
- Impress your colleagues
- Eat snacks

All on company time.

MEETINGS - The practical alternative to work!

However, meetings perform a number of useful functions in emergencies, including:

- sharing of information;
- discussion and consultation;
- decision making and ratification of decisions;
- review of previous decisions and actions taken.

At an inter-agency meeting you are a representative of your agency and will be viewed as such by others. Expect to be asked to give an opinion on an issue, even outside of your area of expertise. If you are not briefed on an issue, it is better to admit it and defer comment until you have discussed the issue with your manager. Present the information you have prepared in an interesting way, particularly when representing other people's concerns and activities.

Preparation increases the efficiency of meetings. As part of your preparation, consider what you want from the meeting and ensure that the meeting is conducted properly, that is, it covers the agenda points, stays on course and details action points and who is responsible for them. 'Minutes' or notes of what took place at the meeting are important to refer back to and to inform non attendees. These need to be available to everyone soon after the meeting. A manager needs to call regular meetings of the team and will have the most opportunities to manage the proceedings. Demonstrating a planned and organized approach to meetings will help you to influence the outcomes. Box 3.12 suggests ways to make meetings more effective.

Negotiations

There are many types of negotiations that have to be made in any emergency. These range from negotiations over employment terms and conditions, to the types of services the project will provide. A participatory approach will mean an increase in negotiations. How will you react with a community when they identify food, better security or a football pitch as of greater priority than hygiene promotion activities? When communities really feel they have a stake in the programme they may be quite vocal in expressing their negative views. For example, disgruntled people in Goma, in DRC, who were not targeted as part of the sanitation programme, marched to the NGO offices and demanded to be heard.

The key to effective negotiations is preparation. Prepare carefully for important negotiations. Be clear in your own mind what you want out of the negotiation. A useful exercise is to sit down and draw up a 'shopping list', including your 'ideal' and 'worst possible' outcomes for the negotiation. When you have done this for yourself, think yourself into the position of the other party and ask yourself what they want out of the negotiation. The areas of overlap between the two 'shopping lists' will be the area where the negotiation can take place and agreements reached. Role plays are effective tools to develop and practice negotiation skills. A description of how to use role-plays to improve negotiation skills can be found on pages 223–24 of the Appendices.

Coordination

The importance of trying to coordinate and work alongside other agencies, especially government ministries and officials, cannot be over emphasized. In some instances, government bodies may

---

Box 3.12 How to hold effective meetings

- Hold meetings regularly and select a suitable location. Actions agreed at previous meetings should be followed up and progress monitored. The location should facilitate discussion. Avoid noisy or dusty areas or places where one or more attendee can be called away. Switch off mobile phones!
- Have an agenda drawn up before the meeting. Give participants the opportunity to see the agenda before the meeting so that they can also prepare for it. At the end of the meeting, ask for agenda items for the following meeting. Set time limits on agenda items so that it is clear from the outset how long the meeting will take.
- Arrange the seating – make sure the seats are in a circle.
- Start the meeting on time. Agree at the beginning the finishing time – this focuses everybody on the task ahead.
- Introduce everyone. Ensure that everyone knows everyone else's name and role.
- Appoint a chairperson and minute taker. These people should be informed of what they are expected to do in advance. The chairperson is normally responsible for making sure the agenda is followed, and the purpose of the meeting is clear, as well as trying to encourage participation from all members and drawing attention to points of agreement. The minute taker should briefly but accurately note outcomes, action points and persons responsible for those actions and the time frame in which those actions will be done (including when the minutes will become available). It is good to rotate these roles so that everyone has a chance to develop these skills and the tasks can be shared out more evenly.
- Provide some refreshments if people have come a long way or the meeting is more than an hour in length.

Source: Adapted from Davis and Lambert, 1995; and Hubley, 1993.

Box 3.13 Some points to bear in mind when negotiating

○ Consider where the negotiation is to take place, who will conduct it, who will be present, and the time frame.
○ Ask lots of questions. This will help you to discover more about the other party's needs, it slows things down (which provides new thinking time) and shows that you are interested in their point of view.
○ Let people know your motives. This helps the other party to understand why you are making a certain suggestion and avoids guessing and suspicion. Try to understand their motives.
○ Repeat your key offers or demands regularly – repetition will encourage the other party to believe that you are serious.
○ Avoid using irritating expressions such as 'reasonable' and 'fair' or 'generous offer' – the implication is that the other party is being unfair, which does not make for a cooperative atmosphere.
○ Avoid verbal defend/attack spirals.
○ Avoid diluting good arguments with weaker ones. Quality of argument is better than quantity of reasons.
○ Be prepared to walk away if you are not satisfied. Avoid making large concessions simply to obtain a settlement.
○ People may return with new demands if they feel you are a weak negotiator.
○ Flag behaviour changes. Use phrases such as 'I'd like to suggest...' or 'Could I ask if ...'. They are clear and request the listening and perception of the other party.
○ Saying 'I don't understand' or 'I don't know' gives you time, and the other party may think they have an advantage.
○ If someone tells you that you will have to do better, ask 'How much better?' Encourage them to be specific.
○ Broaden options. Be innovative and be prepared to consider the unusual.

Source: Davis and Lambert, 1995.

be overwhelmed by the influx of foreign aid workers who, in their eagerness to act, may not listen to their local knowledge and may undermine their authority and position. On arrival in another country or district, introduce yourself to the national and local officials and seek their advice. Attend any meetings that they invite you to attend. If possible discuss your plans with the respective authorities and try to involve them in what you are doing. They may be not be able to do their work effectively, not because they are not fully capable, but because they do not have the resources that they need, such as transport or computer facilities or even salaries. International agencies cannot take on the payment of salaries for government officials but they may be able to facilitate the work of government staff in other ways such as providing fuel or temporary vehicles to carry out an assessment or immunisation campaign. The implications of any support that is offered should be thought through carefully before commitments or obligations are made.

Information collection and analysis

Information collection and analysis are an important basis for assessing the situation at the start of the project, deciding on project activities and monitoring changes over the project period. These aspects are detailed in Chapters 1 and 4.

Working with community members to identify problems and solutions to those problems can be

Box 3.14 Aspects of information collection and analysis in emergency hygiene promotion projects

○ Working with community members to identify problems and solutions to those problems.
○ Identifying the common high-risk hygiene practices and those individuals or groups who practise them.
○ Identifying who and what motivates people not to practise those risky hygiene behaviours.

done using the participatory needs assessment tools outlined in Chapter 1 (e.g. mapping, focus group discussions, key informant interviews, ranking exercises). Identifying the common high-risk hygiene practices and those who practise them can be done using participatory hygiene assessment tools (e.g. focus group discussions, key informant interviews, observations, pocket charts). Identifying who and what might motivate people not to practise those risky hygiene behaviours can be done by interviewing those who use improved hygiene practices to find out what motivates them to practise better hygiene. WASH motivator forms have recently been developed for use in a water and sanitation project in Ethiopia and these can be used to support problem identification and setting priorities with communities. Objectives for desired changes in the community and/or household are represented in pictures. The community facilitators discuss with each household what changes they want to see and how they might achieve these changes. An example form is on pages 205–6.

Share your findings with the community. This can be done in community meetings and with charts and tables and also with written reports and notices posted on information boards, large trees or health centre walls. This information should be updated regularly. The information collected then provides the basis of other hygiene promotion activities and also provides information against which changes can be meas-

ured. Collection of information and analysis of that information are ongoing processes and time should be made available for these activities throughout the project. It is important to realize that in an emergency, the project cycle can not always be followed in a simple linear fashion and you will often have to keep returning to a particular stage to fill in the gaps.

Campaigns, education and social marketing

Campaign activities, especially those involving education are more traditionally associated with hygiene education. The key elements of campaigns are listed in Box 3.15.

Selecting key hygiene promotion messages requires analysis of the collected information through discussions with staff, volunteers, community leaders, government officials and other influential stakeholders. This is covered in more detail in Chapters 1 and 2 of this manual. Effective communication methods and materials are detailed next.

Selecting effective communication methods

Methods that have been used successfully in hygiene promotion campaigns in previous emergency hygiene promotion projects are listed in Box 3.16.

The selection of methodologies will depend on the numbers of people involved, the size of the budget, the time available and of course, the

---

Three-pile sorting was used as part of the training for facilitators to work with internally displaced persons in Sierra Leone. The trainee facilitators were very surprised that the participants knew so much and the participants were also surprised that some of their traditional remedies such as the use of coconut water with a pinch of salt were considered to be useful remedies to help rehydrate people with diarrhoea! Unfortunately the sessions were not taped and inadequate notes were taken. It was difficult to make the facilitators understand that it was the detail of what people said that was interesting and useful.

Oxfam, 1998, personal communication

Box 3.15 Key elements in a hygiene promotion campaign

o Selecting key hygiene promotion messages.
o Identifying and selecting effective communication methods.
o Preparing communication materials (dramas, puppet shows, radio programmes, posters, leaflets, newspaper articles, announcements).
o Spreading the hygiene promotion messages.

Box 3.16 Hygiene promotion methods used in emergency hygiene promotion projects

o Announcements.
o Posters (on paper, card, cloth or walls).
o Street theatre (drama and puppets).
o Slides, films, video presentations.
o Radio broadcasts.
o One-to-one communication, including home visits.
o Large and small group discussions.
o Skills development.
o Learning through enquiry.
o Games, for example, snakes and ladders.
o Drama.
o Role play and simulation.
o Story telling, songs, concerts.

project objectives! It will also depend on what you found out during the assessment activities. As discussed in the Introduction, education techniques range from participatory to didactic. There is no single 'correct' way and different methods may be appropriate in different circumstances. Sometimes, especially in an acute emergency, the community may be looking for basic information about hygiene; participatory approaches may appear to be taking too much time. Usually though, dialogue between learner and educator is essential if learning is to be translated into action and hence every opportunity to incorporate participatory methodologies should be explored. This can be done without precluding the use of more didactic techniques where necessary. The best possible mix of methods should be selected according to the situation.

Large and small group discussions, skills development, learning through enquiry, games, drama, role play and story telling have been considered previously. Campaigns, posters, street

The momentum created by the learner directed approach can pave the way for better utilization of messages being disseminated by more didactic means.

Srinivasan, 1990

theatre, puppet shows, one-to-one communication and mass media are detailed in the next sections of this chapter.

Information campaigns

A campaign is usually focused on a specific topic over a short time span and uses a number of universal messages targeted at large numbers of people. A sophisticated social marketing campaign involves careful research to analyse the needs and preferences of different segments of the population and then tailors the message to suit those segments. In an acute emergency setting, however, the priority will lie in finding effective ways to convey essential information aimed at encouraging rapid compliance with specific behaviours in an effort to avoid epidemics. In more stable conditions, campaigns may be used against a backdrop of other education methods to draw attention to particular issues, for example, to promote specific hygiene practices in conjunction with the installation of new water or sanitation facilities using the positive messages of the social marketing approach. A campaign often makes use of the mass media as a means of reaching a large audience. This can be backed up by other communication methodologies, such as folk media, posters, public meetings and one-to-one communication. National campaigns have been used successfully in this way in a number of countries to promote the use of oral rehydration solution and the uptake of immunizations.

Communication campaigns should be directed where the intended audience will see or hear them. The most vulnerable people often have the poorest access to useful information, so ensure that they are being reached. A communication campaign should: *attract attention*; people should be drawn to look, listen or participate. It should be *understood* by the person who is targeted to receive it. Simple verbal language that focuses on the desired change is better than the provision of complex and descriptive information. Written words should be used only if most of the target population can read them. Visual aids such as posters should be tested with pilot groups to ensure that their meaning is clearly understood or can be easily learned by the receivers. The information conveyed must also be *acceptable*

Box 3.17 Planning steps for organizing a campaign

o Begin by setting objectives. Which key messages are to be communicated?
o Who are the primary, secondary and tertiary target audiences?
o Communicate with the key people who will be involved and others who may offer their support.
o Decide on the channels of communication to be used – mass media will usually have more impact if backed up by person-to-person communication and discussion, so consider how to combine the two as soon as the situation allows.
o Plan and pre-test any materials to be used – mass media channels do not allow for feedback from the audience so the materials and messages need to be tried out in advance.
o Train those who will be involved in the implementation, focusing in particular on people from sectors who are used to communicating with the public, for example, health workers, extension workers, teachers.
o Ensure that a meeting is arranged following the first day of the campaign to allow campaign workers and facilitators to voice any concern or problems they faced. Further follow-up meetings should be arranged frequently.

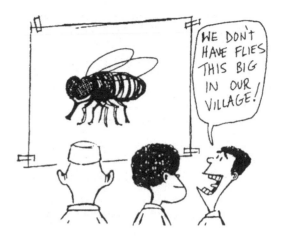

Posters

Posters created in the local area in collaboration with local people will be more effective since immediate feedback will reduce the risk of misunderstandings.

When there is no time or opportunity to do this, professionally designed posters can be used, if they have been pre-tested, to ensure that the content is understood. Where you require new posters, local artists can be brought in to develop materials on site and pre-test them with pilot groups in the community. School children can also be asked to design posters, perhaps on a particular theme as part of a competition. Information about how to make posters is included in Box 3.18 and on page 209.

to and accepted by the recipient. This is more likely if the message is in line with the beliefs of the recipient and is delivered or endorsed by a person they trust and respect. Positive messages such as, 'washing hands with soap after contact with faeces makes your hands smell nice and you feel good when you feel clean' are often more likely to change behaviour than messages about health benefits, child diarrhoea, doctors or death. The information must be *accurate*. Wrong information will undermine confidence and will not bring about the desired health outcome. It should also be *feasible*; people should have the means to be able to act on the information they are given.

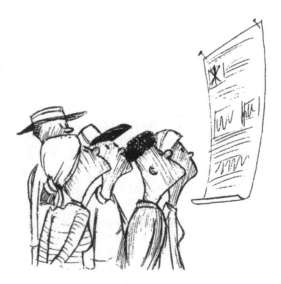

Box 3.18 Guidelines for making posters

o Keep the details in the poster to a minimum and communicate one message at a time.
o Make sure that the pictures are as accurate as possible and are familiar to the audience.
o Do not distort the size of an object and try to avoid using sections of the body out of context as it may cause confusion.
o Avoid using abstract symbols, especially if people are not literate as they are unlikely to understand them. Similarly, trying to indicate movement in a picture may not be understood in the way it was intended.
o Do not assume that a sequence of activities that makes sense to you will necessarily be understood by the viewer.
o Write words only if most of the target population can read. If words are to be included, use them sparingly and keep the message clear and simple. Try to convey positive messages whenever possible.
o If using colours, try to make sure that they resemble the real colour of the object they are depicting, to avoid confusion.

Box 3.19 How to copy or enlarge a picture

o Draw lines to form squares on the original drawing.
o Draw the same number of squares but larger on the surface you want the copy on.
o Copy the drawing square by square.

Copying and/or enlarging pictures from other sources, such as the ones included in this manual, may also be helpful. If the programme budget allows, purchase a digital camera and use it to take pictures of the local environment. These can be used to start focus group discussions or for three-pile sorting activities. Help participants in training workshops to take pictures as they learn to identify public health threats in the local environment.

Further details on making visual aids can be found in some of the books listed in the Annotated Bibliography, particularly Linney (1995), Werner and Bower (1982), IT Publications (The Copy Book) (1988) and Röhr-Rouendaal (1997 and CD version 2006).

Films and videos and radio broadcasts

Films, DVDs and videos are entertaining ways of passing on information to large groups of people at one time. Projectors can show them to audiences of a few people or to as many as one thousand at one time. They can be played to people who have gathered for the purpose of seeing the show or they can be shown to groups who have gathered for other reasons, for example, hospitalized patients or people queuing in reception centres. Where conditions permit, films can be shown outside after dark by projecting onto large white walls or using a sheet as a screen. Mixed audiences are likely to attend, including those from disadvantaged and minority groups. Videos and DVDs can be shown to audiences of 30–40 people on a standard TV screen. Larger screens can accommodate larger audiences. Many towns and large villages in Africa and Asia have film venues and it may be possible to persuade the owners to show material that promotes public health. Films, videos and DVDs are available on a variety of

The lack of artistic ability does not have to be a major constraint to the production of effective visual aids, especially if pictures or posters are used in an interactive way. Teaching people to make their own materials is a more empowering approach to use and communities can then develop their own materials as required instead of using the same set of standardized pictures. Posters made by members of the community are less likely to be ignored or misunderstood. However, people who do not have any formal education may find it difficult to 'read' pictures initially. Linney (1995) suggests that visual literacy can be learnt in a few hours and this is why discussion is important when using visual aids. Stand alone posters often do not have the desired effect of stimulating action but can provide information. Posters can be made on paper, card, cloth, billboards and walls – or any other blank surface.

Box 3.20 Points to remember when showing films, videos or DVDs to large audiences

○ Choose a suitable site to show the film, video or DVD.
○ Obtain permission from the relevant authorities to show the film.
○ Request the assistance of police to assist with crowd control if you are inviting many people.
○ Publicise the show, including the topic of the film, by loudspeaker or notices.
○ If you have something important to say – say it before the show so that the audience can leave immediately after the show.

development topics. *Prescription for Health* is an animated film produced in Thailand by UNICEF and although it looks at a rural scene in a development context, it depicts the faecal–oral route of diarrhoeal disease transmission very clearly and has been used effectively in a broad range of cultural contexts in Africa and Asia. When showing films or videos remember the points in Box 3.20.

With small audiences, discussions about the material can be facilitated after the show. With large audiences, people prefer to be entertained and to leave immediately after the show rather than sitting around discussing with a large group of strangers. Government information officers may also have equipment and films/videos/DVDs that could be utilized.

Radio broadcasts can include news, spot announcements, slogans and jingles, discussions, phone-in or write-in programmes, interviews, talks and documentaries, drama (short or long, series and soap operas or one-off radio plays), music, quizzes and panel games. Many people have access to radios, although men may have more access than women and children. At certain times of the day, radio programmes may be listened to by a whole family or a whole neighbourhood. They can be used as an opportunity for people to meet, listen and discuss together. Radio broadcasts are most effective when they are clear, brief, lively and entertaining. More voices are easier to listen to than just one. They should catch people's attention and end with something that people will remember. When recording a broadcast, it is best to think of the person listening to the radio as a friend you are talking to.

Street theatre

Street theatre has its roots in story telling and can be used as a learning tool and as a way of passing on hygiene messages. Street theatre is short, lively and spontaneous and is flexible enough to allow audience participation. Equipment for street theatre is minimal and productions can be put on anywhere and literally in the street. Street theatre can be carried out as dramas with actors or with puppets acting out the scenes. Box 3.21 outlines things you can and cannot do effectively with street theatre and page 207 explains how you can develop and use a street theatre drama. Street theatre has been carried out in a number of settings, including refugee camps to promote safe water use and the maintenance of water points.

Puppet shows

Puppets can be used to give theatre performances or with small groups to encourage discussion. They are especially helpful for communicating with small children as they will often talk directly to a puppet although they may be too shy to talk to an unfamiliar adult. Puppets are also able to do things that actors or ordinary people physically or culturally cannot do. Details of how to make

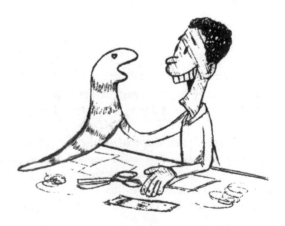

Box 3.21 Dos and don'ts for street theatre dramas

Dos:

o Men dressed as women;
o Comic village stereotypes, for example, drunkards, 'lads', obsequious servants, simpletons, beggars, traditional healers, dishonest merchants, religious leaders;
o Exaggerated characterization;
o Villain/hero conflicts ('goodies' and 'baddies');
o Macabre incidents, for example, ghosts returning, death, white sheets;
o Dance and song;
o Asking the audience questions ('Where is she?') and getting them to reply ('She's behind you!');
o A few simple messages;
o Frequent repetition of the messages;
o Messages made clear through actions rather than words;
o Audience participation (asking members of the audience to come into the performance area and join in with certain tasks);
o Spontaneous and lively with a minimum of characters and props.

Don'ts:

o Long gaps between scenes;
o Fast speech;
o More than one person speaking at one time;
o Scenes involving sitting or lying down;
o Long speeches or dialogues without action;
o Lecturing one actor by another;
o One actor playing different roles that may be confused, for example, dishonest pharmacist and doctor;
o Complicated plots and detailed scripts.

Box 3.22 Dos and don'ts for street puppet shows

Dos:

o Short simple plots:
o Stock characters, for example, traditional healer, beggar, villain;
o Speaking animal characters, for example, fly, worm, louse;
o Interaction between puppets, for example, beating, carrying, embracing, (especially those interactions that human actors cannot do)
o Swift changes between scenes;
o Very loud, slow speech;
o One character speaking at one time – the puppet should move or nod when speaking;
o Music and dance;
o Comic sound effects, for example, baby going to the toilet;
o Character moving when speaking.

Don'ts:

o Long monologues by single puppet;
o Messages conveyed through words alone rather than words and actions;
o Puppets asking the audience questions during the show, unless someone ensures puppeteers can hear them.

puppets can be found on page 209 and Box 3.22 outlines the dos and don'ts for puppet shows.

One-to-one communication and home visiting

This is perhaps one of the most traditional ways of carrying out health education. Home visits are usually made to families in their home environments by community facilitator, health worker or hygiene promoter. These visits offer an opportunity for the health worker to assess the domestic environment and to tailor hygiene promotion to the specific needs of that family. Home visits can also be useful for those people who find it difficult to take part in discussion groups because they are given the opportunity to talk about sensitive issues and to clarify and reflect on their situation in a more personal environment at a time that suits them.

Home visiting is popular and can be very effective but it does have its limitations. It can sometimes be seen as threatening to a family and visits need to be handled with sensitivity. The facilitator or promoter needs to develop good listening skills and learn how to engage people in dialogue. Lack of confidence and experience can sometimes lead them to provide too much information at one time

A camp for Burundi refugees at Maza in Rwanda was divided into sectors of approximately 2,000 inhabitants with each sector having two voluntary hygiene animators, one male and one female. They carried out a programme of home visits in the morning and late afternoon, arranged in conjunction with community members. They also implemented opportunistic group discussions and drama performances at water points and communal meeting places. The home visitors/ animators chose two representatives from among their number to act as coordinators who were responsible for liasing with community leaders and organizing monitoring activities. Discussions during home visits focused on water storage, hand washing and safe excreta disposal (especially the faeces of small children who were not considered capable of using latrines). Any reported incidents of diarrhoea or other illnesses were referred to the camp medical centre by the animators.

In Angola, groups of men and women carried out daily activity profiles to identify the best time for home visiting and meetings. They then examined each others' profiles and the men acknowledged the amount of work that the women had and agreed to arrange meetings for when it most suited them.

Norwood and Mears, 1993; Oxfam, 1995

Health promoters used digital cameras to take photos for three pile sorting activities in refugee camps in Chad. These proved very effective on the whole but as the photos were taken in the camps, the images sometimes proved distracting for the participants who were more interested in working out whose donkey appeared in the photo than trying to determine which of the pictures represented positive or negative health seeking practices. The same participants later drew their own pictures to represent health risks in the camp as they perceived them and though the facilitators could not easily interpret the pictures, other refugees had no difficulties understanding them.

Oxfam, 2004, personal communication

Visual aids in the form of flipcharts or picture cards can sometimes be useful to promote discussion but their novelty value can mean that they easily become the focus of the discussion rather than an aid to communication. The promoter should check that the householder shares his/her understanding of the visual images if these are used and should try to evaluate the impact of the visit.

The timing of visits needs to be carefully planned. People in camps may be in and around the camp for much of the day or their time may be taken up in securing the basic essentials for survival. In village settings, houses are often empty for much of the day when people are cultivating or attending to daily chores. They may not mind

or turn the contact into a lecture. A one-to-one approach with its focus on the individual can lose sight of the external pressures influencing a person's hygiene practices. Home visits are also time consuming. On average one health worker can visit six to ten households in one working day but would need to be remunerated for such intensive work. If the health worker works six days a week, that worker can cover 180 households in a month. An average refugee camp of 25,000 people would require 28 home visitors in order to cover all the households once a month. This would be insufficient in an acute situation. If it is decided to have volunteer workers, at least three times this number would then be necessary.

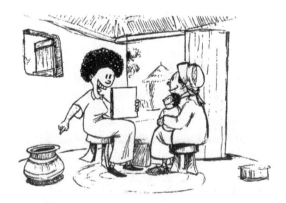

being interrupted at home but there may be times that are inconvenient.

Home visits are often used for gathering baseline data and monitoring, as described in Chapters 1 and 2. They can provide useful insights into the effectiveness of hygiene promotion at the household level.

Operation and maintenance of water supply and sanitation facilities

Experience has shown that the long-term operation and maintenance (O&M) of water and sanitation installations should always be taken into account, even in emergency situations. This is especially important where permanent water supplies are being constructed or renovated. People will not automatically assume responsibility for keeping the system functional and paying for its use in the longer term. They may think that these things will be taken care of by the agency that organized the construction or repair. The community may well have 'participated' in the construction work but this does not automatically mean that they feel a sense of ownership for the completed project or a willingness to pay for its upkeep. Hygiene promotion projects in previous emergency water and sanitation programmes have included a range of activities, some of which are included in Box 3.23.

Discussions with the various groups in the community should be started as soon as possible. The advantages and disadvantages of all possible technical options, including costs, should be discussed with them to identify com-

---

Box 3.23 Hygiene promotion activities for operation and maintenance of water and sanitation facilities

○ Consultations between the community and engineers about appropriate designs of drinking water sources, excreta disposal, hand washing facilities, laundry and bathing facilities, solid and liquid waste disposal facilities.
○ Consultations between the community, engineers and planners regarding appropriate locations for each water and sanitation facility.
○ Organizing appropriate mechanisms for the construction and maintenance of water and sanitation facilities with community members, planners and engineers.
○ Training of water and sanitation committees.
○ Organizing workshops with local or national staff from government ministries and local NGOs to talk about strategy for future support and maintenance.

---

munity preferences and their intentions for managing repairs to the system when it breaks down. It is important to remember that it is often unrealistic to expect a community to manage its facilities without any outside support from the government or a local NGO and every attempt should

---

In Maza camp for Burundi refugees in Rwanda, the community identified problems with children not using latrines. Hygiene promoters assisted the community to develop latrine designs for children. These had smaller squat-holes so that the children could not fall down them, and wooden railings for the children to hold on to.

Oxfam, 1994

Following the Tsunami at the end of 2004, sanitation engineers in one project designed communal shower and toilet blocks for the temporary settlements. Unfortunately the dirty water from the showers drained onto the washing slab at the end of the blocks and women did not like this and often went elsewhere to wash their clothes. As the engineers did not speak the local language and did not have access to interpreters, the design went unchanged until the evaluation discovered the mistake.

Oxfam, 2005, personal communication

be made to link communities with potential, future means of support.

Agreements need to be negotiated regarding community contributions for labour and construction materials (preferably in line with host government policies and practices) and preferred options for maintenance and long-term financing (combinations of self maintained, community-managed or private enterprise).

Ensure that issues of financial accountability are also discussed. The availability of spare parts for pumps or other systems will also need to be

In the Dadaab Refugee Programme in Kenya, there were some technical problems with the initial latrines. Some filled up within a month. They were also smelly. The refugees voiced complaints through the health educators who promptly fed back this information to the engineers, who produced new designs. Similar innovations were required for the disposal of children's excreta, which was otherwise being disposed of in drains. A trial was underway with carefully designed children's latrines with no shelters and smaller squat-holes. The hygiene promoters became closely involved with the latrine building programme. They taught and discussed latrine use, the importance of keeping latrines clean and how to do this. Most importantly, they allocated latrines to refugee groups. No one was allowed access to new latrines until ownership had been settled. User groups guarded access to their latrines, most employed caretakers to keep the latrine clean. Each day, in turn, one family would provide the caretaker with half a kilogram of cereals in payment for their work. The hygiene promotion component was flexible, participatory and changing. It was non-directive and enabled the refugees to take responsibility for their latrines, their drains and their shelters. If one group had dirty latrines, the hygiene facilitators would encourage discussion and offer solutions, but if the refugees chose not to do anything about the problem, they were allowed that liberty.

CARE, 1997

researched and viable systems identified. Identify a feedback mechanism to make sure that the agreed system is working adequately. Try to ensure open ongoing dialogue about the project. It is important to remain flexible and to encourage suggestions from community members on how the project should proceed. Be prepared to construct sample facilities to start with, if time allows, and to use comments from the community to make the designs more appropriate and acceptable to them.

When the parties involved in the consultations have reached agreement, decisions should be formalized and the roles and contributions of each party clearly specified in formal agreements or contracts. An example of a community contract has been included in the Appendices on pages 255–56.

Other practical actions

A range of other practical actions have been initiated and carried out as part of the hygiene promotion activities of various emergency programmes. A list of practical actions is contained in Box 3.24.

Tool loan-and-return schemes
Progress on the construction of latrines and other important facilities for better hygiene is often slow because people do not have access to the tools required to get the job done. Supplying local tools, appropriate for the work will enable more people to get on with that work at any one time. In some emergency situations, sets of tools (one hoe, one spade and one sharp cutting tool) have

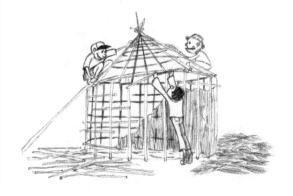

Box 3.24 Practical actions that could be part of emergency hygiene promotion projects

o Organizing distribution/lending of tools for construction of water and sanitation facilities or other things.
o Chlorination of drinking water (at source or in storage containers) and testing of residual chlorine levels.
o Demonstrations of how to make and give oral rehydration solution.
o Distribution of soap, water containers, food storage containers and other essential items for hygiene.
o Organizing lingerie fairs so that affected women can choose their own underwear and menstrual protection.
o Mobilizing for vector control and solid waste disposal.
o Small business development (soap production and marketing, recycling).
o Providing separate meeting centres for men and women and play areas for children.
o Arranging a community festival resulting in community led hygiene initiatives.
o Hygiene promotion as part of a community based care programme for people living with AIDS.

Hygiene promoters worked with Sudanese refugees living in an overcrowded camp in Eastern Chad to help them to organize environmental clean up campaigns. As the refugees had travelled with their animals, large amounts of animal excreta added to the rubbish that was polluting the camp environment. The camp population (approximately 15,000) was divided into sectors based on community groups and meetings were held with the leaders of each of the sectors. They were supported in organizing a series of community meetings to raise awareness about the health risks resulting from the dirty environment and they identified clean up teams within their sectors. Wheelbarrows, shovels and hoes were distributed to each sector leader and they in turn distributed the tools on a rotating basis to the clean up teams. Some of the rubbish was burned and some of it was deposited in locations at a distance from the camp. After much discussion with the camp authorities it was agreed that the clean up activities would be organized using voluntary labour from the community to try to ensure that ongoing responsibility for cleaning the environment rested with them.

Oxfam, 2004, personal communication

been purchased and supplied to the community representatives. These representatives loan out the tools to the households they represent and are responsible for their return and maintenance. Such schemes can increase construction dramatically. When organizing a tool loan-and-return scheme the following points need to be considered:

o Purchase sufficient sets of durable tools, for example, hoe, shovel, pick-axe. One general set may be required for each 20 households and one specialized set of tools for each mason and carpenter;
o Identify persons in the community who are willing and able to give out and collect tools at a local level (without charging a commission);
o Establish criteria on who can borrow the tools and for how long;

o Prepare a system of replacement/repair if tools get damaged or lost;
o Monitor the use of tool sets and the rate of construction of agreed facilities.

Chlorination of drinking water

Sterilization of drinking water may be a useful control measure for diarrhoeal disease outbreaks. The most common water sterilization method is the addition of chlorine to water at the water source or in storage containers. Chlorine needs to react with the water for at least 20 minutes prior to drinking in order to kill any germs that may be present. The following approach may be appropriate:

o Identify sources of drinking water and ways of improving water quality (for example, cordoning off water sources);

○ Identify places where water could be chlorinated and stored for 20 minutes before consumption (directly into water storage tanks or into domestic water storage containers);
○ Discuss with community representatives the need for chlorination and the views of the community about this activity;
○ Request community leaders to inform the community of the decision;
○ If appropriate, identify and train people to carry out the chlorination activities and explain to others the reasons for this being carried out;
○ Organize sampling schedules and samplers for testing levels of residual chlorine.

In many situations where normal water supplies are thought to have become contaminated or where people are obliged to use unprotected sources (for example, floods), chlorine tablets are now distributed to households. It is vital that people are supplied with adequate quantities of chlorine and that they have information on how to use it correctly. Information and demonstrations should be provided at the time of distribu-

---

Recent research has highlighted the extent to which water is prone to contamination during storage and use within the household. Water filters containing ceramic filters have been shown to be effective in improving household water quality in studies carried out in a number of countries. Research is ongoing as to the information and education components which may facilitate the effective use and maintenance of the filters.

Clasen et al, 2004

---

tion as well as a written leaflet giving instructions with accompanying pictures.

Distribution of oral rehydration salts

Dehydration may be the major cause of death in a diarrhoeal disease outbreak. Dehydration of a cholera patient can be so rapid that death can occur within four hours of the onset of diarrhoea and vomiting. Drinking fluids prevents or rectifies dehydration even if the patient continues to vomit. Providing fluid by mouth will rehydrate a patient more rapidly than can usually be done with intravenous drips. Any 'home available fluid' (soup, gruel, cereal porridge, breast milk, tea, water) should also be used to supplement rehydration. In some countries, packets of oral rehydration salts (ORS) are available for mixing with water (see page 236). These contain simple sugar, salt, sodium and potassium. Homemade salt and sugar drinks, especially made with cereal are often cheaper to prepare than shop bought ORS packets. When organizing the provision of ORS the following points should be considered:

○ Identify and train staff and volunteers in the principles of ORS (what is ORS, why give ORS, when, how much and how to give ORS to children and adults, problem solving);
○ Produce posters on ORS to reinforce the information given;
○ Supply volunteers with ORS sachets only with the agreement of local health officials;
○ Identify distribution points at strategic places in the community for ORS distribution (for example clinics, shops);

During the peak of a cholera outbreak in Kampala, Uganda, Red Cross volunteers distributed chlorine tablets to the caretakers of the community-managed springs in the most seriously affected 'slum' areas of the city. Spring caretakers were informed of the risk that the contaminated spring water posed in the spread of the cholera epidemic. They were also instructed to place two chlorine tablets in each of the 20 litre jerry cans used by almost everyone in the community to fetch and store their drinking water. They were instructed to explain to the spring users the purpose of the exercise and the need to keep the chlorine tablets and the water in the containers for at least 20 minutes before use so that the chlorine had a chance to sterilize the water. The intervention was very time consuming but was thought to reduce the number of people infected with cholera during that critical period.

Ministry of Health Uganda, 1998b

> *IDP camps in Western Uganda suffered cholera outbreaks for two years running. Programme evaluators in one of the camps were told by camp residents that deaths from cholera were greatly reduced the second year. The IDPs attributed this to the fact that community volunteers had been taught how to administer ORS and were called upon as soon as anyone had diarrhoea. This was considered important, especially at night since it was not safe for people to leave the camp.*
>
> Oxfam, 2000, personal communication

○ Organize systems to keep these distribution centres sufficiently stocked;
○ Arrange a community-based monitoring system to check that the ORS distribution is working and that volunteers are giving appropriate advice.

Distribution of other items essential for hygiene

Distribution of soap, water containers, food storage containers, sanitary towels for women and other essential items such as mosquito nets are all activities that have been undertaken as part of emergency hygiene promotion projects. To maximize their health promotion potential, the distribution of these items should be timely and closely linked with other hygiene promotion activities. When distributing sanitary towels, it is important

> **The Oxfam Bucket**
>
> *The majority of drinking water contamination takes place at household level during its collection and storage. Jerry cans are often used as water containers but are bulky to freight in large numbers and difficult to keep clean inside. A stackable 14 litre plastic bucket with a removable lid and push-on cap was developed by Oxfam. The containers are easy for women to carry, can be cleaned easily (both inside and out) and are less bulky to freight.*
>
> Bastable, 1998

to find out what women usually use and to work out with them what is most appropriate. Sometimes an extra length of new cloth such as a sarong or towel can be provided in the expectation that this will free up other cloth for use during menstruation.

Distribution systems are often established quickly in a camp situation. When considering the distribution of such items, respected representatives in the community (men and women) can provide useful insights on existing problems with the current distribution system and identify possible solutions. Distribution is often associated with logistical blockages and the misappropriation of items. Flexible approaches to problem solving and community-based monitoring systems may help to alleviate some of these problems.

Lingerie fairs

> *Many women living in temporary settlements in Aceh lost all their belongings during the tsunami. They told health promoters that they had received clothes as part of the relief distributions but they lacked underwear. Arrangements were made for local traders to purchase underwear in a variety of sizes and colours and this was delivered at a pre-arranged time to a secluded area of the camp chosen for the purpose, where the women were able to select what they needed in privacy. A similar arrangement was made for the men at a later date.*
>
> Oxfam, 2005, personal communication

Mobilization for vector control and solid waste disposal

Vectors such as flies, mosquitoes and rats can be a problem in some emergency situations. It is important to try to ensure good drainage at water points and people may need to be encouraged to dig drainage around temporary shelters. In Sub-Saharan Africa, some mosquito vectors can breed even in foot or hoof prints and it will be difficult to get rid of all breeding sites. Large areas of stagnant water can be drained or filled in, but some other form of malaria control intervention will probably also be necessary. Insecticide treated nets or spraying inside walls and ceilings with insecticide may be useful to limit the spread of malaria. Whilst treated nets usually only last six months to one year, the insecticide in long lasting insecticide treated nets (LLIN) may last the lifetime of the net (between three and seven years). If nets are to be provided, careful assessment of the problem will be required as well as intensive promotional work in order to ensure that nets are valued and used. Insecticides are also sometimes used to control flies temporarily, especially where there is a major epidemic of diarrhoeal disease. If insecticides are used, people must be informed about safety procedures and the likelihood of any side effects.

Compost pits can be dug for degradable solid waste or waste may be burnt in pits. However, in a large settlement it may also be necessary to organize a system of disposal and collection for solid waste and appropriate areas for the final disposal of waste will need to be identified so that this does not present a health hazard to those living nearby.

Private sector development

Private sector development, particularly the development of small businesses such as local soap production and marketing, recycling of solid waste and safe water vending may be appropriate hygiene promotion interventions in emergency projects. Ways to develop the local private sector include:

o identifying small businesses already operating locally;
o identifying artisans and other skilled people (such as drama groups) that could operate as small businesses;
o discussing with these skilled people the need for other hygiene-related businesses and ways they can be encouraged, for example, soap making, providing enterprise training for latrine diggers, well-diggers, masons, tap attendants and water source caretakers to include book-keeping, budgeting, tendering, sales and marketing skills, how to obtain and administer start-up grants or loans for hygiene-related businesses if necessary;

In the Somali refugee camps around Dadaab in Kenya, women were offered opportunities to join a sewing project. In addition to classes in sewing, they were also provided with some literacy and book-keeping skills. After completing the course, the refugee women were offered subsidies for the purchase of sewing machines. Items made by the refugee women, such as school uniforms and washable sanitary pads were purchased by agencies and distributed to the refugees as part of the non-food rations.

CARE, 1998, personal communication

The International Development Enterprise worked with Oxfam during the 2003 floods response in Cambodia. They were already working on the production of ceramic pot water filters in Cambodia before the floods and made filter production workshops available to train groups of flood-affected communities. They also carried out social marketing activities which resulted in creating a demand for the filters which were purchased by households, providing an income for the village based producers and reducing the public health risks resulting from contamination of the water sources by the flood waters.

Oxfam, 2003, personal communication

o organizing support groups for people involved in small businesses.

Providing safe meeting centres

Some emergency hygiene promotion projects have found a need to provide separate centres for women and their children and also for men. These centres provide shelter where people can meet together and share experiences and ideas away from the demands of their 'normal' lives. For many people who have endured great hardship or loss, this can be a place where they can share their grief with others and find practical support to help them cope.

Young men and adolescents may become depressed and frustrated in a camp situation where

> *In the Dadaab Refugee Programme in Kenya, special attention was needed to address the mental health of the refugees from the start, but this became a priority only once other more urgent needs had been addressed. Community groups enthusiastically embraced the idea of constructing women's centres. These centres became places where women could relax, do handicrafts and exchange health information.*
>
> CARE, 1997

there is little to occupy their time. By providing meeting places and opportunities for games and activities, their energy can be channelled into constructive projects to support the aid intervention. The selection of the site and management and use of the meeting place should be agreed before construction.

Disability and the elderly

The different needs of elderly people or those with disabilities are often overlooked in emergencies. Injuries resulting from the emergency can lead to long-term disability. In the Pakistan earthquake in 2005, many people were injured by falling masonry that eventually led to the need for their limbs to be amputated. In Afghanistan, Cambodia and Sierra Leone the loss of limbs from injuries due to conflict and landmines is common.

> **Organizing a community festival**
>
> *Beneficiaries of a water and sanitation programme in Southern Sudan were invited to a community festival which continued over several days. Sporting activities and competitions were interspersed with displays, discussions, demonstrations and presentations all aimed at increasing awareness of health and hygiene activities. 'Before and after' monitoring of levels of awareness showed an increase in knowledge. Community action plans for improvements in environmental health had been drawn up by a number of participating communities.*
>
> Oxfam, 2005, personal communication

> **Hygiene promotion in a community-based care programme for people living with AIDS**
>
> *A programme in Malawi where the HIV prevalence rate was about 16 per cent in adults, provided training through partners for voluntary carers in eighty villages to equip them to help their neighbours look after people living with AIDS. Food and non food items including soap, buckets and ORS for treating diarrhoea episodes were distributed. The volunteers learned listening and communication skills and how to care for the sick. The practical support they provided ranged from giving advice on nutrition to digging latrines and hygiene education. Participants felt that the involvement of the voluntary carers reduced the stigma and isolation often experienced by AIDS sufferers and their families in these villages. One participant said 'with the efforts we are making we have very good hope for a better future'.*
>
> Oxfam, 2003

The issue of disability must be covered in any training programme so that team members know how to identify and respond to special needs. Latrines can be provided with handrails for assisting users. Wooden seats placed over the squatting hole will allow pregnant women and older people with weak knees to sit rather than squat. Ramps are often easier to negotiate than steps. Potties or bedpans may allow those who are bedridden to defecate with greater ease and dignity. More information on this important subject can be found in Jones and Reed (2005), as listed in the Annotated Bibliography.

What next?

This chapter has given ideas and examples of hygiene promotion activities from recruitment, training and management of staff, negotiation skills, hygiene education campaigns, operation and maintenance of water and sanitation facilities and a diverse range of other practical actions. Having carried out some of the hygiene promotion activities that you planned earlier, it is now time to monitor the effects of those activities and evaluate what has been achieved.

4

Monitoring and evaluation: How shall we know when we have got there?

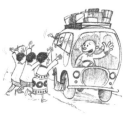

MONITORING AND EVALUATION are essential aspects of the project cycle. Time needs to be made available from the start of a project to consider the information necessary for monitoring the effects of the project activities and evaluating whether the project is making a difference. This chapter explains the purpose of monitoring and evaluation, how to monitor and evaluate, and gives ideas and examples of how monitoring and evaluation could be done in a variety of emergency hygiene promotion projects.

Defining monitoring and evaluation

People frequently ask what the difference is between monitoring and evaluation as the distinction is not always clear. Monitoring is an ongoing process of checking whether the project is going according to plan and evaluation is usually a one-off activity that takes an overview of the total changes that have taken place as a result of the intervention. An evaluation looks at such areas as effectiveness, efficiency, relevance and impact. If there has been no monitoring of the project it is very difficult to evaluate it.

Monitoring

Monitoring is necessary to ensure that the project is doing what it intended to do. It usually looks at individual aspects of the project as it proceeds, concentrating mainly on processes and outputs although outcomes should be considered as well, especially in the emergency context where change is expected very rapidly. It is important that monitoring is not simply seen as a data collection exer-

cise but that the data are also analysed and used to influence decision making.

Evaluation

Evaluation attempts to take an overview of the whole project and the context in which it takes place. It tries to define the extent to which it has achieved its outcomes and intended impact and how and why it has fallen short of them. Evaluation also attempts to assess if there have been any unforeseen consequences of the project activities. While monitoring should take place from the onset of the project, evaluation takes place only after enough time has elapsed for significant change to take place. There is a current trend

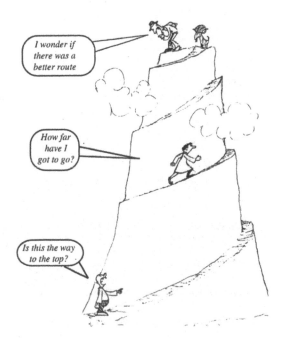

I wonder if there was a better route

How far have I got to go?

Is this the way to the top?

in emergency situations for 'real time evaluations' that seek to identify issues that need to be addressed as they happen.

A large-scale evaluation can be costly and resource intensive and ongoing monitoring may be all that is possible in some instances (Naidoo and Wills, 1994). Indeed, if there has been good monitoring then an evaluation may not always be necessary. However, a good evaluation is never a substitute for monitoring as it is vital to measure the process and how things were done as much as the impact of what was done.

Why monitor and evaluate?

The aim of both monitoring and evaluation is to find out if the actions taken are meeting their intended objectives and to identify weaknesses in the project so that remedial action can be taken, namely, to answer the questions, 'How far have we gone?' and 'How can we do it better?' If the evaluation is conducted at the end of a project, the remedial action will hopefully apply to any future projects and future programme strategy. Monitoring may identify issues that can be dealt with immediately. For example, talking to latrine users might identify design modifications or improvements in the siting of other facilities still to be constructed.

Who will monitor and evaluate?

All project staff should be responsible for some aspect of monitoring and evaluation but it may also be helpful to appoint a monitoring and evaluation officer whose role it is to support others to carry out this necessary work. The roles and responsibilities of all staff with regard to monitoring should be clearly defined in a monitoring plan. An example of a monitoring plan is given later in this chapter.

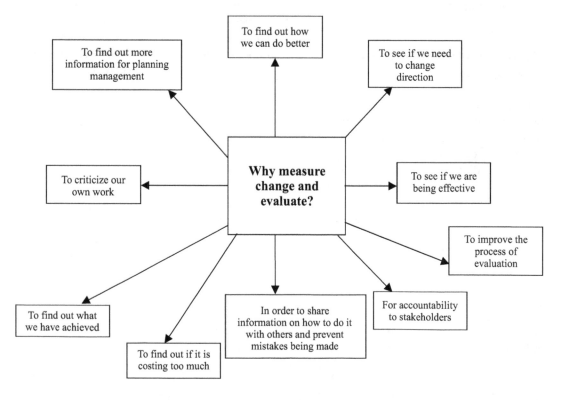

Figure 4.1 Why measure change and evaluate?
Source: Adapted from Feuerstein, 1986.

It is often argued that the ultimate evaluators of a project should be the individual beneficiaries and this should also apply in emergencies. Indeed, involving the community in identifying criteria for success and impact is one of the keys to a successful hygiene promotion project. Some large-scale evaluations benefit from being conducted by outside experts (*external evaluations*). Sometimes an outsider can take a fresh look at the situation and identify strengths and weaknesses that have not been seen before. An exter-nal evaluator is also said to be more objective than inside evaluators, because she or he is independent of the project. However, the presence of an external evaluator can sometimes prove threatening to project staff and can be disruptive to project activities. Although it is sometimes thought that *internal evaluations* are too biased to provide valid results, they can be seen as a way to stimulate learning about the project for the benefit of the most immediate stakeholders. If beneficiaries and the project staff evaluate the project themselves, this can often motivate them to make the necessary changes to improve subsequent outcomes in later stages of the project.

The box on this page provides information from an evaluation of a water and sanitation project in Ethiopia that highlights some of the things that could have been done better. If effective monitoring had been carried out then some of these issues could have been identified earlier.

Information stakeholders

In any project or programme we can identify at least three different levels of stakeholder: beneficiaries, project staff (agency or local government) and donors. They all require specific information on how the project is performing. The information may also be required in a different format for different stakeholders. The following list details some of the perspectives of different stakeholders regarding their information needs:

- ○ *Beneficiaries*: need to know if what they are doing is working and how it can be made to work better.
- ○ *Project staff and managers*: need to have information with which to make decisions on how to improve the project.
- ○ *External agencies/donors*: want to know if the funds they have contributed have been well spent.
- ○ *The wider community outside the project area*: might be affected by an influx of displaced people or by the way in which the project is designed.
- ○ *Other water, sanitation and hygiene projects*: need information to inform their own projects.
- ○ *Government and policy makers*: will have policy guidelines for all water, sanitation and

---

The project succeeded in restoring water supplies and in increasing the quantity of water available above pre-intervention levels. The availability of water for livestock was increased and facilitated by the provision of cattle and shoat (sheep and goat) troughs. Women also reported that more water was being used at the household level. In addition, environmental sanitation was improved through the mass disposal of dead animal carcasses. This was the first time such an intervention had been undertaken and was appreciated by communities especially. There was some increase in awareness of hygiene issues amongst the beneficiaries. In particular several people said that in future they would burn or bury dead carcasses. Several members of the water committees, especially women, were also requesting help to build latrines. However, opportunities were missed to have a greater impact on human health by not maintaining a broad public health overview of the situation, not assessing the needs of specific communities nor the different needs of men and women in those communities; for example an outbreak of dysentery in one village went unnoticed. The identification of specific indicators for changes in hygiene practice would have been useful, for example, for hand washing or covering water containers. Training sessions in hygiene promotion were undertaken but no other follow-up activities were organized.

Oxfam, 2003

hygiene projects and will want to know if these have been adhered to, and issues for learning.

In the past, the information needs of the beneficiaries have often been ignored and donors have appeared to instigate monitoring and evaluation as a means of making the project accountable to the donors only. This type of non-participatory evaluation (especially when carried out by outsiders) is likely to be viewed with mistrust by project staff and the target population instead of being seen as a constructive tool to provide feedback on what works and what does not. When project staff and beneficiaries are involved in participatory evaluation, information becomes available to all stakeholders, but especially to those who need it most (the target population). They are then in a better position to make decisions about the future of the project for themselves. In addition, it is also easier for project staff to accept the negative aspects of an evaluation if they have discovered these themselves. Whatever the choice of approach, feedback should always be provided to staff and beneficiaries so that they can help shape the final conclusions.

Donors often demand evaluations that rely on more formal methods of data collection that yield quantitative data, such as questionnaire surveys, but both qualitative and quantitative information should be gathered and analysed to assess the impact of the project.

Sphere standards

Sphere standards stress the importance of accountability to all stakeholders, especially the population affected by the disaster. The Sphere manual provides a set of minimum standards for emergency response in water, sanitation and hygiene promotion, health care, nutrition, food aid, food security and shelter. It also contains standards common to all sectors that cover the initial assessment, response, monitoring and evaluation, participation and targeting. For each standard there is a list of indicators to allow 'measurement' of the standard. It therefore provides an essential tool in monitoring a water, sanitation and hygiene

promotion programme. The relevant standards and indicators are included in the Appendices on pages 121–26.

What to monitor and evaluate

Monitoring frameworks will be based on the objectives and indicators that have been defined for the project. However, it is also important to measure the process that allowed you to achieve the objectives (or not) such as training activities, problem solving capacity and degree of participation. In an emergency programme, the overall goal of the combined interventions of government agencies and others is usually to prevent unnecessary death and suffering in a way that preserves people's dignity. The specific purpose of the water and sanitation intervention is to ensure that people have access to and use water and sanitation facilities in an optimal way in order to help prevent the spread of diarrhoea. However, diarrhoea is affected by many variables (for example, presence of other disease and availability of food and health services) and although the failure of a water and sanitation project to deliver on its objectives may lead to disease outbreaks, it is not possible to conclusively attribute a decrease (or increase) in diarrhoea cases to the provision of water and sanitation facilities unless we can control all of the other variables. It is therefore usual to use what are known as proxy or substitute indicators to measure the success of a water and sanitation project. These are, for example, the use of clean drinking water or the consistent use of latrines and hand washing facilities by all sections of the community. Health trends should, however, still be monitored by talking regularly with health clinic staff and communities so that potentially harmful changes can be picked up quickly and acted upon but this data must always be interpreted with care.

The logical framework details the indicators for the different levels of objectives, as shown in Box 4.1.

Another model suggested by Narayan (1993) looks at three main areas indicating change in water and sanitation projects: sustainability,

> **Box 4.1** Hierarchy of indicators
>
> The *INPUTS* include resources utilized (people, materials and equipment) and *ACTIVITIES* such as training courses held, plans prepared and the number of people carrying out hygiene promotion activities.
>
> The *OUTPUTS or RESULTS* include a better informed and organized community, increased capacity and intention to take action to improve health, increased self-confidence and problem solving capacity, the number of water and sanitation facilities constructed,
>
> The *INTERMEDIATE GOAL, PURPOSE or OUTCOME* relates to the objectives of improved hygiene practices, improved and increased use of latrines, increased use of improved water sources, evidence of other preventive measures taken.
>
> The *FINAL GOAL or AIM* refers to the decrease in the incidence of water-borne and sanitation-related diseases and a better quality of life, namely, the impact on people's lives.

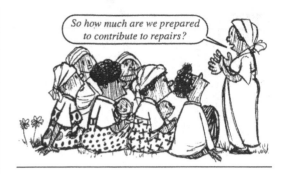

effective use and replicability – which together result in capacity building.

Sustainability

- *Reliability of systems*: quality of water sources, number of facilities in working order, maintenance arrangements.
- *Human capacity*: management abilities, knowledge and skills, confidence built in all socio-economic groups.
- *Local institutional capacity*: autonomy, supportive leadership, systems for learning and problem-solving.
- *Cost sharing and unit costs*: community contribution, agency contribution, unit costs.
- *Collaboration among organizations*: planning joint activities.

Effective use

- *Optimal use*: are the facilities being used to obtain their maximum benefits or are they used by only a few beneficiaries? Are all children's faeces being disposed of? Are hands being washed at key times? Are increased quantities of water being used? Is water being wasted? Do people with physical disabilities also have access?
- *Hygienic use*: are the facilities kept clean and maintained? Are measures taken to prevent contamination of water stored for drinking, or food stored before eating?
- *Consistent use*: are the facilities used all the time and all the year round? By all socio-economic groups of people?

Replicability

- *Community ability to expand services*: additional water/latrine facilities built, upgraded facilities, new development activities initiated.
- *Transferability of agency strategies*: proportion and role of specialized personnel, institutional framework, documented administrative/

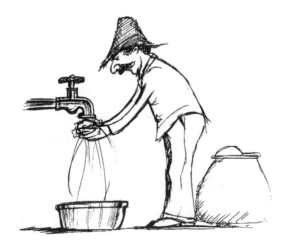

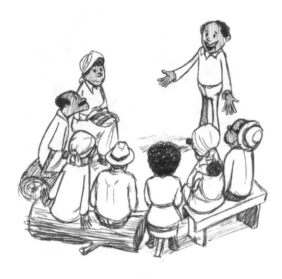

> *In one water supply project, the change from the use of unprotected wells to the use of protected wells and a windlass pulley system was very successful. However, the more successful it became the longer the queues at the water point became and this led to people using their own, sometimes dirty buckets to draw water, thus contaminating the water source.*
>
> Boot and Cairncross, 1993

implementation procedures, other special unique conditions.

Narayan's indicators can be adapted for the emergency context according to the length of the project and the urgency of the water, sanitation and hygiene intervention.

Measuring change

Change rarely takes place in the ordered and linear way that many planning models assume. A project may have very positive outcomes in terms of increasing people's self-esteem, for example, but this may not be measured by the evaluation as it was not a focus of the original objectives. The outcome of the evaluation will thus be dependent on the original objectives, what is actually measured and the choice of indicators.

Monitoring and evaluation attempt to measure progress against the baseline data gathered at the beginning of the project as well as to identify faults in project design and unnecessary or unrealistic objectives.

When to monitor and evaluate?

As discussed previously, monitoring needs to be instigated as soon as the project activities begin and continue until the end of the project but an evaluation will usually be a one off event. The

project cycle often indicates that evaluation takes place at the end of a project but a mid-term review is possible and some agencies have introduced the idea of 'real time evaluations' that occur relatively early on in a large-scale project.

A one-off evaluation will require more planning and personnel to ensure that the evaluation activities take place within the defined timescale. The best time to conduct the evaluation will have to be discussed and the following issues may need to be taken into consideration. Is there a time of the year when people are less accessible, for example, harvest time? Will the onset of the rains make access to some of the areas difficult? Are there times of the day when people, especially women, are more willing to attend meetings or will be at home to answer questions? Are there special events or festivals that might make people too busy? Might there be elections that could influence the process of the evaluation? Do project staff have particular work commitments that prevent them from taking part in the evaluation? When is the optimum time for evaluation results to be available for planning purposes? There may be similar time constraints to carrying out monitoring activities and these will also need to be scheduled in, following discussions with men and women in the community.

Participatory monitoring and evaluation

By being actively involved in the process of gathering data, participants are more likely to learn from the experience and are in a better position to use that information. By looking more closely at why certain conditions exist, ways to solve them can be identified. Progress and achievements can also be monitored and this can generate further involvement in reaching project objectives – particularly when those objectives have also been set by the beneficiaries. Evaluation then becomes a part of the participatory process. It does not exclude the possibility of external evaluation but provides a more dynamic way to measure progress. It differs fundamentally from conventional data collection methods because its main aim is to enhance community-level problem solving. Participatory evaluation respects the knowledge that people already have and aims to build on this, allowing new knowledge to be generated by the group, rather than imposed from outside.

Narayan-Parker (1989) compared the use of participatory techniques with more objective forms of evaluation. The results indicate that in all cases the participatory techniques had four advantages:

1. They were more 'fun'. They generated great enthusiasm, got people emotionally involved and brought people together; the old, the young, men and women, the somewhat educated and the non-literate.
2. As a result of everyone's involvement and emotional engagement, the activities brought forth perspectives, findings, and issues not revealed by the more direct, individual, private interviews.
3. In most cases, self-evaluation ratings coincided with those given by external 'experts'.
4. They increased people's confidence in themselves. Their awareness of unresolved problems led to their taking immediate initiatives

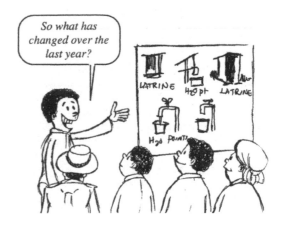

for follow-up action. Within the agencies, the same effects could be seen at all levels.

In summary, evaluation tools are more effective when put back in the hands of local people. Their disadvantage is that participatory processes are often more time consuming. However, this will be time well spent if it means that people are more in control of the process and take more responsibility for the outcomes of the project.

Community indicators

Community groups can also suggest their own indicators for measuring change and decide for themselves when to monitor or assess their activities. These community indicators may not be the same as those suggested by the project team. For example they may feel that the success of a water and sanitation project is not the decrease in diarrhoea but the fact that their daughters are more marriageable because they come from a village with better services. They may decide that a latrine project is successful because it improves the level of dignity amongst women who can go to the toilet in private rather than because it improves health. There has recently been renewed interest in defining community indicators and in involving beneficiaries in the process of monitoring and evaluation.

Measuring participation

It is very difficult to measure an abstract term such as participation and the obvious first step is to try to define exactly what is meant by the term

> *Evaluation is a process of collaborative problem-solving through the generation and use of knowledge. It is a process that leads to corrective action when all levels of users are involved in shared decision-making.*
>
> Narayan and Srinivasan, 1994

The success of the Rohinga Refugee Programme's Hygiene Promotion Project was a major factor in making it possible to leave maintenance of the drainage and garbage disposal and routine care of the latrines to the refugees. A significant part of the hygiene promotion centred on drinking water and the water supply system. As a direct result there was no threat to the quality of the water sources that were used to supply the camps. The water system in Nayapara neither needed guards nor outside operators, unlike the other camps without the hygiene promotion component.

Herson and Mears, 1992

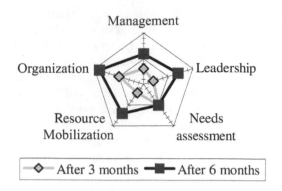

Figure 4.2 Spider gram/evaluation wheel/radar chart

before any attempt is made to measure it (see Introduction). How many people attend meetings, who doesn't attend and why, are all issues that can be raised in group discussions. People can also rate their own degree of participation on a spider gram (see next section). A matrix that allows different aspects of, for example, participation to be measured on a scale of one to five can also be drawn up and used with the spider gram. It is easier to think of more specific aspects of participation, such as the degree to which women or other marginalized groups are involved in decision making and who is involved in the planning and management of projects. However, increased community participation may initially lead to an increase in conflict or confrontation between different groups and this may be seen as a negative aspect of participation.

Spider gram
Rifkin (1988) suggests the use of a spider gram (or radar chart) as a tool to measure community participation. It can also be adapted to measure issues such as sustainability. Different aspects of participation are considered, such as the involvement of women in site selection for facilities or the degree to which the elderly and disabled are considered in appropriate sanitation designs. A matrix is drawn up with criteria for each level of the matrix. Project staff and beneficiaries can be asked to rate each individual indicator along a scale from zero to five by assessing the extent to

which the criteria fit the current situation. This can be done as a group activity and is likely to provoke much discussion and debate (see Appendices, page 254 for an example of a spider gram matrix).

How to do monitoring

As has been stated, each member of staff working on a project is responsible for some aspect of monitoring, from ensuring that project vehicles are in good working order to working out performance development plans (see example Table 4.1). Many aspects of monitoring are undertaken as a natural course of events. However, many agencies struggle with trying to ensure that project processes and outcomes are systematically measured. A first step to successful monitoring is to compile a monitoring plan. Table 4.1 provides an example of a monitoring plan.

Monitoring tools and presenting findings
The type of monitoring tools you choose will determine the type of information you collect. The following sub-sections provide details on some of the choices of tools available. It is important to record the information in as systematic a way as possible and this is why it is useful to devise monitoring forms. Example monitoring forms can be found on pages 230–32 and 205–6. Individual monitoring forms will need to be collated into a 'master' monitoring form and the data should be

Table 4.1 Example project monitoring plan

Who	What	How/With Whom	Format	How Often
Project manager	Overall humanitarian situation	Agency/government meetings	Minutes from meetings	Weekly
	Overall responsibility to ensure monitoring and evaluation carried out	Collation of information from team and observation/discussions during field visits and with Team leaders	Progress Report	Three monthly
	Staff performance		Performance appraisal	Yearly
	Donor reporting		Narrative report	Monthly
Water and sanitation team leader	Overall water and sanitation status/strategies	Coordination meetings	Minutes	Weekly
	Staff performance	Engineers and hygiene promoters	Performance appraisals	Yearly
	Collation of data from engineers and hygiene promoters	Observation/discussions with community members and staff	Project monitoring forms	Weekly/monthly
	Overall progress of project	Monitoring forms, reports, discussions, field visits	Monthly reports	Monthly
Engineers/technicians	Construction outputs and quality of work	Field observations Team meetings	Project records Monthly reports	Monthly
	Water quantity and quality at source and household level	e.g. Delagua (water testing) kit Source and household measurements/observations	Water quality testing forms	One off testing for faecal coliforms and other chemical tests if possible
	Functioning systems, design suitability	Discussions with users	Monthly reports	Weekly/as necessary
Hygiene promoters	Use and maintenance of facilities, hand washing, use of ORS, user satisfaction (safety, privacy etc.), participation, training of facilitators and committees, other promotional activities, protection issues/incidents, health status	Mini surveys Focus group discussions with men, women and children Pocket charts, demonstrations, observation, Clinic records and discussions with clinic staff Team meetings	Survey monitoring forms, Hygiene promotion action plans, Monitoring reporting form	Weekly/monthly 19 households
Community facilitators	Use and maintenance of facilities, community hygiene actions and risks	Discussions, household visits Observation Meetings with hygiene promoters and engineers	Verbal reports, Pictoral latrine monitoring form, WASH motivator form	Weekly/monthly 10 households
Community members	Community defined indicators	Observation, discussion	Verbal reports	As time allows
Monitoring and evaluation officer	Project indicators and processes	Facilitation of use of above methods and feedback to community	Project report	Monthly
	Training on monitoring and evaluation	Training evaluation	Evaluation forms	After each training

When water availability is estimated/measured by dividing the output of the source by the number of users, this should be checked through discussions with users at the household level as access may be affected by the lack of containers, disability or distance to the water point, etc.

discussed and analysed in a written report. If possible it is useful to also try and present the data in a pictorial form. The information gathered should then be shared with the wider community through the existing channels of communication (for example, community leaders, local religious establishments, notice boards, radio) in order to stimulate renewed action. Box 4.2 suggests three ways of presenting monitoring information to reach more people in a meaningful way.

Monitoring meetings

Informal monitoring can and should be done on a continual basis to identify problems as they come up. For example, it may become obvious during the course of the project that community management meetings are organized but very few people attend. In this instance, it is very important to find out why and to see what can be done about it, otherwise the project will obviously fail to meet its objectives. It would be good to ask people to explain why they do not like attending meetings. If a small focus group were organized close to where people live, they might be more willing to attend. If not, then it may be wise to visit people in their homes – they may be prepared to invite their neighbours for the discussion.

Assessment tools

Similar tools to those used for baseline data collection can also be used at intervals to collect monitoring data (Chapter 1). Qualitative and quantitative information should be collected and the number of indicators selected should be limited to avoid overburdening staff with data collection. Be careful also that the gathering of data is not

---

seen as an indicator of staff performance or this may encourage cheating and bias the results.

Focus group discussions

Participatory tools and approaches that are a key element of hygiene promotion activities also lend themselves well to monitoring activities. Communities can be asked whether changes have occurred during focus group discussions. Voting activities can provide some indicative data, for example, as to whether improved water sources or sanitation facilities are being used and if not, the reasons can be explored in group discussions.

Records should be kept of the views expressed during group discussions and these should be collated and summarized in a monitoring form. The monitoring form should indicate who and how many people were involved in the discussion and what changes have occurred since the previous discussions. This data can be used later to inform evaluations. An example of the findings of a focus group discussion on water, sanitation and health needs is provided on page 229 in the Appendices.

Self-monitoring forms

Hygiene promotion activities might involve the use of 'self-monitoring' forms, for example for latrine use and maintenance or to gain an impression of community perceptions of changes in their health status. Each participant is given a form to fill in over the following two-week period. The results are then collected and discussed at a subsequent meeting, asking people whether they found the exercise useful, what they learned from it and what thoughts they have about changing their living conditions (such as making their own latrines better). The results do not have to be shared with the rest of the group in a way that might cause embarrassment. If anonymity is desired the facilitator could simply collate the results as numbers. Examples of self-monitoring forms are on pages 230–32. The WASH motivator form (also on pages 205–06) can be used in a similar way to envisage change and monitor progress. Project staff also need to monitor their own activities. Through regular reports and team review meetings they can record their activities and discuss problems and successes. It may also

---

> **Box 4.2** Presentation of monitoring information
>
> Information is often more appealing and receives more attention if it is:
>
> o discussed orally;
> o summarized on not more than a couple of pages;
> o illustrated with graphs, figures and pictures.

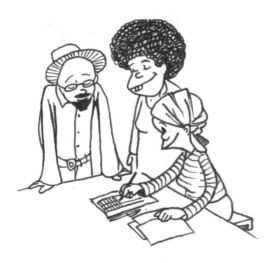

be helpful to compile an action plan each week to record intended activities and subsequent problems encountered or particular achievements.

Many of the participatory methods of data collection can be adapted for use in assessing staff progress. Focus group discussions may be used to try to identify some of the particular problems encountered and some of the possible solutions to these problems. Self-monitoring forms to assess the development of facilitation skills can be used at all levels and provide a visual representation of progress.

The type of monitoring process employed, indicators used, and the frequency of use are also open to being evaluated and changed.

Trainers' assessment forms

Training workshops need to be monitored to assess whether the learning objectives have been achieved and whether the quality of the learning experiences can be improved upon. It is important for the facilitator to evaluate how the training session went. The usefulness of the training sessions from the participants' perspective can be rated on a spider gram (or radar chart) such as the one shown on page 94. If people are unable to read, a list of aspects of training can be read out loud and participants asked to circle the appropriate face (see page 98).

Observation/exploratory walks

Exploratory walks can be used to monitor whether facilities are being used and maintained and

---

Box 4.3 Children's monitoring activity (see pages 231–32)

Identify a maximum of twelve children and the area in which the monitoring will take place. Divide the children into pairs. Give a monitoring form, a pencil and a rubber to each participant. Ask the children what they see in each picture to ensure they understand the photograph properly. Explain to them that they will walk around a specific area to assess the practices related to water and sanitation. If they find similar situations to the one in the pictures, they must count how many times they see this and write the number below each picture (they can make tally marks below each picture). For example, they should count how many latrines they see with open lids, how many uncovered water containers etc. Assign each group a zone to monitor that includes latrines and give them a certain time for this task (around 15 or 20 minutes) depending on the area to be monitored. Summarize the total number of the identified situations when they come back and write them in a new form. Discuss the most problematic situations: why certain practices are a problem and what they can do to improve or resolve it. Agree on some actions that will be done during the week that includes sharing this information and survey form with family members and friends. Arrange to meet the group again after one week to discuss progress on the actions decided. After some time the exercise can be repeated in the same place to compare results.

Source: Veronica Kloster, 2005, personal communication

---

individual discussions held with users at water points or in their homes. Hygiene promoters will need to be trained to observe particular risk factors and it is helpful if they all agree beforehand the criteria for their observations of a 'clean' water container or 'well maintained' toilet. For example a 'clean' toilet might be one that:

o is free from flies;

> *Weekly reports produced at each level of the project structure were collated and findings fed back through the health education network to the community and through the health education coordinator to the engineers, camp authorities and other agencies, as appropriate. The health education checklists and supervisors' reporting forms were the basis of the monitoring system.*
>
> Oxfam, 1993

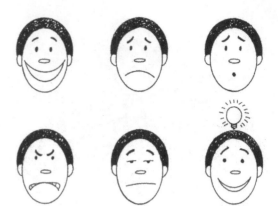

Box 4.4 Some problems encountered with monitoring

o Indicators are not developed from recorded baseline data making it difficult to infer change.

o Indicators are not realistic or measurable.

o Terms used are general and open to interpretation, for example, raised awareness or correct usage.

o Process indicators are not developed.

o Indicators are measured too frequently to detect change.

o Monitoring tools are not specific enough about the data to be collected so different people using them will probably measure different things.

o Large amounts of data are collected but not regularly analysed and used to adjust project activities.

o Data collection becomes a burdensome task and detracts from health promotion and community mobilization activities.

o Qualitative methods are used to collect quantitative data and vice versa.

o Qualitative data is not recorded or analysed as people are unsure of how to go about this.

o has no evidence of excreta on the slab;
o has no smell.

Checklists

Questionnaires (such as the one on pages 119–20) can be used as a type of checklist for monitoring or evaluation. This checklist could be used every two to three months on a sample of households in the community. However, it must be remembered that this information will need to be collated and analysed and this can become very time consuming. It is important that the time for promotional work with the community is not undermined because too much time is being spent analysing data in the office.

Table 4.2 provides examples of some indicators and the methods used to measure these indicators. The potential constraints of these methods are also highlighted. Morbidity and mortality data are included as indicators but they cannot be used on their own or without careful interpretation.

Accessing clinic data to monitor health trends

Morbidity and mortality data generated by clinics and hospitals may be useful for tracking health trends though this data should be treated with caution. Inadequate facilities and long queues or distances to travel may dissuade people from attending the health clinic. In many countries traditional healers or market vendors will be visited first when illness strikes. Where aid is distributed on the basis of the number of people per household, families may be reluctant to register a death that has occurred at home. In refugee camps an outreach system is often established and sick people encountered during home visits are referred to clinics for treatment. The data may therefore be more reliable in this setting.

Talk regularly with clinic staff about the trends they are seeing and their interpretation of the data

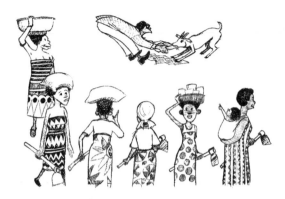

they are collecting; does it indicate a need for a more water and sanitation activities or a hygiene campaign in a specific location? Communities can be asked about their perceptions of disease trends: what do they think are the common health problems affecting men, women and children? Is the situation better/worse than last month/the same time last year? How closely do their impressions correlate with the clinic data?

Community-based monitoring systems

Community-based monitoring systems can be very effective ways of monitoring services. Systems can be set up in consultation with the local community to monitor the quality or frequency of services provided.

> *In a camp for Sudanese Refugees in Koboko, Uganda, the distribution of water during the acute phase of the emergency was a considerable problem. River water was treated in one location and taken by tanker to 10,000 litre water tanks in different parts of the camp. The tankers were seldom working, often because the truck fuel was misappropriated. A token system was set up, where one woman living in the shelter next to each tank was provided with a number of tokens. She would provide the driver of the tanker with a token only after he had completely filled up the water tank. The tanker drivers could receive their salaries and fuel allowances only when they submitted the correct number of tokens to the camp manager at the end of each day.*
>
> Morgan, 1994a

Carrying out evaluations

There are numerous frameworks for evaluation. The main questions that most evaluations try to answer can be grouped as follows:

○ *Appropriateness*: Are the activities the right ones? Do they address the most important problems? Do they provide a solution to these problems?
○ *Effectiveness*: How well are the different activities carried out? What are the effects and impact of the project?
○ *Efficiency*: What does the project cost? Are the available resources used in the most effective way? How does the approach of the project compare to other projects in terms of cost?
○ *Participation*: Who attends meetings? Who doesn't attend and why? What nature and characteristics do they have? How often do they attend? Do different stakeholders in the community feel that they have had an opportunity to be involved in the programme? How has community management of the facilities been initiated and what is the level of people's commitment to it? What actions have the community initiated themselves?
○ *Sustainability*: What potential does the project have to continue after external support has stopped?
○ *Unintended outcomes*: Are there outcomes that were not intended? Are they positive or negative?

The logframe approach tries to assess the inputs, activities, outputs, intermediate and final goals.

The indicators chosen for evaluation will depend on the phase of the emergency, the outcome of the baseline data collection and the objectives and indicators that have been identified in the project plan and by individual community groups.

The following activities need to be scheduled into an evaluation:

○ Decide what you would like to find out (you need to reach a consensus with all the

Table 4.2 Indicators and methods for their measurement

Indicator	Method	Recording Data	Constraints
Morbidity and mortality data	Communicate with health centre staff to get reports on disease trends or collect self reported data from communities	Summary of clinic data or reports from coordination meetings Focus group discussion reports	Clinic data may be unreliable or incomplete Data must be interpreted with care
Improved sanitation according to Sphere guidelines	Latrine inspection by community and public health promoters Focus groups with men, women and children Exploratory walks to look for signs of open defecation Pocket voting with children Picture drawing for children Photographs	Picture forms for community members Checklists Written analysis of focus group discussions	Concepts such as 'clean' need to be defined Taking photographs may not be acceptable (especially if they are embarrassing to adults)
Access to clean drinking water and adequate quantities of water	Water testing at source Water point inspection Jerry can inspection at water points Household visits to look at water storage containers and estimate quantity of water used Testing of water containers Mapping of water points for equity of access	Water point monitoring forms Household visit forms Maps of water points used for different purposes and during different seasons	Some communities object to someone being posted at the water point with a form – it is seen as 'spying'
Increased knowledge of hygiene and improved hygiene practices	Inspection of hand washing facilities at the latrines – noting whether they are there or if the soap/sink/ ground is wet Focus group discussion Household visits Observation of hand washing by children Pocket voting with children Three-pile sorting of habits that have changed Quizzes and competitions for children Observation of ORS demonstrations Exploratory walks around the camp or community or at communal latrines Timelines and seasonal calendars for disease prevalence	Household visit forms Written analysis of focus group discussions Pocket voting results recorded	Hand washing is hard to monitor any other way than direct observation as people tend to tell you what you want to know: triangulation of data is important Children are good at observing their own family behaviours and tend to be more honest
Gender and increased community participation	Focus group discussions Exit interviews after committee meetings Observation at committee meetings	Written analysis of focus group discussions Spider grams (see above)	Having women on committees is not enough, there must be evidence of their actual participation in decision making

stakeholders, which might take lengthy negotiations over several weeks).

o Identify people to undertake the investigations (this can also take several weeks and will depend on their availability and willingness to help).

o Organize logistical arrangements (including making sure that the people who need to be interviewed and the necessary reports and information are available at the appointed time with interpreters/translations if necessary).

o Guide and review findings with the investigators (this may need to be coordinated through a review committee, comprising key representatives from the different stakeholder groups).

o Feed back the findings of the investigators and report (different presentations, meetings and reports will probably be needed for different levels of stakeholders) and agree the next steps.

Control groups

Some evaluations attempt to compare the type of intervention with either no intervention or other types of intervention. This uses what is known as a 'quasi-experimental' model because it tries to be like a laboratory experiment using control groups. These control groups should 'match' the experimental group as far as possible in terms of socio-economic variables such as education, income, or occupation. For example, an intervention in a rural area in Rwanda cannot be compared to an urban area in Rwanda (let alone another country). A community where there are predominantly young people under the age of 15 could not be matched with a community where there is a very large proportion of elderly people. Such evaluations are sometimes difficult to conduct because it is hard to control all of the variables. The intervention may have had an effect because of the characteristics of the hygiene promoters rather than the intervention itself, or the intervention group may have had contact with the control group, thus biasing the results. It may also be unethical to provide health benefits to one group but not to another, especially during an emergency. In recent years researchers have been promoting the use of the case-control study

method as a more statistically reliable and a more ethical approach to measuring the impact of an intervention than the with-and-without approach. The method compares differences within the same population instead of differences between different populations (see Chapter 1). A smaller sample size is acceptable because differences between the populations are reduced.

Lot quality assurance sampling

The LQAS method of sampling (see Chapter 1) is being used by many NGOs as a way of measuring the effectiveness of health promotion programmes. It uses a smaller sample size than is usual (19 per supervision area) but is seen to provide a 'good enough' assessment of how well the project is performing and therefore is more likely to be employed by busy project staff. The method also allows for comparison between different project areas and it can identify where to target limited resources to best effect. Detailed information and training modules can be found on the CORE website (see page 265 in the Appendices).

Statistical analysis

Results from any type of questionnaire or participatory survey can be tabulated by hand to produce a rough picture of the disease-causing practices, such as in the charts on pages 36–37. This is probably the best way to analyse the information and to identify general trends. If you have access to a computer, statistics software such as SPSS or EpiInfo (see page 35) can be useful to investigate whether the differences are due to chance or are truly or 'statistically' significant. With the right tools, some statistical knowledge and enough time available you can analyse your information in more detail. However, the reasons for carrying out a statistical study should be clear from the beginning, for example, if you want epidemiological proof that your intervention had an impact on the prevalence of waterborne disease. Statistics can be very useful but are easy to misinterpret and should always be used with caution. More information about statistics can be found in most standard statistics texts. Rowntree (1981) is a useful textbook on statistics and is written in a way that is relatively easy to understand (see Annotated Bibliography).

Explaining the findings of the evaluation

There are numerous evaluations that indicate that hygiene promotion is better than no hygiene promotion (DFID, 1997a). Experience suggests that more interactive ways of working are usually more effective in terms of making people aware of the issues and enabling them to take positive steps to improve their health. Even if resources are available to use a quasi experimental study design, some of the data should be gathered using participatory approaches to maximize the opportunities for listening to the views of beneficiaries.

Learning about evaluation

There is no fixed formula for evaluation. Participatory evaluation has emerged only recently into the water and sanitation sector and has yet to be employed consistently in emergency projects. The only way to learn is through experience. The questions to keep asking are:'Does this process give us the information we need to solve the problems we have identified?', and 'Are we using methods that increase our capacity to solve other problems in the future?'. The style adopted in the project for evaluation must be flexible enough to allow changes in the way information is collected and analysed in order to make the process increasingly useful. Other projects will be keen to learn from your experience – both good and bad. Where possible, share the information you have collected so that practice can be developed

using your ideas. After all, there is no sense in reinventing the wheel!

How can we do it better next time?

This chapter has reviewed the process of monitoring and evaluation. It has emphasized the importance of monitoring and evaluation in the project cycle, provided tools and methods that can be used and suggested ways of analysing and sharing the information so that your project and other projects can benefit from your experience and improve on what you have done.

And finally

The final sections of this manual comprise the Appendices. They contain more useful materials and references to help you to promote better hygiene.

If you have enjoyed using the manual or would like to see some changes, please contact the authors through Peter Lochery at CARE International, 151 Ellis Street NE, Atlanta GA 30303 – 2440, USA

The original edition of this manual has been produced as an interactive CD ROM. Both the CD ROM and the original manual have been translated into Spanish and French. Peter Lochery is collecting comments from the French and Spanish editions also. These versions are available on the web.

A three week training course linked with this manual was held by CARE in Zambia. The training course, including detailed session plans, can be found on the internet (see page 265).

APPENDICES

APPENDICES

A1

Assessment tools

How to conduct a community mapping exercise

Mapping is a useful exercise through which you can learn from community members what they feel is important about where they live and promote discussion about their lives, including their hygiene practices. A mapping exercise is usually a public activity and can be initiated simply by approaching a small group of people. It can also be conducted in a prearranged session if you want to maintain a homogeneous group.

To conduct a community mapping exercise:

○ Have a clear idea in your mind of the possible things that might be identified on a map, such as church, market place, water points;
○ Identify possible resources that might be used for the map such as stones or leaves, but allow people to make their suggestions as you go along;
○ Explain who you are and that you would like their help in conducting the exercise;
○ Explain what you hope to find out and how the participants might go about making a map;
○ Allow plenty of time for discussion of the idea of making a map – many people may be sceptical about their ability to do this because they have never been to school;
○ If necessary, begin the process yourself with a central landmark using a stick to draw on the ground. Try to 'hand over the stick' as much as possible to other participants;
○ Listen carefully to what people say and allow free discussion and debate among participants;
○ Keep a record of who took part, when and where;
○ When the map is finished, offer to transcribe it or get one of the participants to transcribe it on to paper. Ask the participants to decide where they would like the map to be kept, or who will keep it.

It might also be useful to compile quantifiable data from the mapping exercise. A table showing the quantities of each thing that has been drawn on the map (for example, numbers of latrines, protected and unprotected water sources) can then provide a baseline for subsequent quantifiable evaluation or for the triangulation of results from questionnaire surveys. This can also be displayed with the map, for those who can read.

How to conduct a focus group discussion

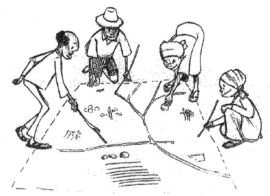

Focus groups are useful for conducting detailed discussions on selected topics with a targeted group of people. They work best when the group members are from the same socio-economic group, such as poor elderly men, middle-class young mothers or users of a particular water source. With careful facilitation, focus

groups can provide insights into the
thoughts and practices of the members of
the group for the facilitator and the group
members.

To conduct a focus group discussion:

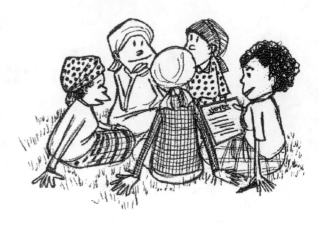

○ Prepare a framework of questions to
probe a particular issue. The questions
should be as open-ended as possible.
Sometimes it may be easier to refer to
someone in the third person, for example, rather than say 'what do you use
for soaking up blood during menstruation?', ask 'what do women use to soak
up their blood during menstruation?'.

○ Invite suitable participants to attend the meeting at a venue and time identified by them. Six to
twelve participants is ideal, but do not turn people away.

○ Introduce yourselves to the group and explain very clearly the object of the exercise and that you
hope that everyone will learn from each other. Explain that there are no wrong or right answers to
the questions. Stress that people should try not to interrupt others when they are talking and that
everyone's point of view will be valued.

○ Do not interfere too much in the discussion or put your viewpoints across. As the session proceeds you will need to formulate new questions in response to what has already been said. If
people ask for your opinion say that you will participate more once you have heard their views.

○ Take notes of the proceedings; preferably this should not be done by the facilitator. The recorder
should try to take as many notes as possible. All of the conversation can be recorded on tape if a
machine is available and if the participants are comfortable with it. Transcribing the session takes
a lot of time, which can be done later but the taping may not be sufficiently clear to make out the
whole session, hence notes should be taken at the same time.

○ Bring the session to a close when you feel that the subject has been exhausted (maximum 1.5
hours). If problems have been identified, try also to get people to consider any possible solutions
and how they intend to implement them.

○ Briefly sum up the group discussions. Thank the participants for their time and ask them if they
would like to be involved in any further discussion groups or if you could meet up with them again
to discuss any further conclusions you have come to or anything that was not clear. The findings
should be included in the project records.

If a large group turns up, carry on with the discussion explaining the reasons why a smaller group
was invited. At the end of the session ask whether people were able to discuss things freely or if only
the most confident ones spoke.

Focus group discussion sample questions

Water use

○ Where do you collect your water (drinking, washing, cooking, watering gardens)?
○ What do you think of the water (taste, quality, distance, colour)?
○ Who collects the water? What do they collect it in?
○ Do you transfer water to another container for storage?
○ What do you store your drinking water in?

○ Where do you do your clothes washing?
○ What do you wash your clothes with?
○ What do you wash yourself with?
○ If with soap, where does the soap come from?
○ What do you do with the water after washing?
○ What is the most important use for water?
○ Where does the water for beer-making come from?

Latrine use

○ What type of latrines do you have?
○ How do you find the latrines (structure, cleanliness, privacy, smell)?
○ Why do you use a latrine?
○ Do you use a latrine at night? If not, what do you do?
○ Do young children use the latrines? From what age do children start to use the latrine?
○ What happens to the stools of young babies?
○ Does everybody do this?
○ Who made the latrines?
○ Who cleans, repairs, empties the latrines?
○ Do young children wash their hands after using the latrine?
○ Do adults wash their hands after using the latrine?
○ What is the health problem that is of greatest concern to you at the moment?
○ What do women do to take care of menstrual blood?

How to do key informant interviews

Interviewing people is a very good way of obtaining their view on a subject. General and specific information can be gathered by asking questions informally but systematically. Key informant interviews are a useful way of meeting and obtaining support from different individuals, but people may only tell you what they think you want to hear rather than what they actually do or understand to be correct. You can use these interviews to find out which hygiene practices are considered ideal or acceptable and why. A written interview schedule should be prepared for the interviewer to study beforehand. Interviewing may require some specific training of the study team to enable them to learn or improve their interviewing techniques, decide on possible lines of questioning, and the exact wording of any required translations. Try to avoid leading questions such as 'When do you wash your hands with soap?'. Use open questions instead, such as 'What do people do when they have used a latrine?'.

To do key informant interviews

○ Select the people you wish to interview. These could be community leaders, health workers, government officials, women's representatives or children, depending on what you wish to find out.
○ Make an appointment at a suitable time for them.
○ Prepare beforehand what you want to find out. This could be written down, but try not to read out questions during the interview.
○ Take notes of their answers, or ask someone else to take notes.
○ At the end of the interview, ask the person being interviewed whether they have questions to ask you. Be prepared to answer these as best you can, and when you do not know the answer, offer to find out and come back to them with the response.

○ Summarize what you have discussed and agreed at the end of the interview.
○ After the interview, check your notes, add important details that you did not have time to mention during the interview, make sure that the name (and position) of the person interviewed and the community from where they come are recorded.

Include the notes in the project records. An interview should not go on for more than one and a half hours, if you have not found out all that you need during the interview, then ask them for another appointment at a later date.

Source: Adapted from Almedom et al, 1997.

How to carry out observations

Observation is a useful technique to back up or crosscheck information gathered through other methods. Observation is not always as easy as it sounds and some training will also be required to avoid the common pitfalls of observer bias, inconsistency and partiality. Simple techniques of systematic observation may need some practice to refine and standardize them. It should be remembered that the actual presence of the observer can affect the behaviour observed.

Observation must be done with sensitivity and should not carry value judgements with it. For example, a dirty latrine may produce a very negative reaction in the observer, which may embarrass the person being observed and alienate them from the work of the project.

How to do structured observations

Structured observations are used to assess how common particular risky hygiene practices are in a community. The information they generate can be used to design hygiene promotion projects and provides useful quantitative data for evaluation purposes.

To do structured observations:

○ Select the sample households. Depending on how big and how varied your project area is you may need to cover 100–200 families (see pages 30–31). Observe only in households with small children under three years of age. Ask families for their permission and explain that you are trying to find out about health problems. If anybody does not want to participate, thank them and try another house.
○ Work preferably with female fieldworkers. Observe for a standard period, for example, from 6 am to 9 am each morning. Test the observation formats and revise them to suit the circumstances. Train fieldworkers carefully so that they all fill in the forms in the same way. Make a list of instructions.
○ Arrive at the household at getting-up time, greet people politely and then sit down in an inconspicuous corner (if possible) where you can see what is going on. Keep conversation to a minimum.
○ Supervisors should try to visit regularly to ascertain if there are any problems. Hold frequent team meetings to decide what to do about unexpected observations and to encourage the team.
○ Tabulate the results by hand or computer. Consider how much people may have changed their behaviour because there is an observer present. The findings should be included in the project records.

Structured observation checklist for child defecation

1. Did you see the child (0–5yrs) defecate during the observation period? (Yes/No)
2. Approximate age of child (months)

3. Where did the child defecate? (On a pot/ on the ground in the house/ on the ground outside the house/ in nappies/ in pants/ in trousers/ in the latrine/ other – specify)
4. Did someone clean the child's bottom after it had defecated? If yes, who? (Nobody/ the child itself/ mother/ sister/ other relative/ other (specify)/ not seen)
5. What happened to the stools? (Thrown in the latrine/ left lying on the ground/ thrown outside/ taken to the rubbish heap/ washed off/ not seen)
6. What happened to the water used for washing child or nappy? (Thrown in the latrine/ thrown on the ground outside/ thrown on the rubbish heap/ not seen)
7. What did the person do after cleaning the child's bottom? (Wash both hands with soap/ rinse both hands with water only/ rinse one hand/ not wash hands/ not seen)

Source: Adapted from Curtis and Kanki, 1998.

How to do an exploratory walk

Exploratory walks can help to explore and observe life in the community. They can be used to raise issues and prompt discussion on those things observed during the walk, including sanitation conditions and hygiene practices. They can be carried out alone or undertaken as an activity for a group of people, for example, baseline survey team or participants in a training course.

To do an exploratory walk:

○ It is preferable that the walk is done in conjunction with members of the community. Try to identify key informants who are willing to join you.
○ Spend about one to two hours (if there is time) walking round the settlement, discussing the issues of interest with the key informants and with those you meet along the route and making observations on issues of particular interest (a checklist may be useful to remind you of issues to look at).
○ When the walk and discussion are over, the main ideas or issues can be summarized. The findings should be included in the project records.

How to do behaviour trials

Behaviour trials are a social marketing technique that enable health workers and community representatives to work together to design replacement practices for those that are putting people at risk. You can also use them to find out about behavioural motivation by asking what people like and dislike about the new practices and any other consequences of practising them.

To do behaviour trials:

○ Find a number of women who are not using your target safe practices. Invite three or four groups of about 10 to local meetings. Make sure that they are roughly representative of your primary target audience. At the meeting, discuss the results of the observations and your analysis of practises that are putting children at risk. Ask for their suggestions as to what could be done to improve the situation. Ask for volunteers to work with you to try out safer behaviours. Offer physical support, such as soap or potties, so the trial does not require them to spend their own money.
○ Fieldworkers should visit each volunteer at home and work with her to adapt the target practices to her individual circumstances. They ask her to do her best to carry them out for two weeks.
○ Each volunteer is visited every day at first (every two days in the second week) to work with her, help solve problems and find alternatives. After several weeks most mothers will have developed

workable replacement practices, and you will have useful ideas for scaling up the intervention. Key questions to ask at each visit are:

- Did you manage to adopt the new practice?
- What difficulties did you have? How did you solve the problems?
- What else could be done to make it easier?
- Did you like the new practice? Why? Why not?
- What were the costs (time/money)?
- What were the benefits?
- Were there any other consequences?

o Keep track of the progress made by each participant by using forms like the one below. At the end of the trial, summarize the exact sequence of events that go to make up the target practices, the problems encountered, the solutions found by the participants, the advantages that participants felt that they got from the new practices and any other consequences of the new behaviour.
o Meet with the women again to check what you have found, and feed back the results.
o Finally, write up a statement showing the risk practices and the target practices such as:

- Risk practices – 13 per cent of mothers wash their hands with soap after cleaning a child's bottom, 20 per cent of child stools are left on the ground;
- Target practices – 30 per cent of mothers use soap to wash their hands immediately after cleaning a child's bottom and throwing away the stools, 90 per cent of child stools are thrown into a latrine or buried.

| Date | Carer | Child | | | Problems, solutions, advantages |
Household identity number		1	2	3	of new practices
Where did they last defecate? Latrine in yard = 1 Neighbour's latrine = 2 In a potty = 3 On the ground = 4 Other (note) = 5					
How were hands washed after stool contact? Not washed = 1 Plain water = 2 With soap = 3 Other (note) = 4					

Box A1.1 Recording format for behavioural trial

How to do Venn diagrams

Venn diagrams can be used to explore perceived relationships between different things. Circles of different sizes are drawn to represent different structures or organizations.

These circles are drawn so that they overlap, depending on the degree of contact that the structures have with each other. For example, they can be drawn to represent different stakeholders and their relationships within a community or a project. A Venn diagram can be done in a public setting but it works better as an activity with a small group.

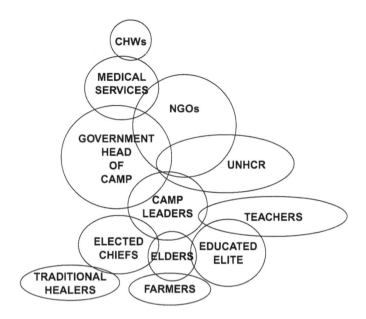

Figure A1.1 Key power structures in an imaginary refugee camp represented in a Venn diagram

To do Venn diagrams:

○ Explain to the participants that the purpose of the activity is to explore how the settlement works in terms of who makes the decisions and how organizations and/or groups relate to one another.
○ Suggest that participants first experiment with different sized circles and how they relate to one another. For example, ask them to consider the following structures: host government, international agencies, non-governmental organisations, community leaders, teachers, traditional healers, medical services, refugees as a whole group, elders, children, female heads of household, educated élite, community health workers, host population.
○ Ask them how these structures are inter-related and the degree of influence that one has over another.

The findings should be included in the project records.

How to do flow diagrams

Flow diagrams can be used to explore the causes of various problems or to examine how systems function. They might also be used to try to predict the possible negative or positive consequences of an intervention. For example, they can be used to show the causes and effects of an illness such as diarrhoea. Again, they are better used with smaller groups.
     To do flow diagrams:

○ Ask participants to consider a particular problem in the camp or settlement. Draw a circle or use a symbol such as a stone to represent the problem.
○ Ask people why this is a problem: reassure them that all answers will be useful and will be included in the diagram. Draw another circle and/or select a symbol to represent this new problem (such as eating bad food).

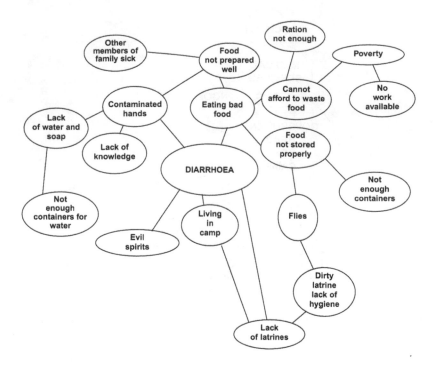

Figure A1.2 A flow diagram

○ Ask participants if they want to take over the drawing. Try not to influence the activity by imposing your perception of how things are, but allow the participants' ideas to guide the process.
○ Continue to ask 'why?' until all the possibilities have been exhausted.

The findings should be noted and included in the project records.

How to do a voting activity

Voting activities can be used to discuss preferences or practises within a community and explore options for taking action. Pocket charts (see Figure A1.7) can be used for voting activities. Alternatively you might like to use pots or jars on the ground. The voting may need to be done in secret if, for example, hygiene practices are to be considered, so it's a good idea to use a screen or turn the pocket chart away from the participants or ask participants to wait outside the meeting place before coming in to vote.

To do a voting activity:

○ Prepare the voting tokens from paper or card or use bottle tops or small stones. It is a good idea to prepare different types of voting slip for different groups, for example, men and women or children or elderly if the group is mixed.
○ Hang the pocket chart on a wall so that everyone can see it. Explain to the participants what the purpose of the activity is, for example, to find out about the frequency of various illnesses or of certain hygiene practices.
○ Allow people to discuss the pictures first to ensure that everyone sees them in the same way. This discussion may also highlight other issues of concern. A trial vote with two or three people might be a good idea to begin with.

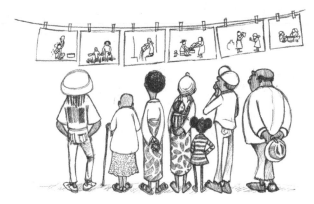

Figure A1.3 Pocket chart voting

o Hand out the voting tokens to each participant and explain that each person will vote in turn. If considering the most common diseases, only one or two voting tokens need to be given out per person. If looking at hygiene practices, as in the example, hand out a token for each different practice. If several tokens are handed out it is a good idea to conduct each vote separately and count the votes before the next practise is considered.
o When each person has voted, count out the votes in front of the whole group. The voting chart could be placed on a table and the voting tokens lined up in front of each picture.
o Get people to discuss the significance of the results and what action might now be taken.

Remember to record the results for the project records and for possible further discussion with other groups (obtain permission first). A project evaluation will be able to compare these results with future results.

How to do matrix and pairwise ranking

Matrix and pairwise ranking can be used to prioritize problems or compare preferences, for example, to compare the perceived effectiveness of different treatments for diarrhoea, or for establishing which health problems are the most common or serious. This is most effectively done in small groups.
   To do matrix and pairwise ranking:

o Ask participants to brainstorm the issues in the camp or settlement that you are going to compare, for example, 'Which diseases are people in the community most worried about getting?'.
o Decide on symbols or pictures to represent these issues. Place one set of these in a row along the top and another in a column along the side to form the matrix (see Figure A1.5).
o For each square in the matrix, ask participants whether the symbol at the top of the column is more important or less important than the one at the left of the row. Stop when each symbol has been compared with each of the others. (Only the top half of the matrix will be filled in.) Keep a tally of each choice in the relevant box.
o When the participant has made his/her choices, try to get each person to give the reasons why they were chosen.
o The scores can then be added up to find which issue is the most important. In this example, people were most worried about contracting diarrhoea.
o This should be followed by further discussion on the outcome of the scoring exercise and what can be done about the problem.

The findings should be included in the project records.

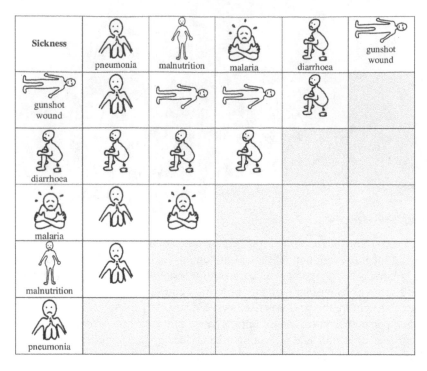

Figure A1.4 Example of a pairwise ranking matrix
Note: Ranking Order: 1st diarrhoea (4), 2nd pneumonia (3), 3rd gunshot wounds (2), 4th malaria (1), 5th malnutrition (0).

How to do timelines

Timelines are the visual representation of the history of an individual or community. Subjects can include almost anything from trends in local beliefs or incidence and severity of diseases to population movements and trends in education. They can be done with elders to get a history of the area or of local practices and with different groups to consider how things have changed in their lifetimes. They can be used with the affected community to find out what hygiene practices have changed and what caused those changes.

To do timelines:

o Explain the purpose of the activity and that it is a way to discuss some of the changes that have taken place in the community and whether things have improved or not.
o Draw a line on the ground with a stick. Ask participants to try to recall the earliest event they can remember. Mark this on the timeline (with a symbol if participants feel this is a good idea).
o Other significant events that the group can recall should be marked on the line to show changes over the passage of time.
o Ask the participants to try to recall other things from this time: how the village was organized, what people grew and ate, and anything else they can remember.
o When the timeline and discussion are finished, the main ideas can be summarized and comments made.
o Transfer the line on to paper in order to preserve it and decide who will keep it and where it will be kept.

The findings should be included in the project records.

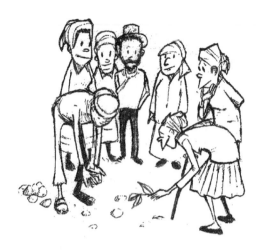

How to do pie charts

Pie charts can be used to represent proportions or percentages. They can be used to determine proportions of anything, including relative proportions of people suffering from particular diseases, or proportions of water used by a household from different water sources. Pie charts are easy to understand and simple to construct. They can be made by dividing something familiar and round, for example, a piece of fruit like an orange, or a pancake, or can be drawn on the ground with a stick. Alternatively, a pile of small stones can be used.

To do a pie chart:

○ Explain to the participants that the circle, orange or stones represents the total number of people or communities that conform to given criteria or hygiene practices.
○ Ask participants to draw lines on the circle or divide the orange or stones according to their relative proportions. There will usually be some discussion before a consensus is reached.
○ Record the diagrams on sheets of paper for future reference. Agree where to keep the paper record.

The proportions should be included in the project records.

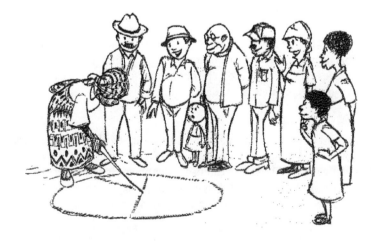

How to do body mapping

Body mapping can be used to explore people's perceptions of how their body functions. This can be particularly useful for exploring the causes of different types of diarrhoea and how treatment works. It is best done with a small homogeneous group.

To do body mapping:

o Maps can be drawn individually or as a group. Give each participant some paper and a pen and ask them to draw, for example, what happens inside a child when she/he has diarrhoea.
o If people have difficulty in drawing individual maps, a group map can be drawn to begin with.
o Once the participants are happy with the map they have drawn, start to ask questions about the map to get a clearer idea of the process involved when a child has diarrhoea.
o Ask if there are other changes to the child and what treatment is available and how the treatment works.
o Once the diagram is completed, it should be transferred on to paper. The participant(s) should decide where to keep the paper and a copy should be kept for the project records.

How to analyse qualitative data

Many people find it difficult to know what to do with the data collected from participatory methods. Below is a brief summary of how to analyse this type of data. However, remember that one of the main reasons why these methods are used is to try to enable the people that you are working with to analyse the information for themselves, in their own way, and to come to some meaningful conclusions.

Qualitative data consists of the words that people say and once collected this will need to be analysed in a logical and systematic way if it is to be used formally in an assessment report. You will first need to state where the data came from, for example, who are the key informants, why did you choose them or who took part in the focus group discussions (without mentioning names), and why they are/are not representative of the wider population, who asked the questions or did the observations, and how many groups you worked with.

There are four basic steps to analysing qualitative data:

o Organize data
o Shape or code the data
o Interpret and summarize the information
o Explain the information

Organize
Put the data into a format that is easy to work with. For example, tape recordings will have to be transcribed onto paper (remembering that one hour of recording is usually about four hours of transcribing). Rough notes will ideally need to be collated and typed up, if possible. You should then have an overall picture of the complete set of data available.

Shape
Read through the data and write down the main themes that are evident or the different categories or types of responses found. Sometimes interesting or unfamiliar terms used by the group studied can form the basis of analytical categories. You can use separate cards or sheets of paper to do this step or simply highlight different themes with different colour pens. Try to separate the data into groups that share similar characteristics. Starting with a large number of categories will make it easier to

allocate all the data. After becoming more familiar with the data and thinking about the relationships between the groups, it may be possible to reduce the number of categories. Compilation sheets may help to categorize the data and once ordered, the data can be presented in a matrix or flow chart to make interpretation easier. The important thing is to use the actual words that people said to back up what you want to say.

Interpret
Do not try to quantify the responses (for example, you cannot use percentages.) Instead look for the range of views expressed. It is possible to say 'some', 'others', or even 'many', but it is better not to say 'most' or the 'majority'. It is important to make sure that all opinions or views are represented in the summary. You can say 'half of the group' or 'two-thirds of the group' if you are referring to a focus group, but you must state how many people there were in the group and make sure that you do not automatically generalize to the whole population.

Explain
When trying to interpret what the information means, it is advisable to discuss it at length with others in the team. It is always better to be cautious about leaping to conclusions or making assumptions. The process of discussion with other members of the team or in feeding back to the community can also help to refine the interpretation and stimulate action. When writing a report, the actual hard data (what someone has said) must be quoted verbatim to illustrate a point of explanation. Remember that qualitative data cannot be assumed to refer to the wider population. Table A1.1 is an example of how the hard data from an assessment might be shaped using a matrix.

A common practise in analysing qualitative data is to do something like a long-hand version of what researchers call 'factor analysis'. Take the first quote from the notes for the focus group. Let us say it was, 'we want to have latrines but we can't afford them'. Then take another quote. Let us say the person said, 'it costs a lot of money to have a latrine but it would mean that we would have less shame'. The issue of cost is the theme running through both of these comments so you would indicate that two people highlighted this. The issue of shame is another theme that should be noted even if only one person mentions it. However, as you proceed, similar concerns with privacy or embarrassment could be included in the same category. You can see that you start to build up a picture of the most common attitudes about sanitation and your analysis sheet could end up looking something like the example given above.

Remember that you cannot count up the tally marks and convert this into a percentage. However, you can say that there were a certain number of responses under a certain category and identify the categories that people mentioned most frequently or least frequently. However, you must then include a couple of quotes to back up your interpretation.

There are several computer programmes specifically designed to analyse qualitative data but these are often costly and are really only useful with large data sets. In an acute situation, you may need to do a very rough analysis of the data until you have time to be more precise. Remember that you should also continue to assess the situation throughout the project cycle, especially in an environment where things are changing rapidly. A part of disaster preparedness activities could also be to ensure that you have a more detailed understanding of some of these issues, such as 'normal' gender divisions of labour, attitudes to hygiene, or approaches to disability before the disaster strikes.

A reporting format such as that in Box A1.2 (see page 118) could also be used to combine the hard data and interpretation of key themes.

Table A1.1 Matrix for focus group discussion on sanitation

Question	Response	Similar Responses
What do young children do?	Go in the compound	||||||
	Use a plastic potty	||
	Use an old tin	||||
	Taken to the toilet by sibling	|||
	Scared of dark latrine	||||||||
	Hole too big in latrine	||||
	Cannot go to the bush as too far	||||||||
What do older people in your family do?	Use bush	||||||||||||
	Use latrine	||||
	Have arthritis cannot bend legs – must stand up to go	||||||||
	Use children's potty	|||
What makes women use latrines?	Private do not expose self to strangers	||||||||
	Convenient	||||||||
	Stop compound smelling	||||
What prevents people from using latrines?	No money to build	|||||||
	Men too busy to dig pit - working or looking for money	|||||||
	Men too hungry to dig pit	||||||
	Not in men's interest to dig – they don't use latrines	||||
How could people be persuaded to build and use latrines?	Force – laws	||||||
	Makes house better	||||
	Good for family health	||||
	Need help with cost	|||

Box A1.2 Reporting format to combine hard data and key themes

Assessment/ Baseline/Monitoring Format (delete as necessary)

Name of village/group:
Number of people in the group:
Male/Female/Age/Special characteristics:
Time spent with the group:

Example

Question	What people said	Summary
I see some of you have latrines here, can you tell me how you decide to build one or not?	It's the men who decide (general agreement among the women) My husband saw one in the market and liked the idea of privacy (two women) The children have one in the school and they kept saying we must have one too (four women) My daughter was attacked one night in a field so I begged my husband (one woman)	The men are important decisionmakers Schools are important starting point Women's safety a big issue

Example questionnaire

Community outreach checklist

Parish/Ward.........   Name of interviewer.........

Village/Zone.........

Name of head of household..............   Tribe...........

Religion................

Date................

Water handling and storage

1. From which source do you collect your drinking water?

    tap / protected spring / unprotected spring / stream / other

2. (Observation) Is the inside of the drinking water storage container clean?   Yes/No

3. (Observation) Is the drinking water storage container kept covered?   Yes/No

4. What do you use to collect drinking water from the container?

    mug / glass / scoop / pour out / other

5. Is a specific mug or scoop reserved for collecting water from container and pouring into mug/ glass for drinking?   Yes / No

6. Who usually serves drinking water from the container?

    mother / female child / maid / anyone / other

Hygiene

7. With what do you wash your hands? (mark appropriate box)

	Soap	Ash	Water only	Other
Before cooking				
Before eating				
After eating				
After defecation				
After handling children's excreta				

8. (Observation) Does the household use a drying rack for kitchen utensils?   Yes/No

9. Is left-over food kept covered?   Yes / No / No left-over food

10. What do you do with raw food before eating it? (e.g. mangoes/guavas/sugar cane/tomatoes)

    Wash before eating / eat directly

11. (Observation) Is domestic rubbish disposed of in a separate compost pit or container?

    Yes/No

12. (Observation) Is waste water disposed of in a pit or trench?   Yes/No

13.   (Observation) Is the home heavily infested with flies?   Yes/No

Diarrhoea and ORS

14.   Do you know how to prepare ORS correctly?   Yes/No

15.   Please demonstrate preparation of ORS   Correct/Incorrect

16.   Please explain when you give ORS?   Correct/Incorrect

17.   Why do you think people get diarrhoea? (dirty hands, dirty water, flies, domestic animals, dirty soil)

                                                                                   Correct/Incorrect

18.   Is there anybody else in this area with signs and symptoms of severe diarrhoea? If yes, ask respondent to describe symptoms

                        Profuse diarrhoea without blood / diarrhoea with blood / dehydration / other

Latrine

19.   Is there a latrine for the household?   Yes/No

20.   How many households share the latrine?

21.   Which members of this household use the latrine?

       Children under 5 years (boys or girls)

       Boys
       Girls
       Men
       Women

22.   (Observation) Is their latrine sanitary?   Yes/No
       (Yes - includes a clean squatting hole & slab, a well fitting lid or water seal, or screened vent-pipe, few flies)
       (No – includes filled up pits, dirty hole or slab, severe fly problem)

23.   (Observation) Is the compound free of excreta?   Yes/No

24.   Interviewer asks for water to wash their hands with. Were they:
                                              Offered soap / not offered soap

Community Action

24.   (Discussion) What can be done to prevent the outbreak of diarrhoea in this area?

       ....

A2
Planning tools

Sphere: Minimum standards in water supply, sanitation and hygiene promotion

The Sphere Standards stress the importance of making humanitarian agencies accountable to those they seek to assist. The common standards outline the responsibilities of governments, organizations and individuals when providing protection and assistance. Under the Sphere project, concerned relief organizations have agreed standards for five technical sectors and eight core 'process and people' standards that are common to all sectors. Water, sanitation and hygiene promotion are defined under one technical sector with hygiene promotion as the umbrella for both water and sanitation. The Minimum Standards in Water, Sanitation and Hygiene Promotion, as with other sectors, are a practical expression of the principles and rights embodied in the Humanitarian Charter, as reflected in the body of existing international human rights, humanitarian and refugee law. The standards provide a benchmark by which agencies and governments can measure the acceptability of their interventions in crisis situations. The core standards are: 1) participation, 2) initial assessment, 3) response, 4) targeting, 5) monitoring, 6) evaluation, 7) aid worker competencies and responsibilities, and 8) supervision, management and support of personnel.

The Minimum Standards for Water, Sanitation and Hygiene Promotion are presented below.

Hygiene promotion
Effective hygiene promotion relies on an exchange of information between the agency and the affected community in order to identify key hygiene issues and to design, implement and monitor a programme to promote hygiene practices that will

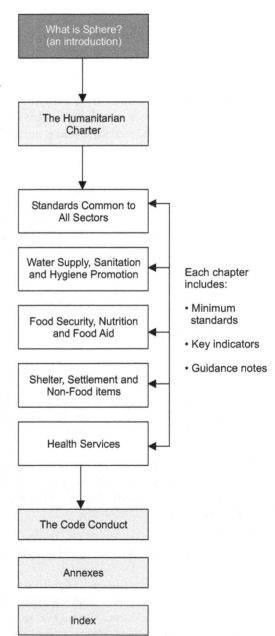

Each chapter includes:

• Minimum standards

• Key indicators

• Guidance notes

Figure A2.1 Overview of Sphere

ensure the optimal use of facilities and the greatest impact on public health. Community mobilization is especially pertinent during disasters as the emphasis must be on encouraging people to take action to protect their health and make good use of facilities and services provided, rather than on the dissemination of messages. It must be stressed that hygiene promotion should never be a substitute for good sanitation and water supplies, which are fundamental to good hygiene.

Three key factors in hygiene promotion in emergencies are:

1. Mutual sharing of information and knowledge;
2. Mobilisation of communities;
3. Provision of essential materials and/or facilities.

Hygiene promotion is an overarching standard with related indicators. It is integral to all the standards and indicators for water supply, excreta disposal, vector control, solid waste management and drainage.

Hygiene promotion standard 1: Programme design and implementation

All facilities and resources provided reflect the vulnerabilities, needs and preferences of the affected population. Users are involved in the management and maintenance of hygiene facilities where appropriate.

Indicators:

○ Key hygiene related public health risks are identified;
○ Programmes include an effective mechanism for representative and participatory input from all users, including in the initial design of facilities;
○ All groups within the population have equitable access to resources or facilities needed to continue or achieve the hygiene practices that are promoted;
○ Hygiene promotion messages and activities address key behaviours and misconceptions and are targeted for all user groups. Representatives from these groups participate in planning, training, implementation, monitoring and evaluation;
○ Users take responsibility for the management and maintenance of facilities as appropriate, and different groups contribute equitably.

Water supply

Water supply is essential for life, health and human dignity. In extreme situations, there may not be sufficient water available to meet basic needs, and in these cases supplying a survival level of safe drinking water is of critical importance. In most cases, the main health problems are caused by poor hygiene due to insufficient water and by the consumption of contaminated water.

Water supply standard 1: Access and water quantity

All people have safe and equitable access to a sufficient quantity of water for drinking, cooking and personal and domestic hygiene. Public water points are sufficiently close to households to enable use of the minimum water requirement.

Indicators:

○ Average water use for drinking, cooking and personal hygiene in any household is at least 15 litres per person per day;
○ The maximum distance from any household to the nearest water point is 500 metres;
○ Queuing time at water source is no more than 15 minutes;
○ It takes no more than 3 minutes to fill a 20-litre container;
○ Water sources and systems are maintained such that appropriate quantities of water are available consistently or on a regular basis.

Water supply standard 2: Water quality
Water is palatable and of sufficient quality to be drunk and used for personal and domestic hygiene without causing significant risk to health.
Indicators:

o A sanitary survey indicates a low risk of faecal contamination at source;
o There are no faecal coliforms per 100ml at point of delivery;
o People drink water from a protected or treated source in preference to other readily available water sources;
o Steps are taken to reduce post-delivery contamination;
o For piped water supplies, or for all water supplies at times of risk or presence of diarrhoea epidemic, water is treated with a disinfectant so that there is a free chlorine residual at the tap of 0.5 mg per litre and turbidity is below 5 NTU;
o No negative health effect is detected due to the short-term use of any water contaminated by chemical (including carry-over of treatment chemicals) or radiological sources, and assessment shows no significant probability of such an effect.

Water supply standard 3: Water use facilities and goods
People have adequate facilities and supplies to collect, store and use sufficient quantities of water for drinking, cooking and personal hygiene, and to ensure that drinking water remains safe until it is consumed.
Indicators:

o Each household has at least two drinking water containers of 10–20 litres, plus enough clean water storage containers to ensure there is always water in the household;
o Water collection and storage containers have narrow necks and/or covers, or other safe means of storage, drawing and handling and are demonstrably used;
o There is at least 250g of soap available for personal hygiene per person per month;
o Where communal bathing facilities are necessary, there are sufficient bathing cubicles available with separate cubicles for males and females, and they are used appropriately and equitably;
o Where communal laundry facilities are necessary, there is at least one washing basin per 100 people, and private laundering areas are available for women to wash and dry undergarments and sanitary cloths;
o The participation of all vulnerable groups is actively encouraged in the siting and construction of bathing facilities and/or the production and distribution of soap, and/or the use and promotion of suitable alternatives.

Excreta disposal
Safe human excreta disposal creates the first barrier to excreta-related disease, helping to reduce transmission through direct and indirect routes. Safe excreta disposal is therefore a major priority and in most disaster situations should be addressed with as much speed and effort as the provision of safe water supply. The provision of appropriate facilities for defecation is one of a number of emergency responses essential for people's dignity, safety, health and well-being.

Excreta disposal standard 1: Access to, and number of, toilets
People have adequate numbers of toilets sufficiently close to their dwellings to allow them rapid, safe and acceptable access at all times of day and night.
Indicators:

o A maximum of 20 people use each toilet;

o Use of toilets arranged by household(s) and/or segregated by sex;
o Separate toilets for women and men are available in public places (markets, distribution centres, health centres);
o Shared or public toilets are cleaned and maintained in such a way that they are used by all intended users;
o Toilets are no more than 50 metres from dwellings;
o Toilets are used in the most hygienic way and children's faeces are disposed of immediately and hygienically.

Excreta disposal standard 2: Design, construction and use of toilets
Toilets are sited, designed, constructed and maintained in such a way as to be comfortable, hygienic and safe to use.
    Indicators:

o Users (especially women) have been consulted and approve of the siting and design of the toilet;
o Toilets are designed, built and located to have the following features:

  – designed in such a way that they can be used by all sections of the population, including children, older people, pregnant women and physically and mentally disabled people;
  – sited in such a way as to minimize threats to users especially women and girls throughout the day and night;
  – sufficiently easy to keep clean to invite use and do not present a health hazard;
  – provide a degree of privacy in line with the norms of the users;
  – they allow for the disposal of women's sanitary protection, or provide women with the necessary privacy for washing and drying sanitary protection cloths;
  – they minimize fly and mosquito breeding;

o All toilets constructed that use water for flushing and/or a hygienic seal have adequate and regular supply of water;
o Pit latrines and soak-aways (for most soils) are at least 30 metres from any groundwater source and the bottom of any latrine is at least 1.5 metres above the water table. Drainage of spillage from defecation systems must not run towards any surface water source or shallow groundwater source;
o People wash their hands after defecation and before eating and food preparation;
o People are provided with tools and materials for constructing, maintaining and cleaning their own toilets if appropriate.

Vector control
Many diseases are carried by vectors. They can be controlled through a variety of initiatives including some simple measures such as appropriate site selection and shelter provision, appropriate water supply, excreta disposal, solid waste management and drainage as well as some measures requiring more specialist attention.

Vector control standard 1: Individual and family protection
All disaster-affected people have the knowledge and the means to protect themselves from disease and nuisance vectors that are likely to represent a significant risk to health or well-being.
    Indicators:

o All populations at risk from vector-borne disease understand the modes of transmission and possible methods of prevention;
o All populations have access to shelters that do not harbour or encourage the growth of vector populations and are protected by appropriate vector control measures;

o People avoid exposure to mosquitoes during peak biting times by using all non-harmful means available to them. Special attention is paid to protection of high-risk groups such as pregnant and feeding mothers, babies, infants, older people and the sick;
o People with treated mosquito nets use them effectively;
o Control of human body lice is carried out where louse-borne typhus or relapsing fever is a threat;
o Bedding and clothing are aired and washed regularly;
o Food is protected at all times from contamination by vectors such as flies, insects and rodents.

Vector control standard 2: Physical, environmental and chemical protection measures

The numbers of disease vectors that pose a risk to people's health and nuisance vectors that pose a risk to people's well-being are kept to an acceptable level.
  Indicators:

o Displaced populations are settled in locations that minimize their exposure to mosquitoes;
o Vector breeding and resting sites are modified where practicable;
o Intensive fly control is carried out in high-density settlements when there is a risk or the presence of a diarrhoea epidemic;
o The population density of mosquitoes is kept low enough to avoid the risk of excessive transmission levels and infection;
o People infected with malaria are diagnosed early and receive treatment.

Vector control standard 3: Chemical control safety

Chemical vector control measures are carried out in a manner that ensures that staff, the people affected by the disaster and the local environment are adequately protected, and avoids creating resistance to the substances used.
  Indicators:

o Personnel are protected by the provision of training, protective clothing, use of bathing facilities, supervision and a restriction on the number of hours spent handling chemicals;
o The choice, quality, transport and storage of chemicals used for vector control, the application equipment and the disposal of the substances follow international norms and can be accounted for at all times;
o Communities are informed about the potential risks of the substances used in chemical vector control and about the schedule for application. They are protected during and after the application of poisons or pesticides, according to internationally agreed procedures.

Solid waste management

If organic solid waste is not disposed of, major risks are incurred of fly and rat breeding and surface water pollution.

Solid waste management standard 1: Collection and disposal

People have an environment that is acceptably uncontaminated by solid waste, including medical waste, and have the means to dispose of their domestic waste conveniently and effectively.
  Indicators:

o People from the affected population are involved in the design and implementation of the solid waste programme;
o Household waste is put in containers daily for regular collection, burnt or buried in a specific refuse pit;

○ All households have access to a refuse container and/or are no more than 100 metres from a communal refuse pit;
○ At least one 100-litre refuse container is available per 10 families, where domestic refuse is not buried on-site;
○ Refuse is removed from the settlement before it becomes a nuisance or a health risk;
○ Medical wastes are separated and disposed of separately and there is a correctly designed, constructed and operated pit, or incinerator with a deep ash pit, within the boundaries of each health facility;
○ There are no contaminated or dangerous medical wastes (needles, glass, dressings, drugs) at any time in living areas or public spaces;
○ There are clearly marked and appropriately fenced refuse pits, bins or specified areas at public places, such as markets and slaughtering areas, with a regular collection system in place;
○ Final disposal of solid waste is carried out in such a place and in such a way as to avoid creating health and environmental problems for the local and affected populations.

Drainage

Surface water in or near emergency settlements may come from household and water point wastewater, leaking toilets and sewers, rainwater or rising floodwater. The main health risks associated with surface water are contamination of water supplies and the living environment, damage to toilets and dwellings, vector breeding and drowning. A proper drainage plan, addressing stormwater drainage through site planning and wastewater disposal using small-scale and on-site drainage, should be implemented to reduce potential health risks to the population.

Drainage standard 1: Drainage works

People have an environment in which the health and other risks posed by water erosion and standing water, including stormwater, floodwater, domestic wastewater and wastewater from medical facilities, are minimized.
    Indicators:

○ Areas around dwellings and water points are kept free of standing wastewater, and stormwater drains are kept clear;
○ Shelters, paths and water and sanitation facilities are not flooded or eroded by water;
○ Water point drainage is well planned, built and maintained. This includes drainage from washing and bathing areas as well as water collection points;
○ Drainage waters do not pollute existing surface or groundwater sources or cause erosion;
○ Sufficient numbers of appropriate tools are provided for small drainage works and maintenance where necessary.

Source: Sphere Project, 2004.

How to use a problem tree to develop a logframe

A problem tree is a useful exercise that can help in the process of developing a logframe. This process takes approximately 1–2 hours.
    To do a problem tree do develop a logframe:

○ In plenary discuss levels of experience of the participants to different planning approaches. Ask the participants if any of them have used the problem tree before (sometimes known as a cause and effect tree) and, if so, what they thought of that experience. Distribute a problem tree diagram (Figure A2.2).

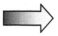

The substantial and direct effects of the focal problem are placed in parallel on the line above it

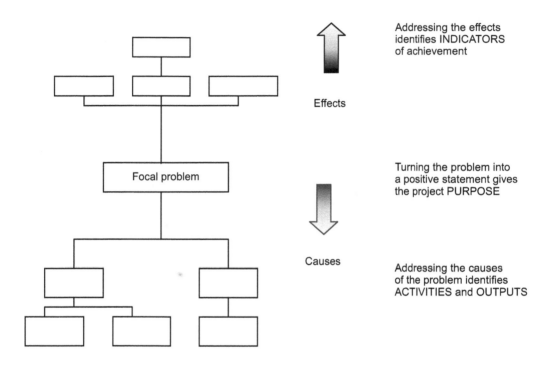

Addressing the effects identifies INDICATORS of achievement

Effects

Focal problem

Turning the problem into a positive statement gives the project PURPOSE

Causes

Addressing the causes of the problem identifies ACTIVITIES and OUTPUTS

Figure A2.2 Developing a problem tree
Source: Toole, 2001.

○ In plenary, work with the participants to develop a problem tree for their particular problem. Identify the problem to be analysed, for example, 'poor hygiene and health in (name of place)'. Write this on paper and stick in the middle of a very large piece of paper (can be made up of flipchart papers, brown paper lengths or newspapers stuck together) placed either on a wall or on the floor.

○ Ask the participants to identify the individual causes of the problem. Ask them to write a card for each of the causes and hand it to yourself as the facilitator. Ask them to be as specific as possible.

○ Place the 'cause cards' below the problem card on the wall (or floor). Start linking the 'cause cards' together identifying clusters and hierarchies (for example, one cause identified may be the result of another). Draw lines between the cards whose ideas are linked together (alternatively use coloured wool or string to show the connections).

○ Once most of the causes are on the wall, ask participants to think of effects of the problem. Again, have them write individual effects on card (as specific as possible) and place them on the wall above the question – also linking effects together. (An example of a problem tree is given in Figure A2.3.)

○ Point out issues that have arisen as both causes and effects (vicious circles), and causes and effects which might not have been immediately associated with environmental health if the problem tree analysis had not been done.

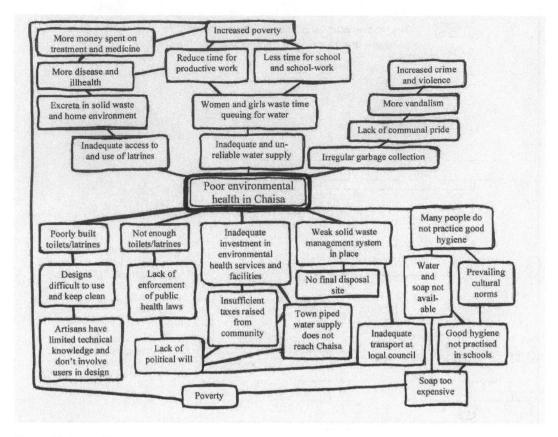

Figure A2.3 A problem tree

○ Discuss with the participants the complexity of the problem and how difficult it would be to work on everything, particularly given limited resources. Indeed, because of interconnections, it may not be necessary to work on everything if 'root causes' can be identified; hence the need to prioritize.
○ With the participants, work out which causes should and can be addressed by the project and in what ways. These become your project outputs and activities to be rephrased and written in your logframe.
○ With the participants, work out which effects can be measured by the project and in what ways. These then become your project indicators and means of verification.

How to do risk assessment

You can use this risk assessment technique to improve your project and develop suitable assumptions for the project logframe. This activity will take approximately 1–2 hours. To do risk assessment:

○ In plenary, discuss how some things outside the control of the project affect whether the outputs, purpose and goal of the project will be achieved.
○ These can be classified as 'risks'. The lower the risk, the more likely the project is to succeed and the stronger the project. If risks are identified, the project can be strengthened by adding relevant activities and monitoring the risks. Stages involved in developing the 'assumptions' column of the logframe include identifying, assessing, managing and monitoring risks.

Stage 1: Risk identification
Identification of risks should take into account:

○ Stakeholder issues,
○ Social and gender issues,
○ Institutional issues,
○ Technical issues,
○ Economic issues,
○ Environmental issues.

Stage 2: Risk assessment
Identify the risks and locate them in the following table according to:
○ Their likely probability,
○ Their likely impact.

Table A2.1 Blank risk assessment table

Probability / Impact >	Low	Medium	High
Low			
Medium			
High			*

Note: *Risks that are considered high probability *and* high impact are 'killer risks' and the project design *must* take such risks into account.

Stage 3: Risk management and monitoring
Discuss how medium to high probability risks or medium to high impact risks can be managed by turning them into project activities and outputs.

Risks that are still medium to high after managing or that cannot be managed by the project should be monitored and inserted into the Assumptions column, reworded as an assumption.

Assumptions checklist
A risk can be reworded into positive language to become an assumption. For example, a risk is that there will be insecurity in the settlement area, the corresponding assumption in the project logframe will be that peace and stability will continue in the settlement area. The logframe assumptions should be checked again:

○ Check the logic of the logframe and revise if necessary (If we do this objective/activity – and this assumption holds true – then that output is reached or goal contributed to)
○ Have manageable risks been managed?
○ Are other risks monitored?
○ Should the project proceed/be redesigned?

Frequently used poor assumptions are to assume that the project will be done! For example, the activity is to carry out a hygiene education campaign, and the assumption is that the campaign will be carried out. You should not assume that your project will be done or that it will work. You need to identify and address the risks that could prevent the activity being carried out or carried out effectively.

Source: Toole, 2001.

Table A2.2 Example logframe for an emergency situation: Acute to intermediate phases

	Intervention Logic	Objectively Verifiable Indicators	Sources of Verification	Risks and Assumptions
Goal	To contribute to the reduction of preventable, communicable diseases and to restore coping mechanisms of affected population	People are no longer dependent on emergency relief Mortality and morbidity data within accepted limits (see WHO) No major outbreaks of communicable diseases in target area X% reduction in communicable diseases as perceived by community members after x months	UN & Government reports Other agency reports Health facility data Community consultation e.g. pocket voting, FGD (Household level monitoring)	Conflict in the neighbouring country does not spill over the border and destabilise the host country. The health centres set up by the other INGO remain operational. UNHCR continue to provide sufficient food rations, shelter, and blankets.
Intermediate Goal/ Purpose	Men, women and children in the target population (x no.) have increased access to, and make optimal use of, water and sanitation facilities, and take action to protect themselves against threats to public health	X no. of people continuously have access to use potable water after x months X no. of people can demonstrate improved hygiene practices after x months* More than 80% of men, women and children are using and maintaining latrines after x months At least 80% of latrines have hand washing facilities that are in use after x months At least 80% of households dispose of solid waste safely¶ At least 80% of community management groups score 4 on Sustainability Spidergram after a year The majority of participants in male and female FGDs express satisfaction about the provision of facilities¨	Information from other NGOs. Focus group discussions Community Monitoring Tools (mapping, pocket charts etc.) Surveys.	

Table A2.2 (Contd)

	Intervention Logic	Objectively Verifiable Indicators	Sources of Verification	Risks and Assumptions
Outputs	1. X no. of men, women and children have access to safe sanitary facilities within six months.	1 latrine constructed per 20 people after community consultation (female/male ratio 2:1) No faecal matter observed in the target area.	Latrine monitoring forms. Reports by latrine assistants. Observation Focus group discussions with women and girls. Random exploratory walk	Government border guards are able to improve security to reduce/ prevent rebel raids. Refugees stay in the camp.
	2. X no. of men, women and children have access to safe drinking water according to Sphere standards within x months	At least 80% of target group accesses at least 15 litres water/ day per person. Maximum distance from shelter/ home to water points is 500m. Water meets international quality standards (Sphere) Queuing time at water sources no more than 15 minutes (on average)	Engineers monitoring and output records. Records from water point attendants. Weekly water testing records Random observation and exploratory walks. (Household level monitoring)	
	3. X no. of men, women and children are enabled to practice safer hygiene in a dignified and culturally appropriate manner	At least 80% of trained promoters are holding at least two meetings/ 10 household visits per week Hand washing facilities are provided at all latrines and a system is in place to replenish them with water and cleansing agent Each household reports the presence of soap (1 bar per week per household) On observation at water points at least 80% of jerry cans meet the criteria of a clean jerry can© All women and girls have access to appropriate sanitary materials and underwear The living area of the project community is free from solid waste and stagnant water	Random observation and exploratory walks. Random household visits Reports from latrine attendants and water point attendants. Focus group discussions,	

Table A2.2 (Contd)

	Intervention Logic	Objectively Verifiable Indicators	Sources of Verification	Risks and Assumptions
Activities	Output 1 – Adequate sanitary facilities in the camp ○ Set up temporary defecation areas. ○ 400 gender-segregated latrines constructed in line with international standards. ○ 40 latrine attendants trained and equipped. ○ Construction of 200 gender-segregated washing facilities. ○ Construction of 80 community washing facilities (laundry). ○ Consultation with female refugees to identify suitable sites for sanitation facilities. ○ Provision of potties for under-fives. ○ Consultation of users on design and locations of facilities ○ Selection of caretakers and committee members Output 2 – Adequate clean water ○ Trucking of water (first phase only). ○ Installation of 32 water points in the refugee camp. ○ Training of four water point attendants in camp.	Means	Costs	Construction materials remain available in adequate amounts.

Table A2.2 (Contd)

Intervention Logic	Objectively Verifiable Indicators	Sources of Verification	Risks and Assumptions
○ Construction of 20 hand pumps			
○ Training of four hand pump attendants in village.			
○ Establishment of a stock of community spares for water pumps in village.			
○ Establishment of water management committee in local village.			
○ Initiate community based monitoring system using tokens			
Output 3 – Improved hygiene practices in camp			
○ Prepare Hygiene Promotion plan based on rapid assessment within 2 days			
○ Conduct more detailed baseline data assessment and modify plan within four weeks			
○ Recruit and train 16 community hygiene promoters in camp.			
○ Order and distribute 3,200 water containers.			
○ Order and distribute 160 community hygiene packs for maintaining latrines etc.			
○ Order and distribute 1,600 household hygiene packs every month for six months (soap, disinfectant, laundry soap, etc, for one family for one month).			
○ Plan radio broadcasts with key stakeholders within six weeks			

Table A2.2 (Contd)

Intervention Logic	Objectively Verifiable Indicators	Sources of Verification	Risks and Assumptions
○ Plan hygiene promotion with children, including hand washing demonstrations in and out of schools			Preconditions National government gives NGO registration to work in the country.

Notes: * These will need to be specified, for example, hand washing at critical times (after defaecation and before eating), safe excreta disposal, safe water storage; ¶ Safely will need to be defined according to chosen disposal system; ˮ Satisfaction will need to be defined in terms of safety, privacy, dignity, accessibility, suitability, adequacy etc.; © A definition of clean: no visible dirt, no cracks, lid intact.

A3

Training exercises

Introductions

These introductory exercises have been selected because they are easy to organize and effective at introducing the participants to each other in an informal way.

Smiley Samuel

○ Everyone sits or stands in a circle, including the course organiser.
○ Ask each person to introduce themselves by their first name and an adjective that begins with the same letter as their name, for example, friendly Francis, smiley Samuel. If the group is not too large, the next person along can be asked to repeat the name and continue like this until everyone has introduced themselves.

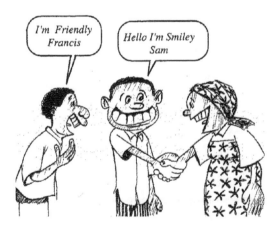

The name game
This can be done after the initial round of introductions, either with or without the 'smiley Samuel' adjectives.

○ The course organizer repeats her or his name and points out another person, asking him to look for a third person, for example, 'my name is Candide, your name is Innocent, can you find Rose?'. Do not look at Rose as you say her name and ask the group not to look in her direction so that Innocent has to try to remember who Rose is by himself.
○ This can be continued until everyone has had a turn.

Favourite animals
Divide the group into pairs and ask them to introduce themselves to one another and tell each other about their favourite animal. This should take only a couple of minutes. Then ask each participant to introduce their partner by first name and to say which animal he/she has chosen.

Names

Stand in circle. Ask participants to remove their name tags. Inform participants that they are to call out the name of a participant and point to them, then they are to call out the name of another person and point to them. If anyone hesitates or points to the wrong person or calls out the wrong name, they are out. Then the game starts again.

Source: Dahar, InterAction, Bangladesh, 2004, personal communication.

Heartbeat

Stand in a circle holding hands. The leader starts by squeezing one person's hand. That person should squeeze the next persons' hand and so on until the pulse stops. At that point, that person is out.

Source: Dahar, InterAction, Bangladesh, 2004, personal communication.

5 s

Stand in a circle holding hands with each other. The first participant calls out 'one', the next calls out 'two', the next calls out 'three', the next calls out 'four', the next calls out 'five' but at the same time tries to slap the hand of the next participant before they remove their hand. If number five manages to slap the hand of the next participant, then the next participant is out. If the next participant gets their hand away from number five, then number five is out. Then the game starts again.

Source: Dahar, InterAction, Bangladesh, 2004, personal communication.

Monkey tail

The participants are instructed that whatever question they are asked, they can only reply 'monkey tail'. One participant starts the game by asking questions of any of the other participants. The one who manages to mention 'monkey tail' without laughing has won.

Source: Mukul, LAMB Project, Bangladesh, 2004, personal communication.

Listening exercises

Nodders and shakers

This exercise can be used to show how body language affects communication. By the end of the session the participants should be able to describe how non-verbal behaviour affects communication, and demonstrate good listening skills.

- Divide everyone into pairs asking them to join with someone they have not yet worked with.
- Ask the pair to hold a conversation for five minutes. During this time one of the pair has to nod his head repeatedly while the other shakes her head. About half way through they should swap around so that she is nodding and he is shaking.
- After five minutes ask everyone to give feedback to the plenary, answering the following questions:
  - Did you feel you were being listened to?
  - Were you distracted by the nodding and shaking?
  - How did making those body movements affect your conversation?
  - Can you remember what was said?
- This can lead on to a general discussion on body language and communication and further role play in which participants practice listening skills.

Source: Adapted from Pretty et al, 1995.

Folding paper game

This exercise will help to show how simple instructions can be misinterpreted. By the end of the session the participants should be able to describe the requirements for clear verbal communication.

○ Ask for four volunteers to come and stand in front of the rest of the group.
○ Give each of them a square sheet of paper and tell them they must close their eyes during the exercise and they must not ask any questions.
○ Verbally give them the following instructions:

'Fold the paper in half and tear off the bottom right hand corner.
Fold the paper in half again and this time tear off the upper right hand corner'.

○ Ask them to open their eyes and show everyone the unfolded paper. (It is very likely that the results will not be the same.)
○ Ask everyone to reflect on how the directions could have been clearer and what words could have been interpreted in different ways. How can people be encouraged to ask for clarification when they do not understand something?

Source: Adapted from Pretty et al, 1995.

Whacky whispers

This exercise can be used to show how information loses its original meaning as it passes through different channels. By the end of the session participants should be able to describe the requirements for clear verbal communication.

○ Ask participants to form a line or circle.
○ Whisper a sentence to the first person in the line and ask them to whisper exactly the same words to the person on their left. Pass the message around in this way from person to person until the last person, who should then tell everyone what he/she has heard. (The last person often says something considerably different to the original statement, especially if this was long or complicated.)
○ Ask everyone to consider how we get feedback in real situations. How can we increase the likelihood that verbal messages are understood?

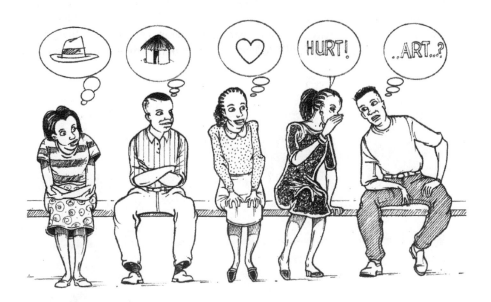

Hygiene learning exercises

These participatory exercises have been selected because they are easy to use and are effective in some situations for encouraging people to learn about their own hygiene practices and about those of others.

Learning about traditional beliefs and practices
The purpose of this exercise is to encourage participants to examine their attitudes to traditional beliefs and practices. By the end of the session participants should be able to discuss the impact of local beliefs and traditions on hygiene practices and suggest how they would deal sensitively with such beliefs and practices as a community facilitator.

- Ask the participants to divide into small groups. Each group should choose two traditional practices or beliefs they have encountered in their own community or in the community they are working with.
- Ask them to discuss who holds the beliefs, and whether it is everyone or only specific groups.
- In what ways do the beliefs/practices have an impact on health?
- Ask them to consider both the negative and positive impacts that this belief might have on health.
- How can facilitators make sure that they deal with these issues sensitively?

Exploring learning styles
The purpose of this exercise is to help participants consider the merits and limitations of different learning styles and identify the necessary requirements for effective adult learning. By the end of the session participants should be able to describe the necessary requirements for adult learning. The exercise uses the series of eight pictures that are pages 139–46.

- Divide the participants into small groups and give each group a set of pictures illustrating different learning environments.
- Ask each group to select three pictures that they feel represent the most effective method of learning and communication. They should also select the three pictures that represent the least effective method of learning and communicating. Ask each group to discuss the reasons for their choices within the group.
- After 15 minutes of discussion within the group, ask the groups to stick their choices on a board or wall, with the most effective pictures on one side and the least effective on the other.
- Ask the groups to give reasons why they chose particular pictures and discuss their choices.
- Ask them how they think they can facilitate learning for group participants in the community setting.

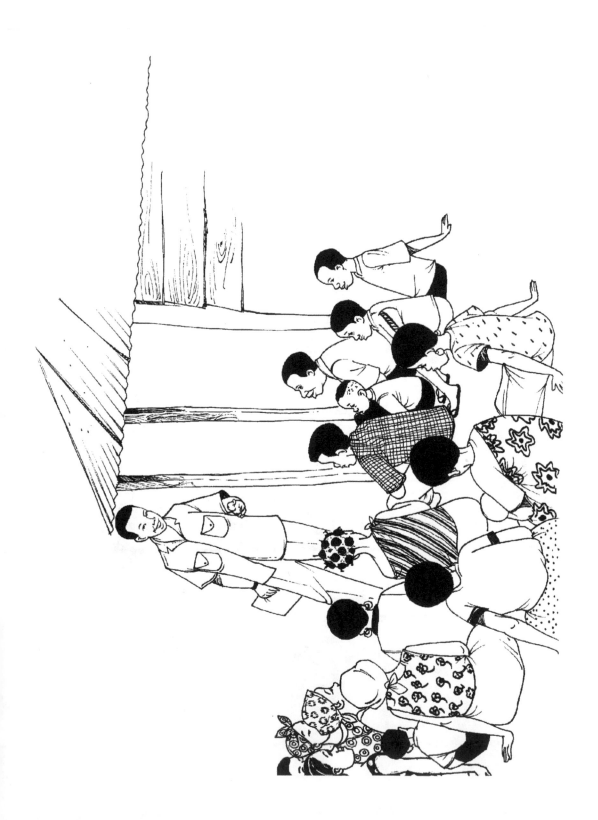

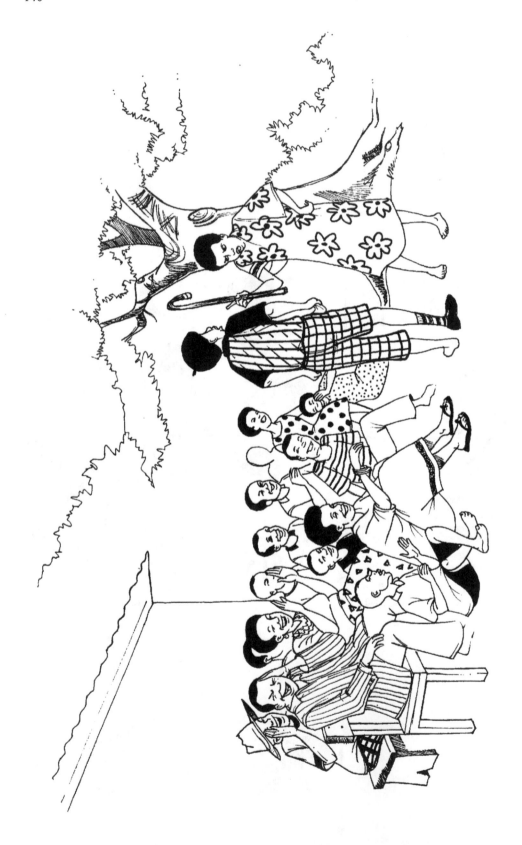

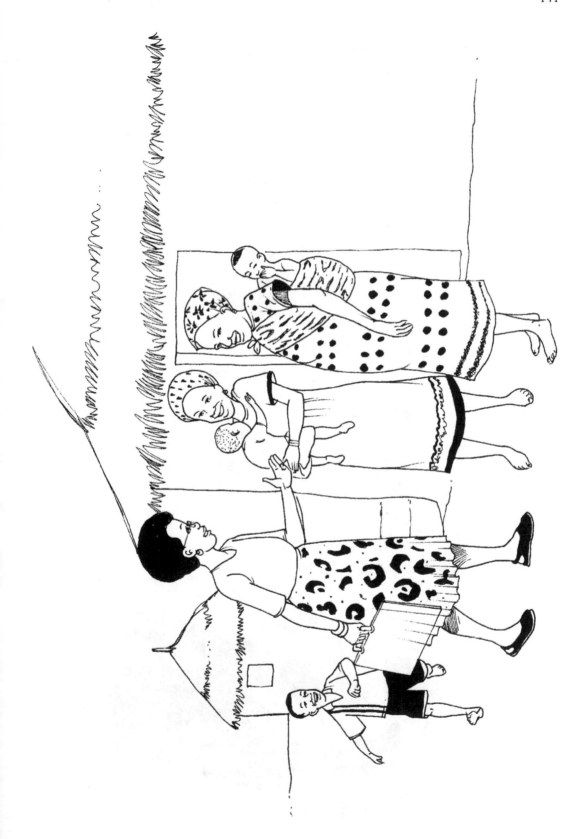

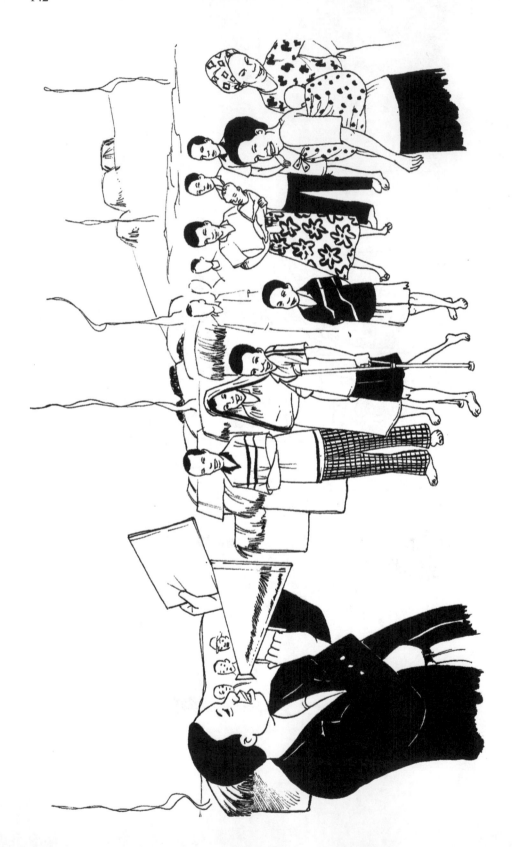

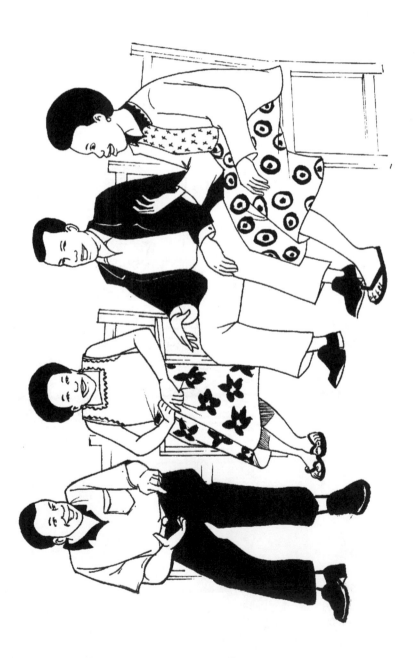

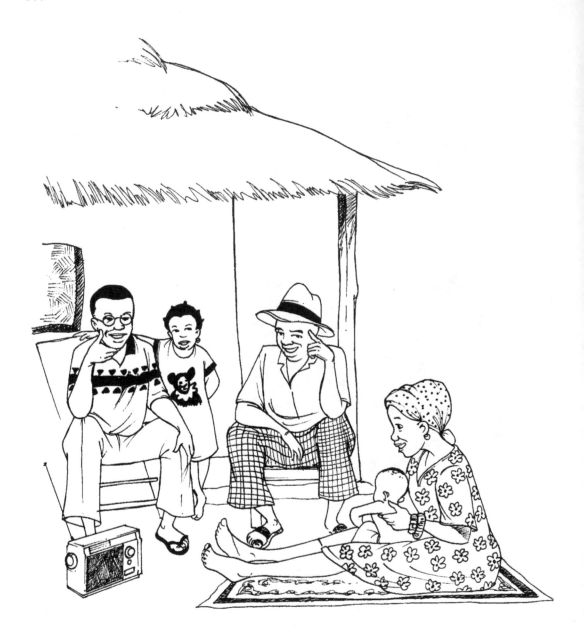

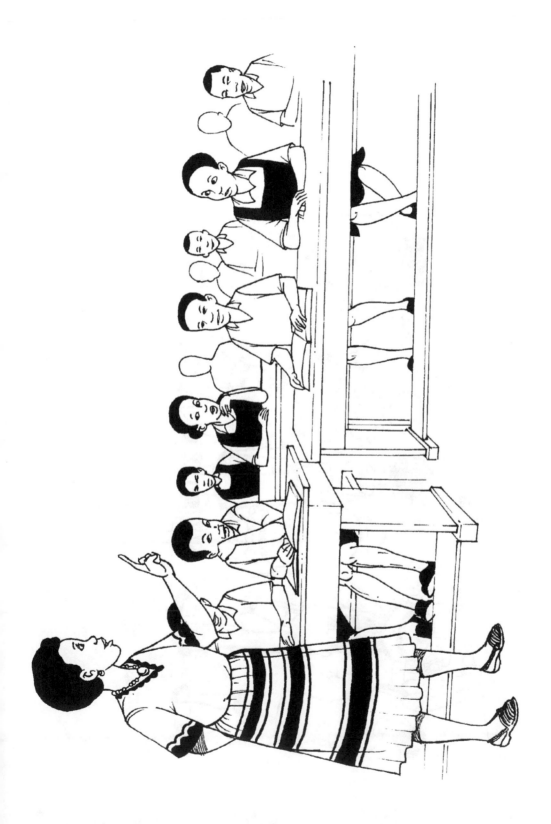

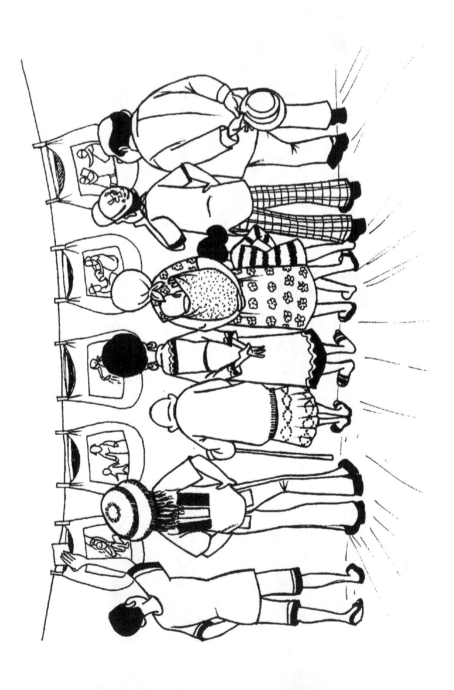

Role play: The disrupter

The purpose of this exercise is to show how communication in groups can be disrupted and to help participants to think about how they might handle different group situations. At the end of the session the participants should be able to discuss the ways in which the behaviour of individuals can influence groups, suggest how they might manage disruptive or distracting behaviour and describe ways of maximizing the participation of less forthcoming individuals.

○ Ask participants to divide into groups of three. One person will be the speaker, another the listener and a third will play the role of the disrupter.
○ The speaker is asked to talk to the listener about some aspect of their life, while the disrupter has to try to interrupt the session (without using violence!).
○ The disrupters can move around the different groups. After a couple of minutes everyone should change roles until each person has had an opportunity to try each role.
○ Discuss with the group afterwards. Ask everyone how they felt about being interrupted and what other experience they have had of this in the past? Discuss ways of dealing with difficult people in groups, for example, ignoring them, confronting them, distracting or diverting them, politely interrupting them. Ask them what other types of individual can help or hinder a group discussion?
○ Debrief the participants and allow them to disengage from their role characters. This can be done by asking each participant in turn to introduce themselves. If this is not done, uncomfortable feelings brought out by the roles and between the actors may cause problems later.

Further role plays could develop from this session. The group could act out how they might help a shy person to participate in the discussion, or ensure that particular people, for example, women or people with disabilities are not marginalized.

Source: Adapted from Pretty et al, 1995.

Drama exercise

To help facilitators learn about drama, the following exercises can be used.

○ Ask participants to divide into small groups.
○ Ask each group to create a dramatic story that they can perform to their colleagues.
○ Suggest that the drama portrays a problem in the community, but stops at a critical point leaving the problem unresolved.
○ Ask the actors to encourage the 'audience' to propose solutions to the problem.
○ Act out one of the solutions as the finale to the drama.

Role play: Teaching styles

The purpose of this exercise is to help participants understand the limitations of didactic teaching methods and encourage them to consider the response of community members faced with this approach.

The course organizer plays the role of the community health worker who has come to the village to give a lecture on diarrhoea. The participants play the roles of villagers.

○ Ask them to split into three groups. Each person should decide on the character they are playing – it can be based on someone they know and each group should choose a variety of people, for example, mothers with children, elderly people, young men and school children. Ask them to share brief details about the character with the other group members. (You could distribute the roles written on cards if you prefer.)
○ Ask the audience to sit in front of the lecturer, who will talk for about 10 minutes on the chosen subject.
○ The lecturer should deliver the lecture in a directive way using medical or technical words or complex diagrams to illustrate the points. Accuse the children of not paying attention and dismiss people if they cannot answer your questions. Use any other tactics you can think of to demonstrate poor communication.
○ After the presentation do not check the understanding of the audience before you dismiss them.

o Following the lecture ask the participants to get back into small groups but to remain in their roles while they discuss the lecture.
o Ask them to consider what they learnt. Did they find it helpful? How could it have been improved?
o What are the barriers to learning as seen from the point of view of their characters in this context?

If any of the participants, or the characters they were role playing, are used to didactic teaching in their own education they might have felt comfortable with the approach so encourage them to discuss how other participants may have felt about the lecture.

o Debrief the participants and allow them to disengage from their role characters. This can be done by asking each participant in turn to introduce themselves again and to share their feelings about their roles and the role play. If this is not done, uncomfortable feelings brought out by the roles and between the actors may cause problems later.
o At the end of the discussion the issues can be summarized. If there is time, the groups could be asked to re-enact the scene using a more participatory style and incorporating the suggestions raised by the participants.

Case study on community participation

The purpose of this exercise is to help participants consider the benefits of community participation in water, sanitation and hygiene promotion projects or programmes. By the end of the session participants should be able to identify the areas where participation is lacking in the case study (Box A3.1) and suggest what action could be taken to increase the potential for community participation.

Box A3.1 Case study for community participation exercise

Jacques was a community participation promoter and had recently attended a workshop in Kigali on sanitary education. It had given him lots of new ideas on how to prevent water contamination and he was eager to pass on his new-found knowledge.

As soon as he returned to work he went on a field trip to a small town called Busoma. By meeting with the leaders and walking round the town and talking with the residents, Jacques realized that few people had latrines and many of these were poorly maintained and dirty. Children did not use the latrines and were allowed to defecate anywhere. Very few people washed their hands with soap before eating or after defecating. The town water supply did not work on Sundays and when the supply was not functioning, people were using water from unprotected springs and wells. Animals were grazing near these sources and were likely to be contaminating them with their excreta. Jacques suggested to the commune leader that a water committee should be formed to encourage the community to protect the supplementary water sources.

He offered to train the committee members about proper hygiene and suggested that they visit other members of the community in their homes to pass on this information. At the same time, he reasoned, they would be able to identify poor hygiene practices and to correct them. The committee members were fired with Jacques' enthusiasm and made several visits to community members and to the primary school. At the school they discovered that there were no hand washing facilities next to the new latrines. They informed the headmaster who said that he would speak to the other teachers, but in fact he was not very pleased that the committee members felt that there was a problem in the school when everyone had worked so hard to get the new latrines constructed.

After visiting a few families, some committee members found that other members of the committee had also visited them. Several families seemed to be resentful of the visitors and later complained to the community leader that they should have been informed about the visits. They said that they did not feel it was right for the committee members to criticize them for not having a latrine when they knew that there were several committee members who also did not have latrines. They also wanted to know why they had been asked questions about when they used soap and water to wash their hands. When Jacques returned to Busoma town he organized a meeting with the committee and was surprised to find how demoralized they all were after having left them in such high spirits. They explained what had happened. The leader, who was also at the meeting, suggested that perhaps they needed to hold a general meeting with the whole village to discuss the problems in the village and to try to find some of the solutions by working together.

Case study 1

The New Vision, Friday, January 9, 1998

Cholera on rampage

By Vision Reporters

KAMPALA City Council has closed five restaurants at the new taxi park and the entire Katimba eating area until they improve their sanitation. The measure is meant to curb the spread of cholera.

Meanwhile, the State Minister for Education, Francis Babu, on Wednesday closed six butcheries in Kalerwe. Several eating places were also shut down.

In a related move, 20 shanty structures, without pit latrines, have been demolished in Mutungo and Kitintale. The move was ordered by LCs early this week in a bid to check cholera.

Kampala Town clerk Gordon Mwesigye said on Wednesday in an anti-cholera meeting at the City Hall, that Owino Market, Kibuye, Shauri Yako and other markets will be closed if they don't clean up.

"We have closed five restaurants in the new taxi park, closed a butchery, and the sale of fresh food in the entire Katimba area," Mwesigye told the meeting, chaired by Babu, who is also

5 taxi park restaurants, Kalerwe butcheries shut down

MP Kampala Central

Sanyu Take-Away, L170 Take-Away, NA Eating House, Budget Take-Away and Dear Restaurant were closed. About 450 food vendors in Katimba, near Baganda Bus Park, are now jobless.

Mwesigye warned: "We cannot go on pretending when people are dying. We shall crack the whip."

Babu advised people to ensure personal hygiene. " From now, houses blocking roads to toilets will request for space from KCC" he added.

Meanwhile, Kampala MPs have embarked on a sanitation programme which begins tomorrow, with a clean-up operation in the Central Division.

MP Rubaga South, Wasswa Lule, said KCC needs support from the cen-

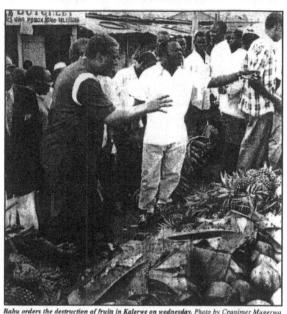

Babu orders the destruction of fruits in Kalerwe on wednesday. Photo by Cranimer Mugerwa

tral government to collect garbage.

Babu on Wednesday closed six butcheries and several other eating houses in Kalerwe in a bid to control cholera. Several other road-side sellers, near trenches overflowing with dirty water, were also ordered to remove their wares immediately. All the affected places were operating under unhygienic conditions.

A number of butcheries, eating houses and shops in the area were given a 24-hour deadline to improve their hygiene or be shut down.

Babu was conducting an on spot tour of Kalerwe in the company of Wasswa Lule, Buganda Minister of Health Robert Ssebunya, the Principle Town Clerk Kawempe Division, Nooh Bukenya and KCC health officials.

Meanwhile, KCC on Tuesday ordered demolition of seven shanty housing structures in Kironde Zone, Kabowa. More than 200 families were left homeless. The move, ordered by KCC, is part of measures being taken to stop cholera which has killed more than 250.

Figure A3.1 Case study 1 on attitudes of health workers

- ○ Read out the following case study material to the group and ask for their comments.
- ○ Ask the group to explain why Jacques' enthusiasm and new-found knowledge were not enough to encourage acceptance of the programme.
- ○ Tell the group that you will read out the case study again and they should try to listen for some of the reasons why Jacques experienced difficulties in getting people to accept his new scheme.
- ○ Ask the group to consider what Jacques could have done to encourage participation.

Case study on attitudes of health workers

The attitudes of health workers towards the communities they work with are vital in determining the effect of their work. These two case studies and questions have been assembled in order to analyse our attitudes to those we work with.

- ○ The first case study (Figure A3.1) should be read by the participants, and then the questions can be discussed.

○ After discussing the first case study (and preferably after reaching a consensus), the second case study (Figure A3.10) should be read and its questions discussed.

○ Conclusions should then be drawn about attitudes to adopt for cholera control measures.

Questions for case study 1:

1. Why did Kampala City Council (KCC) officials demolish those houses?
2. What attitude do KCC officials have to the families who lived in those houses?
3. Why do they have that attitude towards those families?
4. What do you think the attitude of those 200 families will be towards sanitation and hygiene?
5. Does this sort of thing happen here?
6. What other approaches could be used to improve hygiene practices and reduce disease?

Case study 2

The New Vision, Wednesday, January 21,1998

Kotido shuts 24 schools

By Menya Olee

A TOTAL of 24 Kotido primary schools will not be allowed to re-open for the first term unless adequate sanitation is provided, the District Medical Officer, Dr. Louis Okio Talemoe, has directed.

According to the recent sanitation report for 84 schools issued by district health inspectors, 24 schools do not have a single latrine. The report said 16 schools have latrine coverage of below 10% while 4 have a coverage of 50%.

A letter dated 14 January and signed by the DMO, further clarifies that the school with sanitation coverage of below 10% will be allowed to open for one month during which they will be required to increase the number of toilets in their schools to ensure coverage of 50%.

The letter addressed to the DEO, further states that schools with the coverage of over 10% but below 50% will be allowed to open for one term during which they will be required to build more latrines.

" By december 1998, all schools must have sanitary coverage of 100%. I am sure there is no need for me to stress the importance of proper sanitation in schools and other institutions", the letter copied to the ministries of education and health said.

Talamoe also directed that a provision be made for special sanitary facilities for adoloscent girls who require adequate privacy as they manage their menstrual period.

"A small changing room is suggested as latrines are often not clean enough for this purpose", the letter added.

The decision to shut down the schools follows an outbreak of cholera.

Figure A3.2 Case study 2 on attitudes of health workers

Questions for case study 2:

1. Why have the district education officer and district medical officer (DMO) outlined a phased approach to improving school sanitation?
2. What attitude does the DMO have towards the schools in Kotido?
3. Why do you think they have that attitude towards the schools?
4. What else needs to be done to improve hygiene practices and stop cholera from returning?

Source: Ministry of Health Uganda, 1998a.

Three-pile sorting

The purpose of this exercise is to encourage participants to discuss common hygiene practices and explore their attitudes to them. It will also assist the facilitator to learn about community hygiene practices and local attitudes towards them. By the end of the session, participants should be able to identify good and bad hygiene practices and suggest ways in which some of the poor practices could be improved.

This exercise can be done with small groups of about six people to enable everyone to participate. If it is done with a larger group it may be easier to ask for a few volunteers to sort the cards while the others look on and add their comments.

o Volunteers or participants divided into small groups are given a set of picture cards describing a variety of hygiene practices.

o Ask them to sort the cards into three piles according to whether they think the activities depicted are good, bad or neutral in their impact on health.

o Encourage as much discussion as possible. The facilitator can help to clarify the relationship between local knowledge and practice. For example, if people say that boiling water is good, how realistic is this option in terms of scarce and expensive fuel?

o Ask the group to suggest one or two 'bad' cards and to describe what would need to happen and who would be responsible for improving the situation. How can they be involved in making improvements?

o Take note of the discussion points using the local terms. The findings should be included in the project records.

A set of 30 pictures with good, bad and indifferent hygiene practices can be found on pages 152–66.

152

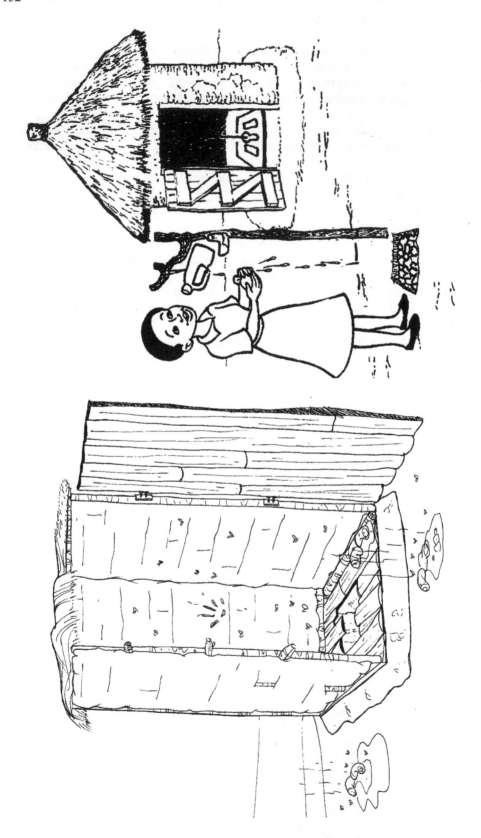

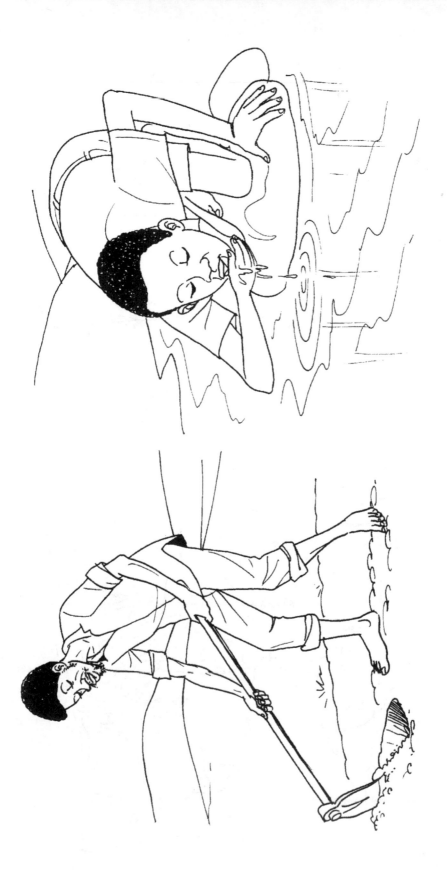

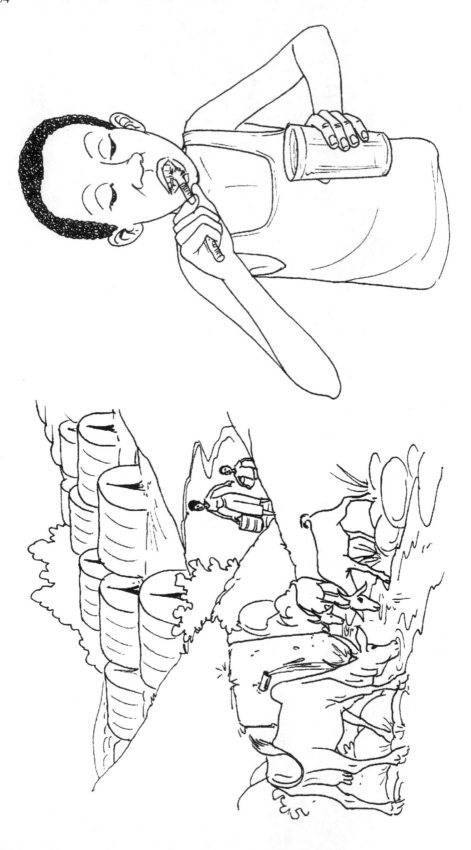

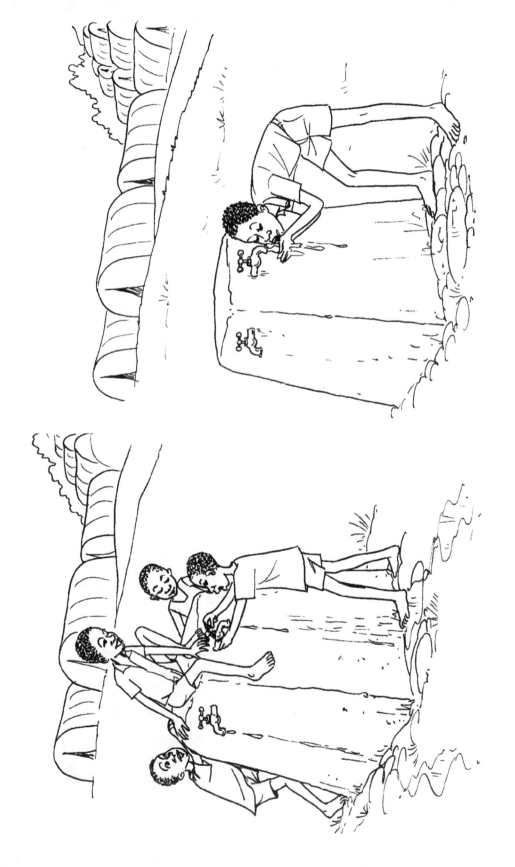

155

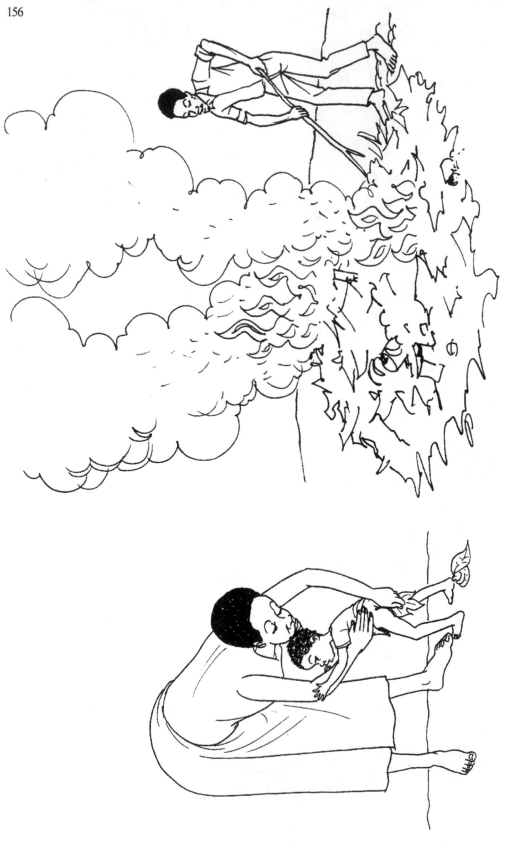

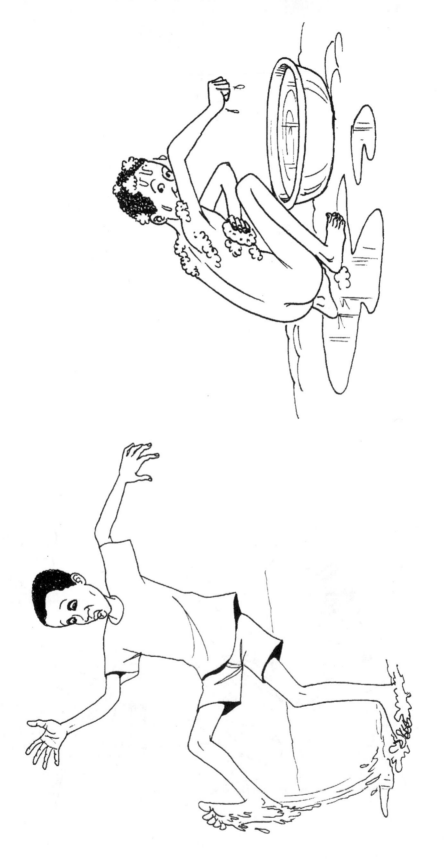

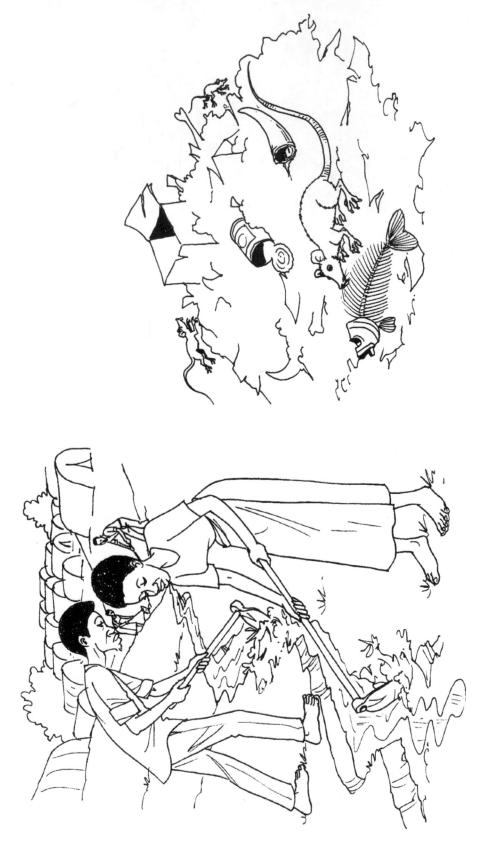

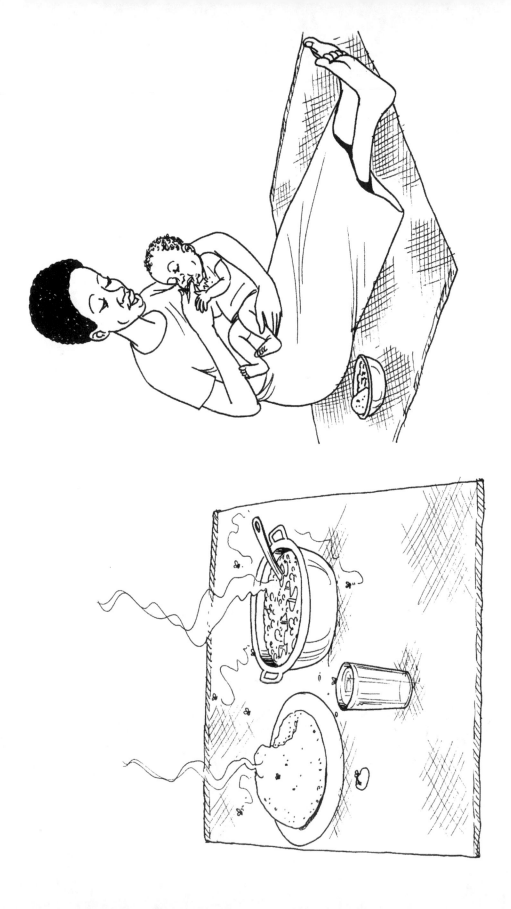

159

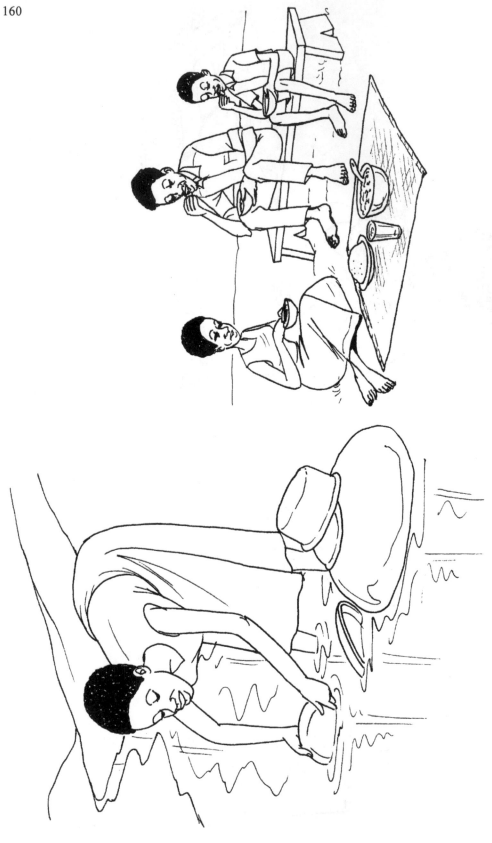

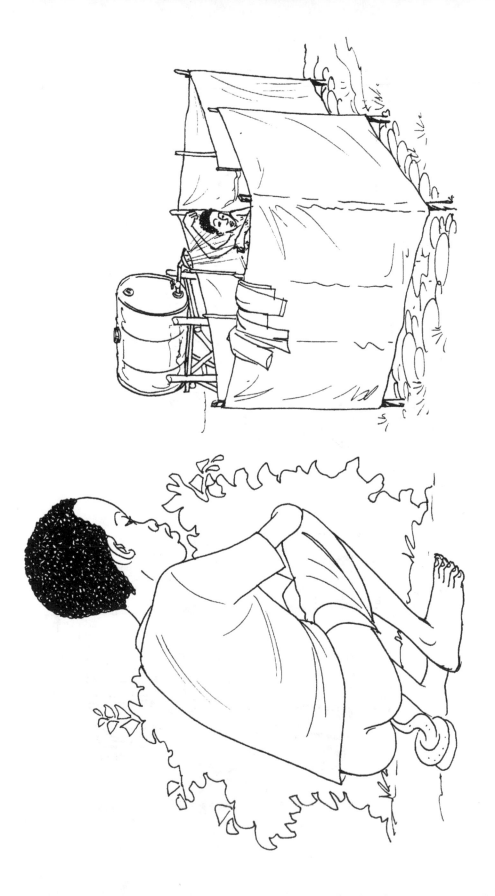

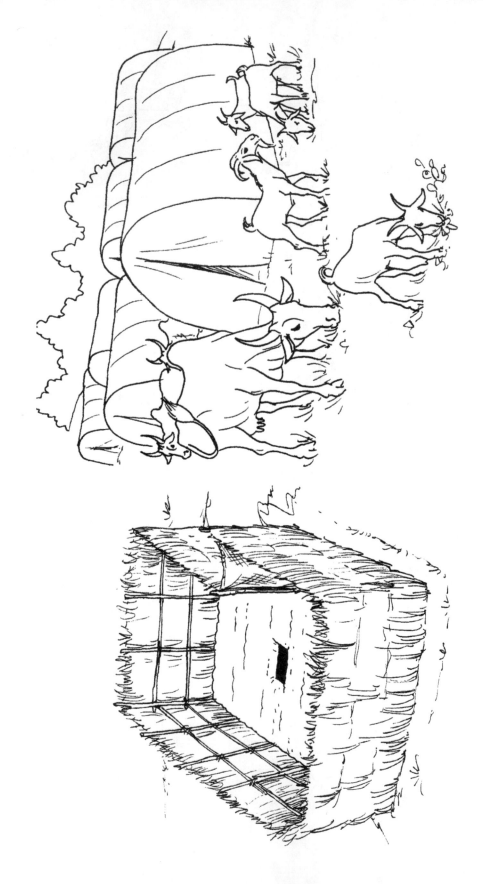

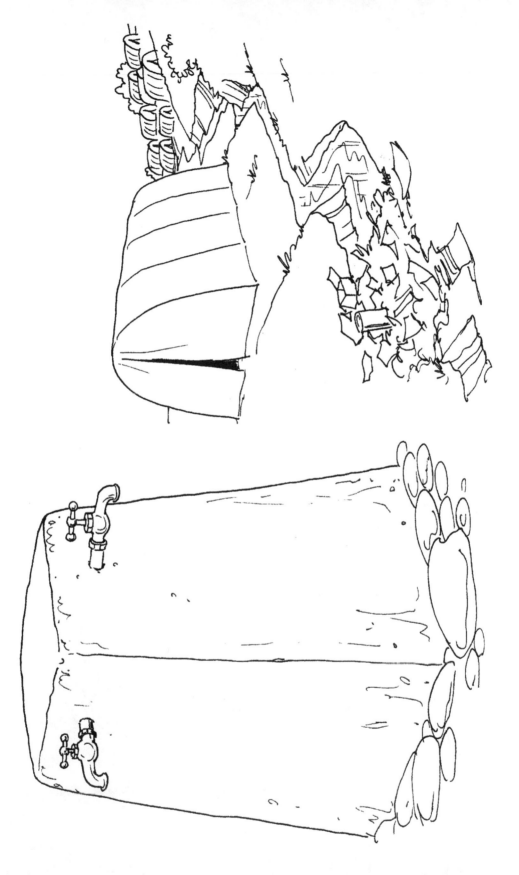

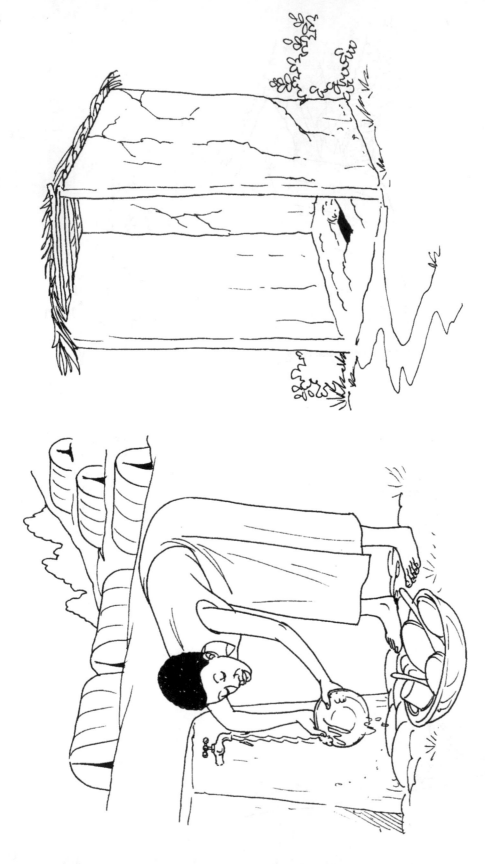

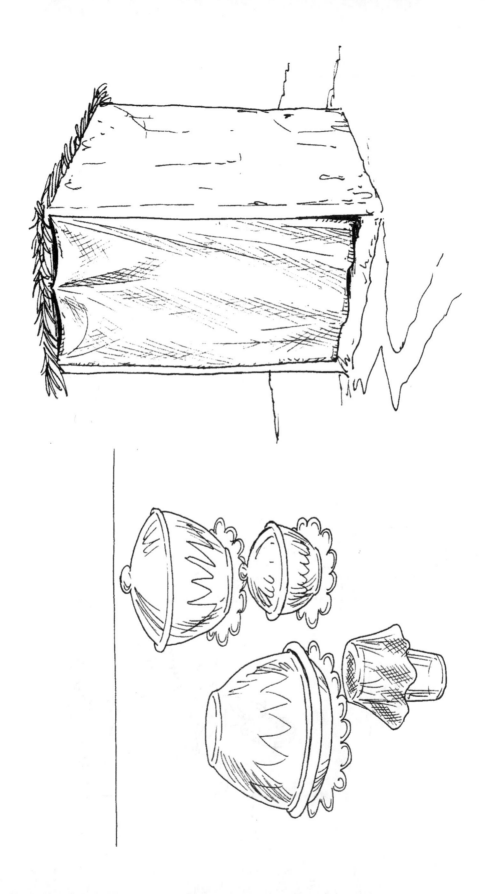

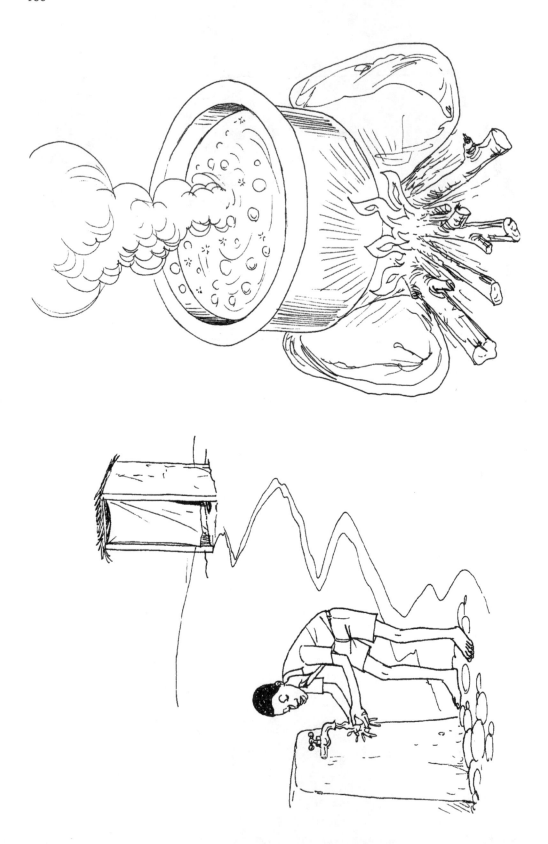

Unserialized pictures

The purpose of this exercise is to promote creativity and discussion about local issues among participants in a group session. It will also help the facilitator to gain insights into the perspectives of community members. By the end of the session participants should be able to identify priority issues in the community and discuss their views on them.

Participants are invited to weave a story around the pictures they select. They give their own interpretation of the events portrayed and in so doing participants and facilitator learn about the beliefs and attitudes of other people and gain useful insights into their perspectives.

○ Divide participants into small groups of not more than six people. Each group is given a set of pictures.

○ Ask them to choose any four of the set and weave them into a story, giving names to the characters and community. Remind them that the story should have a plot with a beginning, middle and end. Allow 20–30 minutes for this task.

○ When all the groups are ready, invite them to tell their stories in plenary session using the pictures to illustrate to the other participants the sequence of events.

○ The main themes and issues in the stories should be noted and included in project records. This can be done by the facilitator or by a community member who is able to write.

○ Give the participants time to discuss the differences and similarities in the stories and the reasons for this. Encourage discussion to enlarge upon priority issues in the community.

A number of pictures that could be used as unserialized pictures to promote discussion around hygiene can be found in pages 167–74.

CLINIC

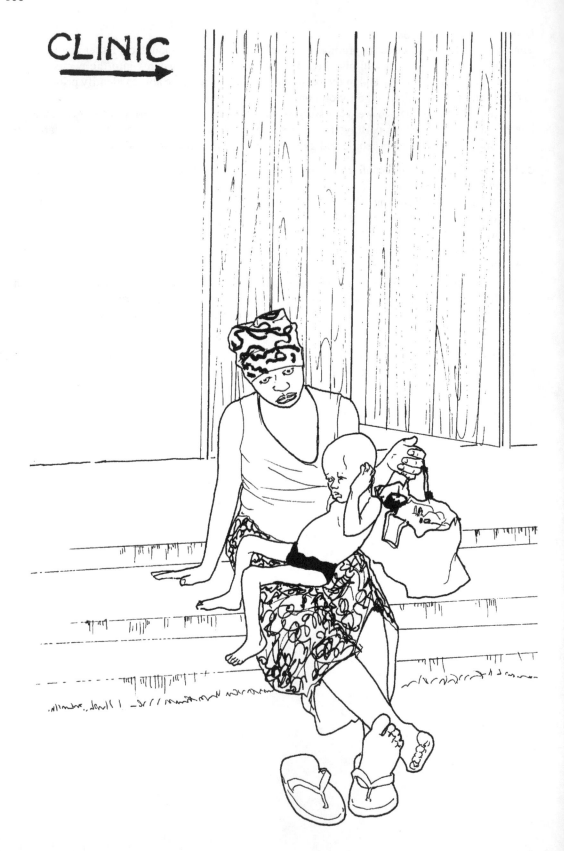

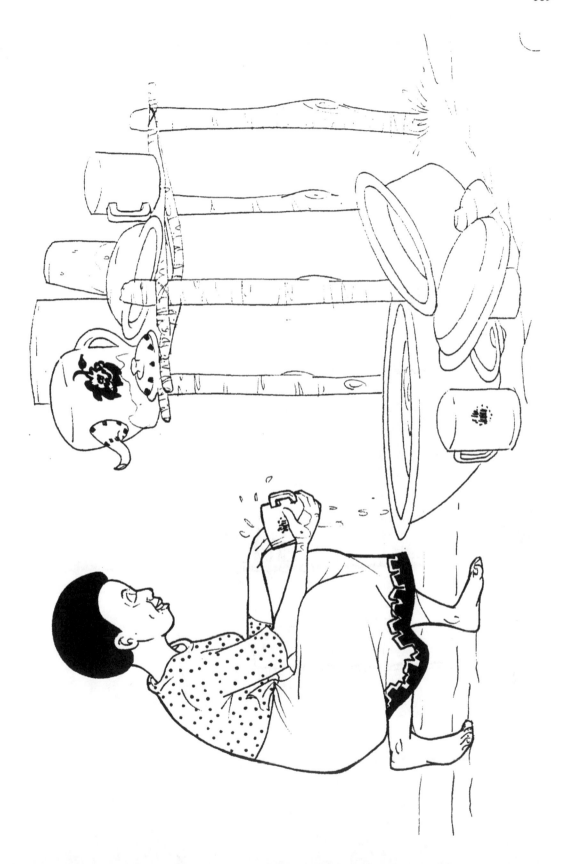

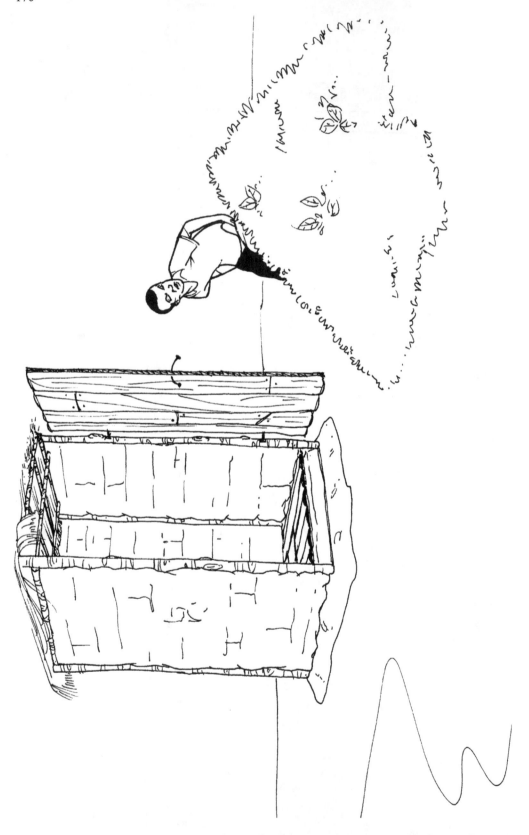

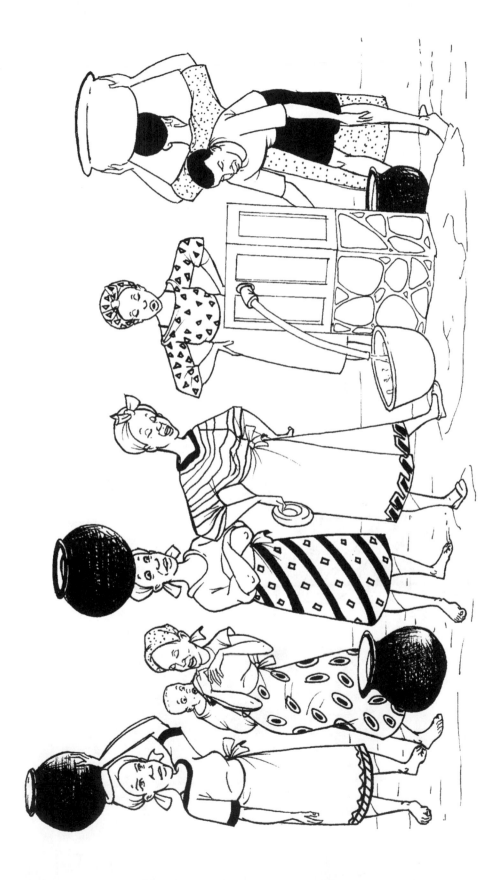

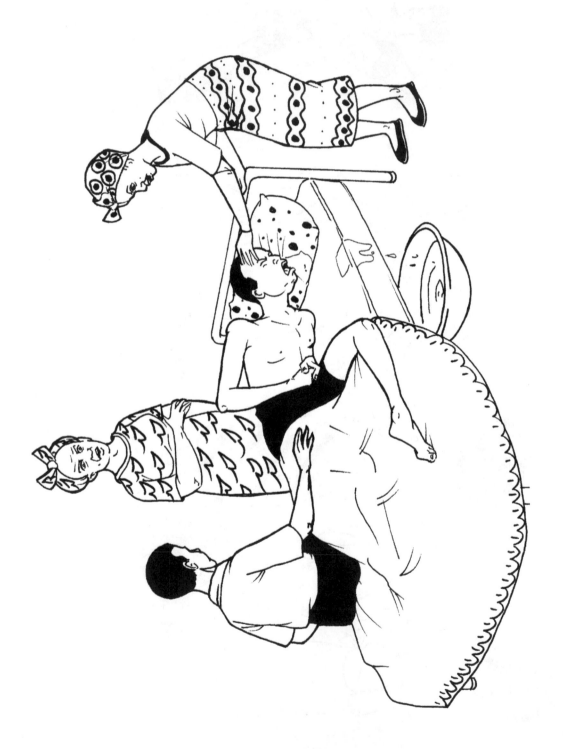

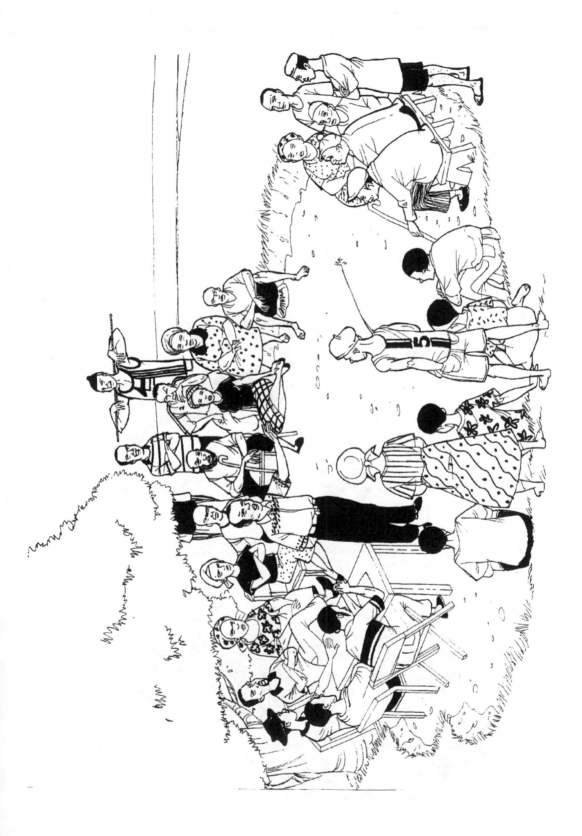

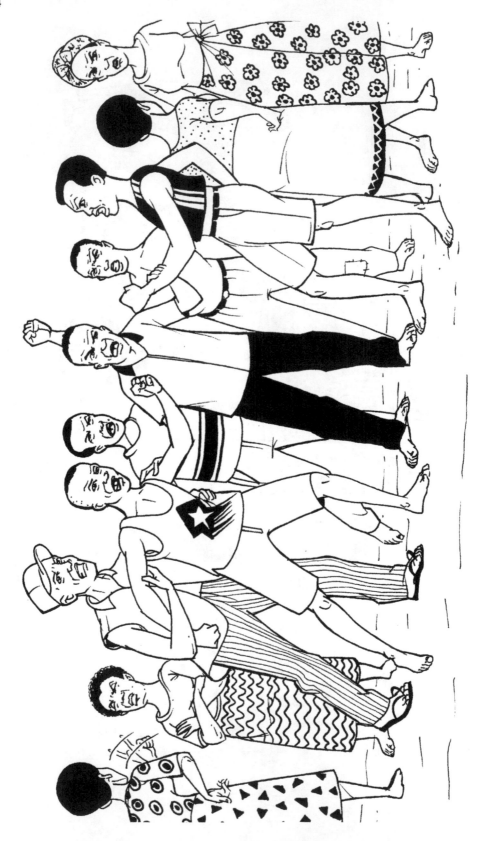

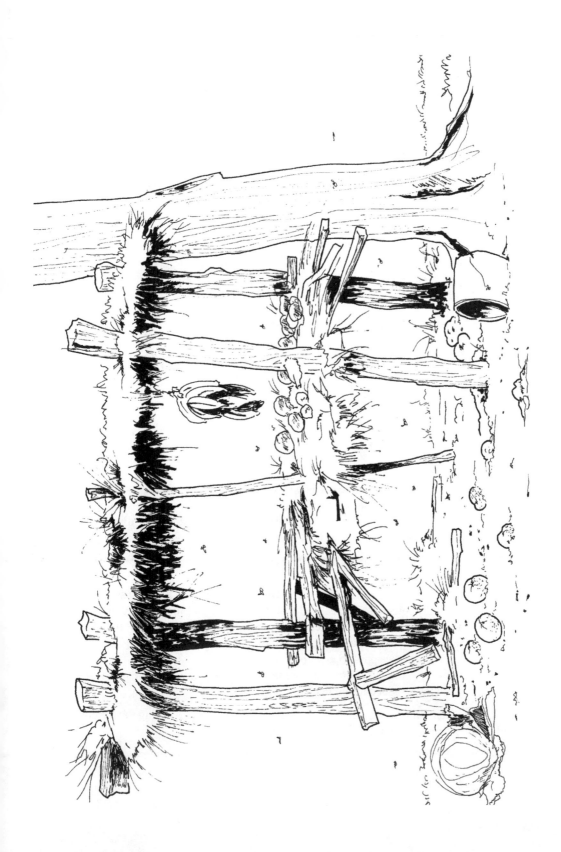

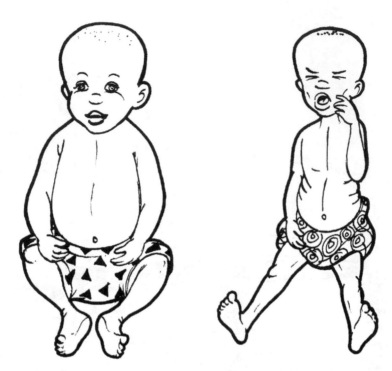

Figure A3.3 Healthy baby, sick baby

Comparative pictures

The purpose of this exercise it to encourage participants to examine some of the good and bad hygiene practices in the community and link them with diseases. By the end of the session participants will be able to identify practices that are likely to cause water- and sanitation-related diseases. It can be carried out with various groups, including groups of mothers who have young children.

○ Place two pictures in front of the participants – one is of a healthy baby and the other of a sick baby (see Fig. A3.3).
○ Divide the participants into two groups. Then present each group with a set of randomly selected 'unhealthy' and 'healthy' pictures. You can select these from any of the pictures in the tool kit.
○ Ask the groups to decide which practices lead to an unhealthy baby and which to a healthy one.
○ Ask one or two people to represent their group's findings in plenary describing the practice and affixing each picture under the appropriate baby.
○ Ask participants how common these practices are in their community and whether they can think of any others that could be added to the list.

Note, ideally the facilitator should have discovered any other practices during the baseline survey and selected or drawn pictures before the session to represent them.

Gender roles

The purpose of this exercise is to encourage discussion about the roles of men and women with a view to enabling women to be more involved in the planning and decision making for interventions associated with water and sanitation and for men and boys to be encouraged to help women and girls with domestic water and sanitation related chores. By the end of the session participants should be able to describe specific activities ascribed to men and women and discuss the skills and responsibilities required for each activity.

○ Divide participants into groups of about six people. If men and women have been invited to the session, ensure that there is an equal mix of both in the groups.
○ Provide each group with a set of activity cards. Ask the groups to sort the cards into three groups according to those activities that are usually performed by men, those usually performed by women, and those usually performed by men and women to the same extent.
○ Explain to the groups that the exercise is designed to encourage discussion and differences of opinion, and that they should be used constructively to gain insights into how the different roles of men and women are viewed.
○ Encourage further discussion by asking the groups to consider what knowledge is necessary in order to perform each task and what decisions must be made before each task can be performed.
○ Finally, ask the group to consider who is responsible for deciding about each different activity.

A series of 12 pictures have been prepared for use with this exercise and can be found on pages 178–89.

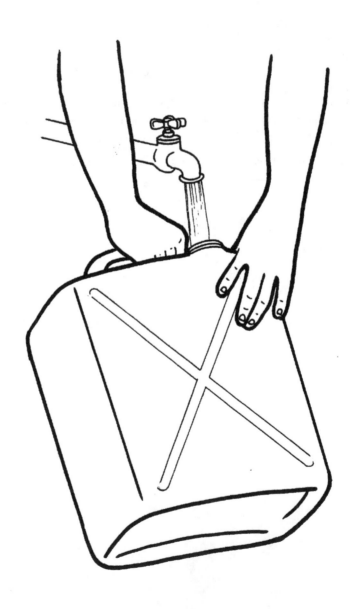

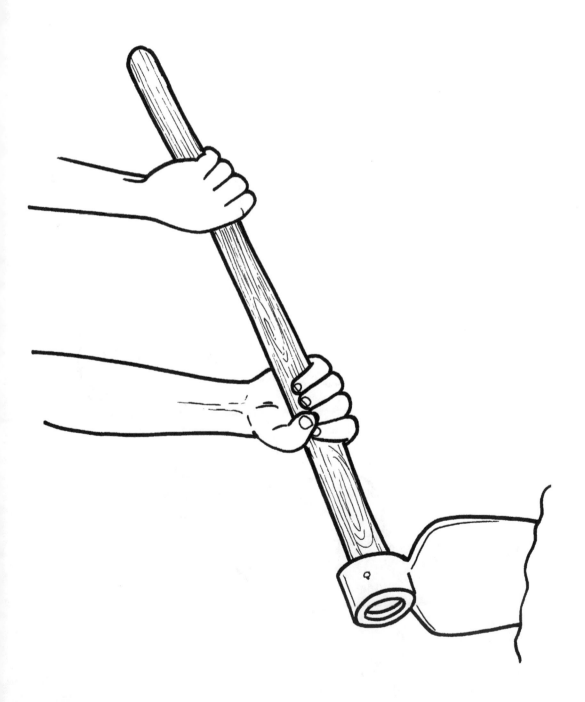

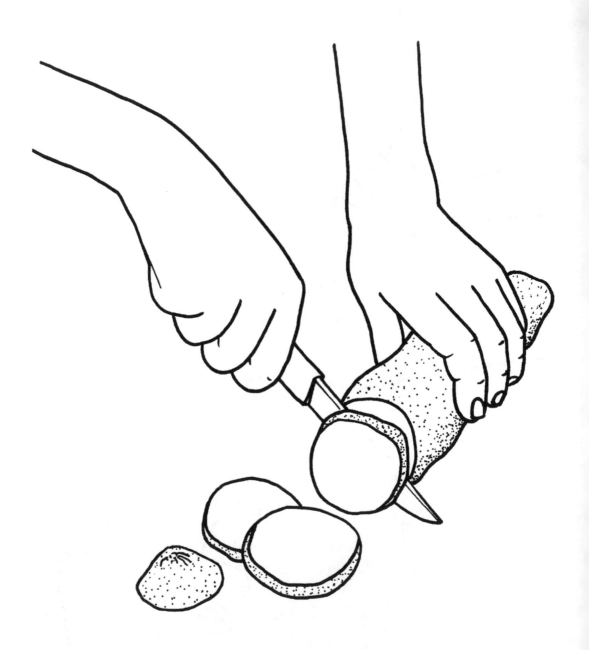

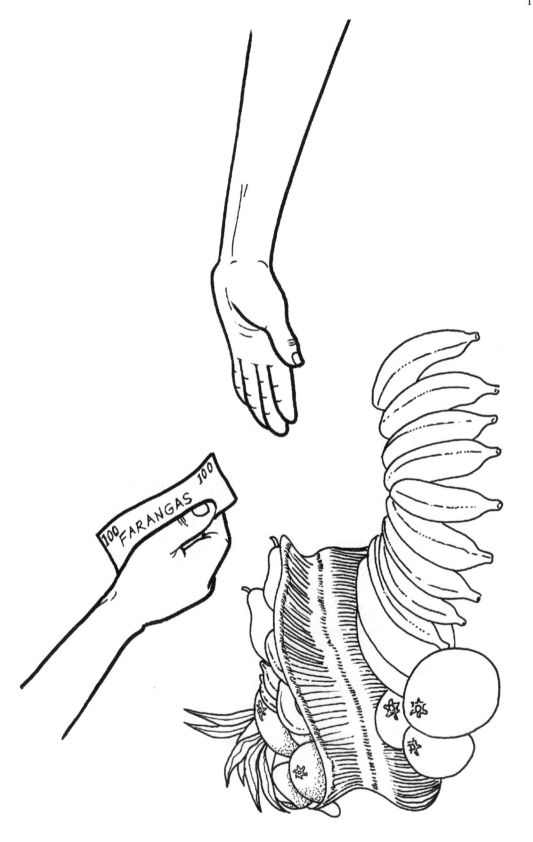

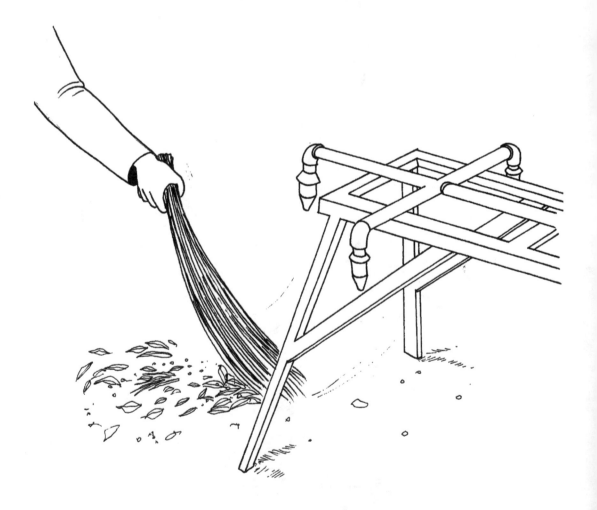

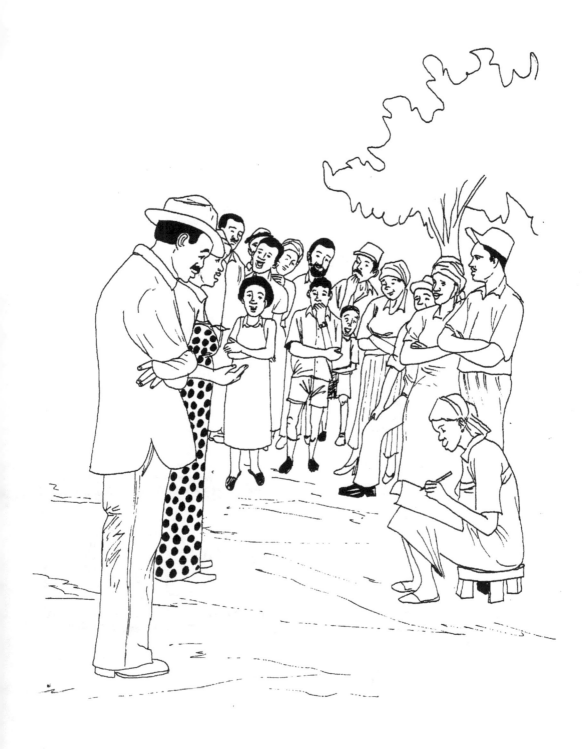

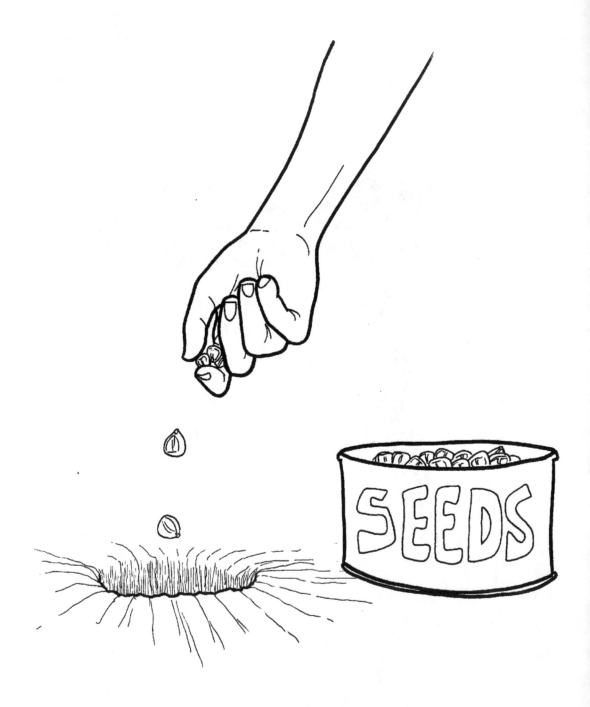

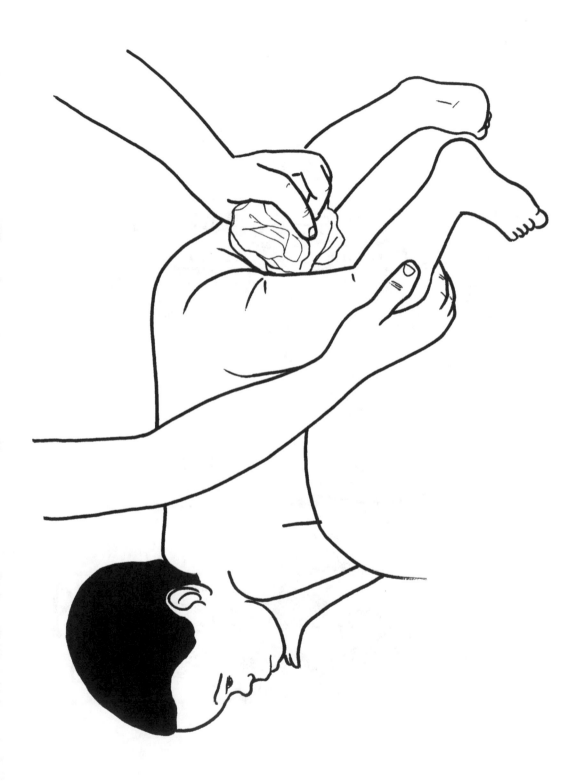

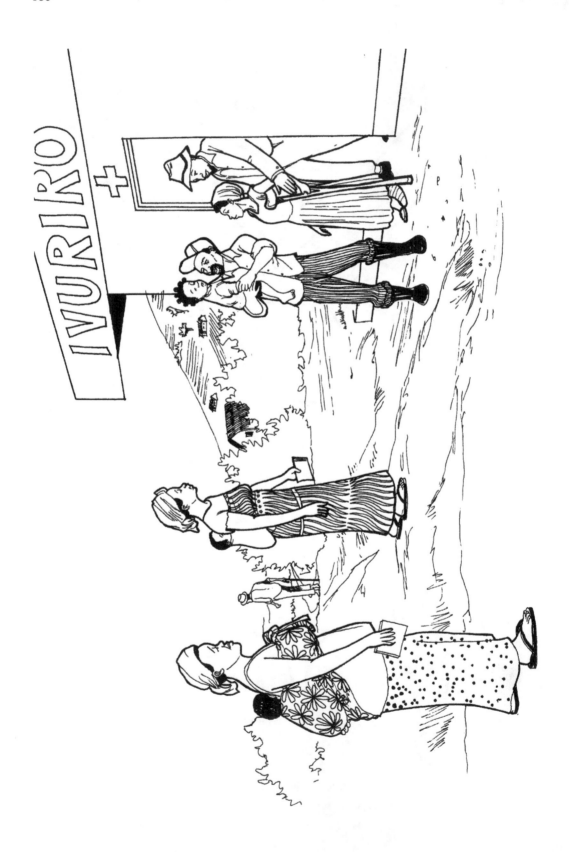

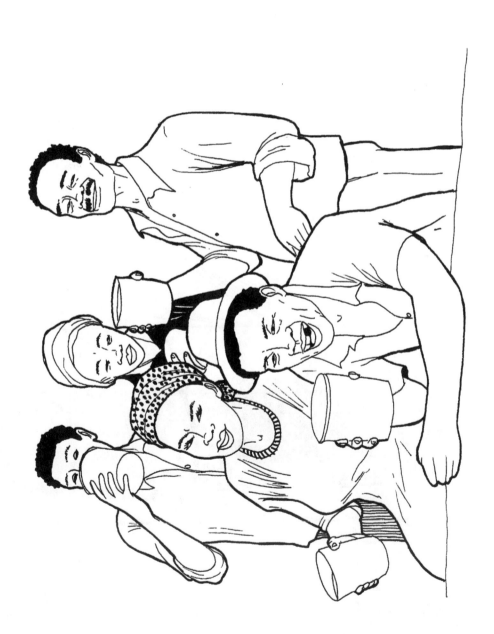

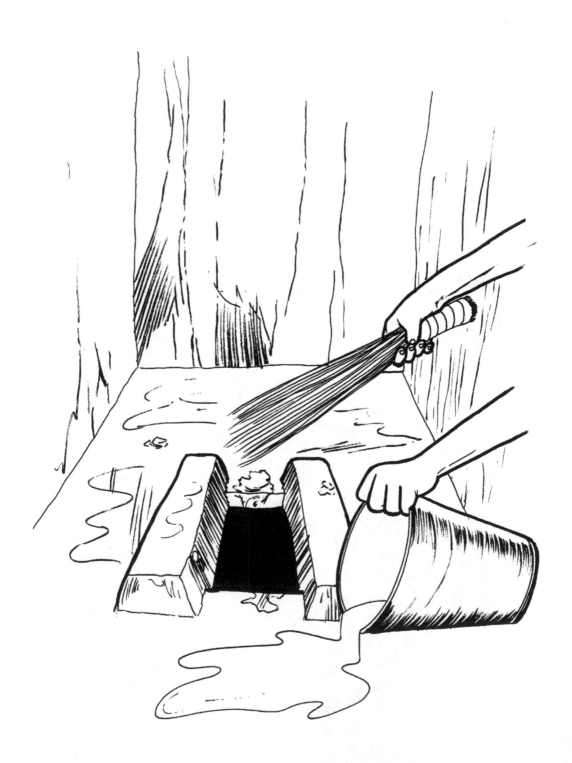

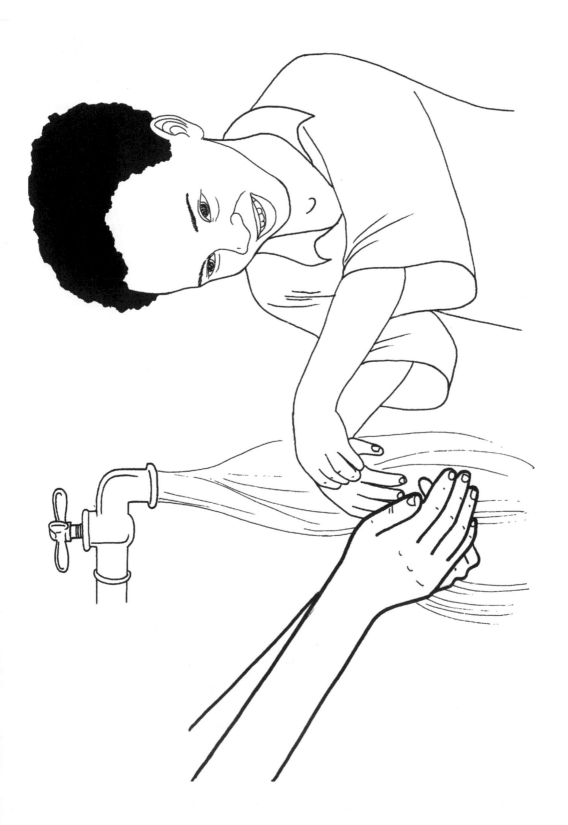

Contamination chain – serialized pictures

The purpose of this exercise is to draw on the participants' knowledge and experience and apply them to problem solving. Local awareness of disease transmission can be explored in this way. By the end of the session participants should be able to describe ways in which hygiene practices are related to the spread of water- and sanitation-related diseases and identify ways of preventing them.

○ Participants divide into small groups and each group is given a set of randomly ordered sequential pictures showing some of the hygiene practices that transmit disease.
○ Ask them to put the pictures into an ordered sequence.
○ Ask them to say why they have made their particular choices and encourage discussion around the issues depicted in the pictures.
○ What action could be taken to improve the situation, and by whom?
○ Ask each group to discuss their findings with the whole group.

A selection of serialized pictures can be found on pages 191–95. Each page has two A5 pictures that should be separated before they are used.

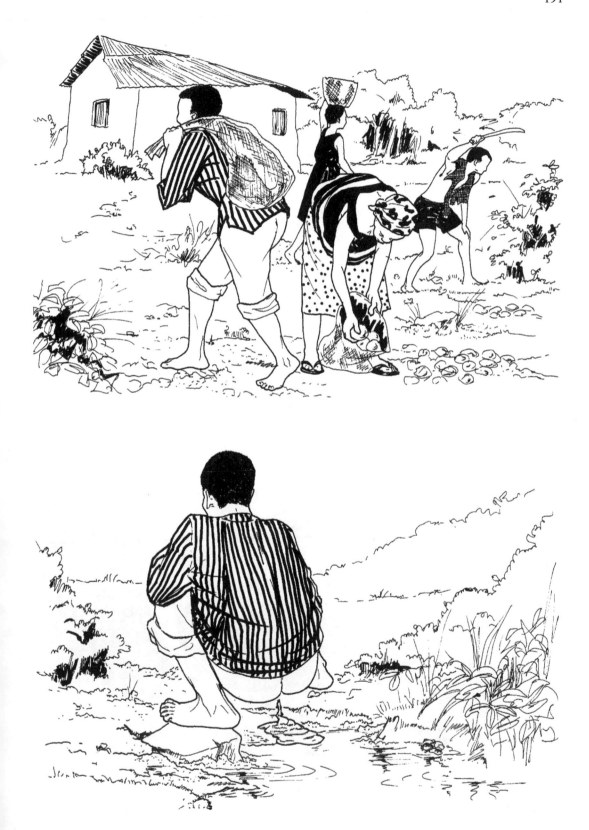

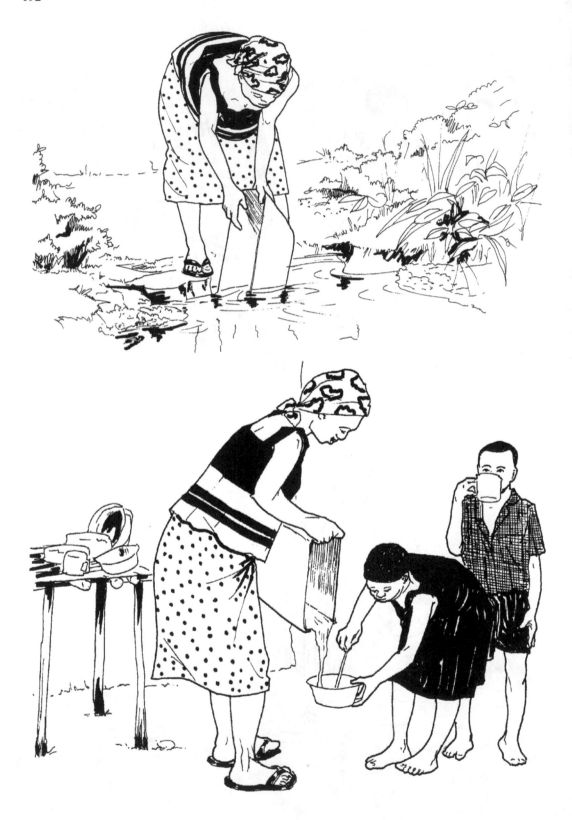

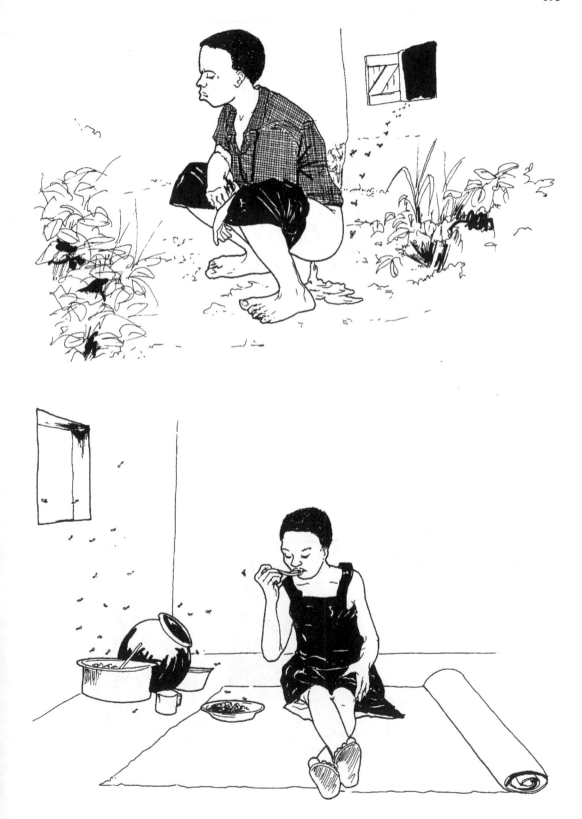

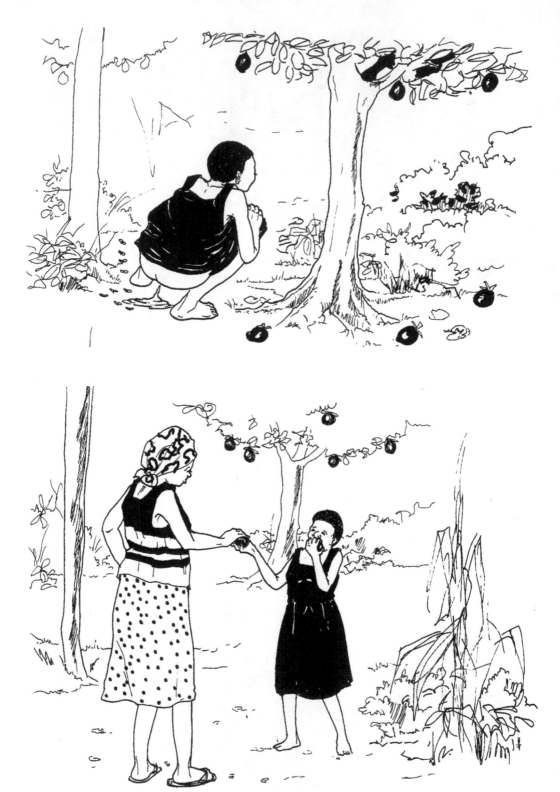

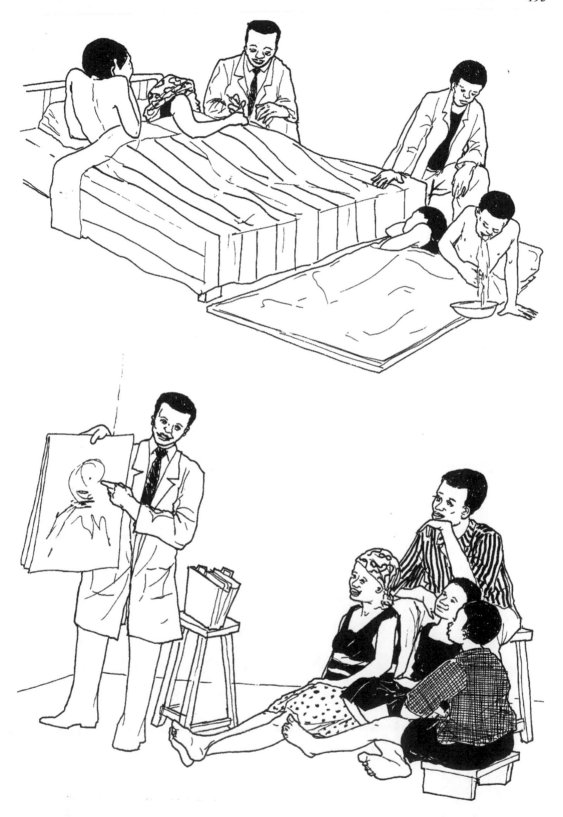

Story with a gap

The purpose of this exercise is to facilitate the participants to become involved in planning water and sanitation activities. By the end of the session participants should have identified local water- and sanitation-related problems and proposed ways of resolving them.

o Divide the participants into small groups.
o Present them with a large poster showing a problem situation (the 'before' scene) and ask for their comments. What has happened and why? The scene can be relayed in the form of a story and the characters given local names if preferred.
o Introduce the 'after' scene in which the situation has improved.
o Ask people to consider how the situation has changed. Who was involved? What did they do?
o These points can be brought out in discussion, or cards depicting the steps can be distributed for consideration. The facilitator can then move the discussion on to consider how the steps can be implemented. What constraints/resources exist within the community? Who will be responsible for taking the actions?

Appropriate pictures can be found on pages 197–200. Each picture is A4-size and takes up a full page.

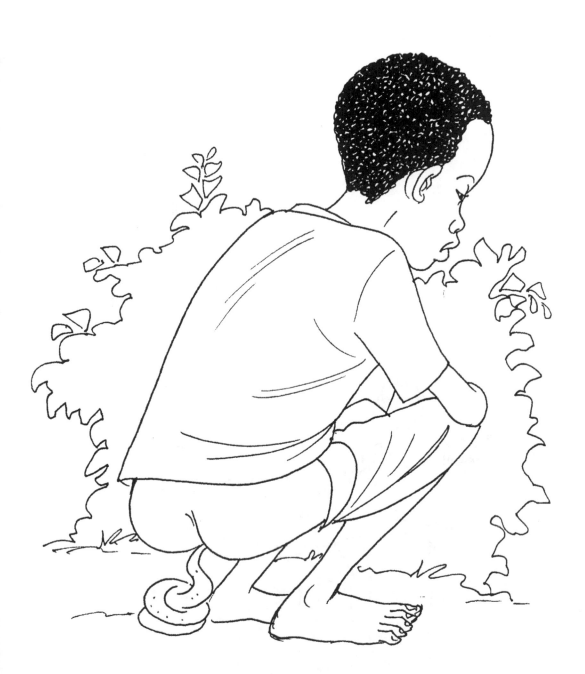

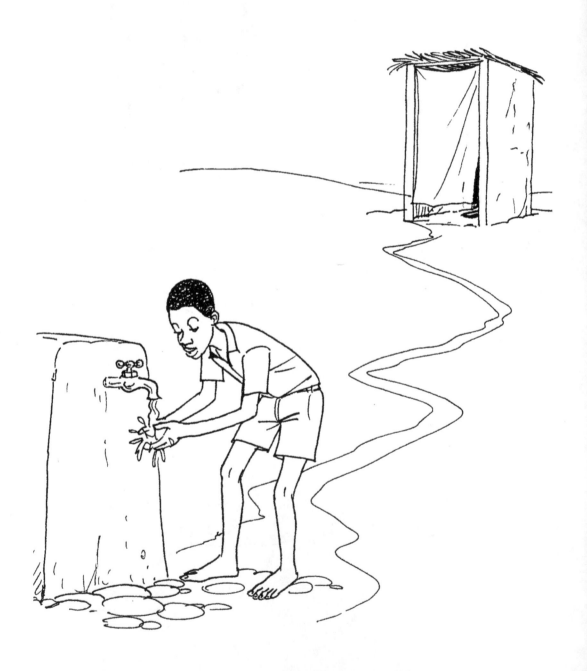

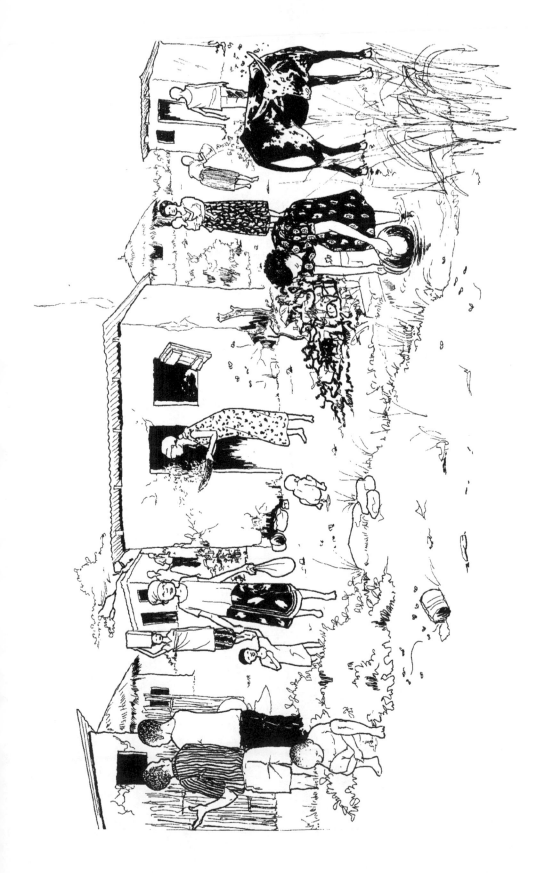

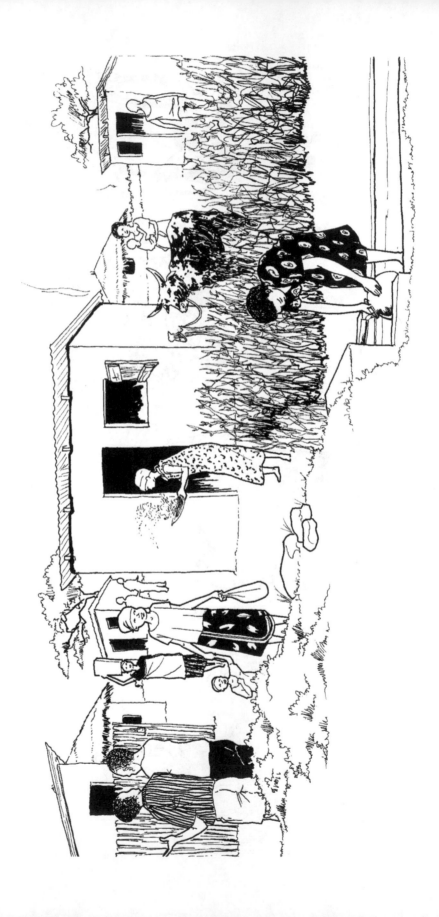

Using flexiflans and flannel graphs

The purpose of this exercise is to facilitate participants to present their views on local issues by illustrating a story with moving cut-out figures. The exercise will also help the facilitator to gain insight into local views and priorities. The figures can be used to start open-ended discussions and are especially useful in working with people who do not have literacy skills to give a visual representation of their views.

Flexiflans are paper or card cut-outs of human figures with flexible arms, legs and torsos joined together with sewing thread or press studs. On the reverse side of their feet, hands and heads they have sandpaper stuck to them. When they are placed on a felt- or flannel-covered board they stick loosely to the board. They can be moved around the board and made to do different things while the person adjusting them tells a story or illustrates a point of view.

Other props, such as cut-outs of houses, animals, trees and household implements are needed for the background context of the figures.

Flannel graph figures are used in a similar way, but do not have the same range of application because the limbs are not articulated. They can be made of paper or card with sandpaper stuck to their reverse sides to use on flannel boards, or they can be made of flannel and stuck on to sandpaper boards (or boards painted with an oil-based paint and covered with a thin layer of sand while the paint is still sticky).

To use the flexiflans and flannel graphs effectively:

○ Present a small group of participants with the flexiflan figures.
○ Ask them to use the flexiflan figures as they like to tell a story about a local issue or describe a point of view.
○ Encourage discussion around the issues.

A series of pictures that can be used to make flexiflans can be found on pages 202–204. These flexiflans need to be made up. Trace the shapes on to a piece of cardboard, change the facial features and the clothing to make them appropriate for your community, and cut out all the pieces. Paint them and join them together with a piece of thread with knots on both sides so that the pieces do not come apart.

Source: Narayan and Srinivasan, 1994; Röhr-Rouendaal, 1997.

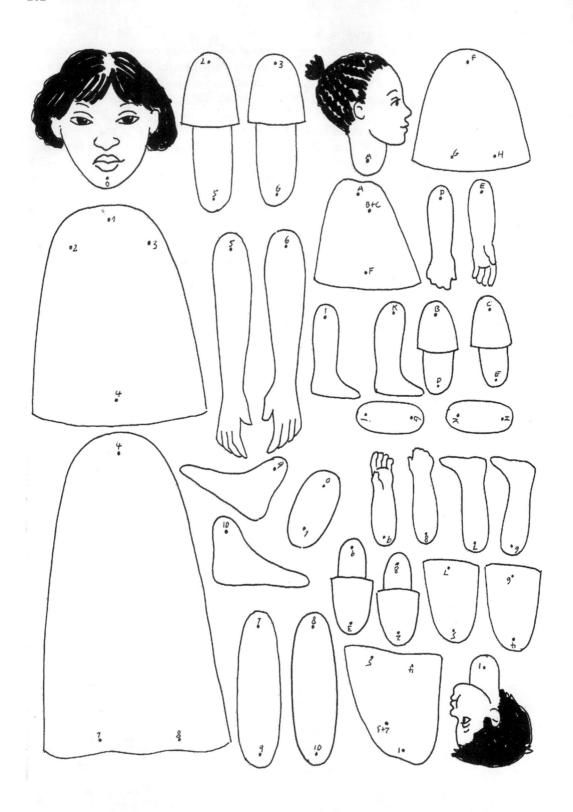

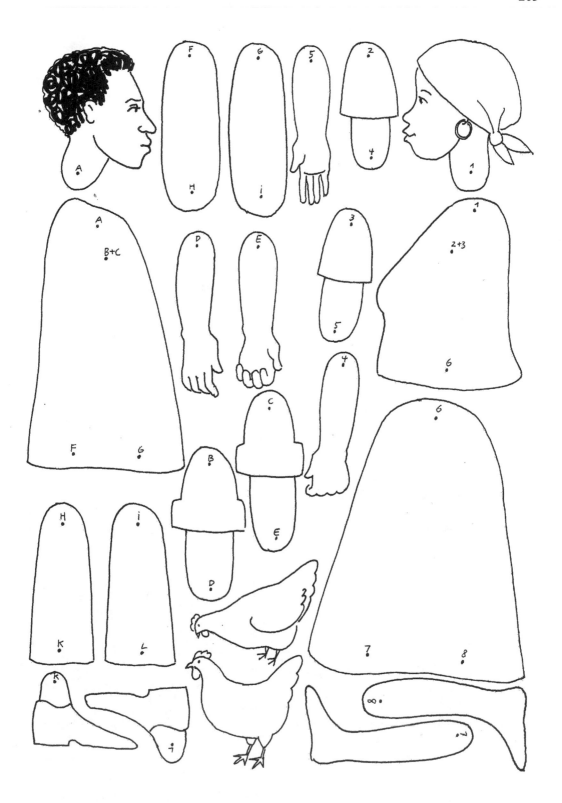

204

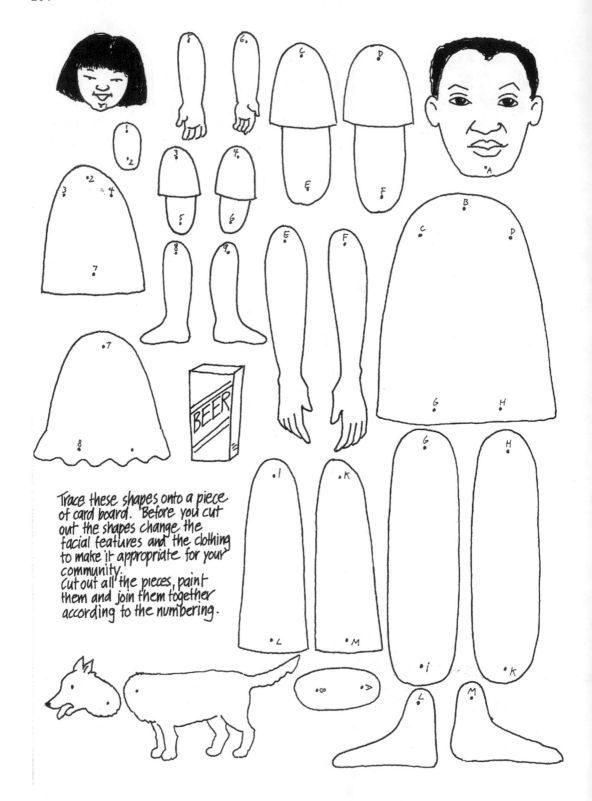

Trace these shapes onto a piece of cardboard. Before you cut out the shapes change the facial features and the clothing to make it appropriate for your community.
Cut out all the pieces, paint them and join them together according to the numbering.

BEER

205

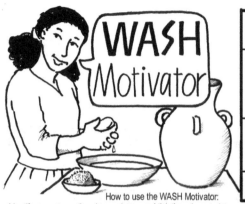

How to use the WASH Motivator:
- Identify current practices in your home and tick the relevant picture.
- Decide the WASH practices you want to change to, then circle those pictures.

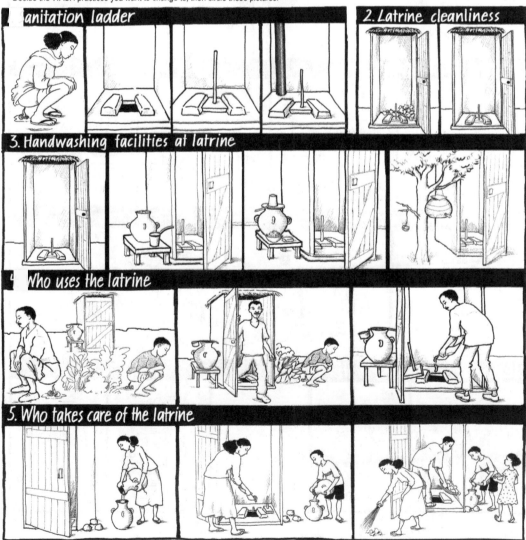

206

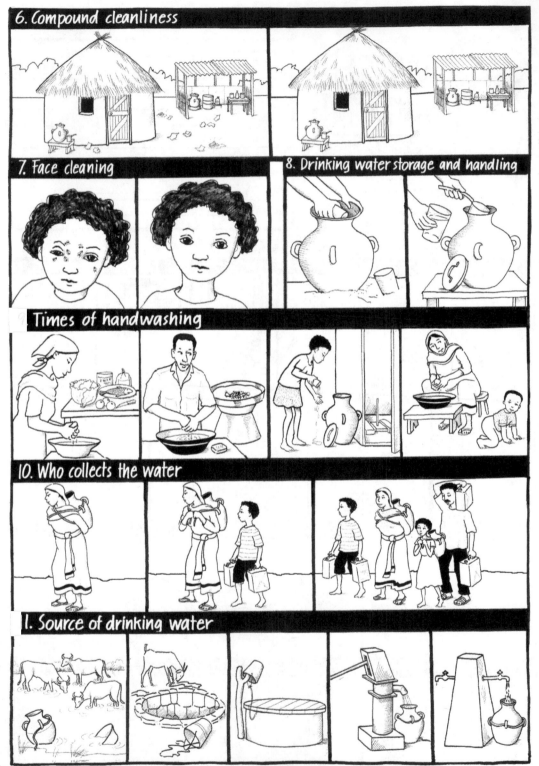

6. Compound cleanliness

7. Face cleaning

8. Drinking water storage and handling

Times of handwashing

10. Who collects the water

1. Source of drinking water

When good progress or innovation is made, inform Facilitator and WASHCO

Example story

Stories can also be used both with adults and children to highlight hygiene issues and stimulate discussion. The story on page 208 was used by several NGOs working in camps for refugees and displaced people in Rwanda. It is important that the facilitator asks questions after reading the story to identify people's reactions and encourage them to think about what they can do to prevent the fly from getting his revenge.

How to do street theatre: Drama

The purpose of this exercise is to promote better hygiene practices in an entertaining way.

○ Brainstorm what makes a good show. The facilitator can suggest these if the participants do not:

- Humour (jokes, men dressed as women, stereotypical characters);
- Drama (hero/villain style, ghosts, death);
- Action (lots of movement, not much sitting/lying down);
- Interesting dialogue/story (clear slow speech, one actor speaking at a time, no long speech by one actor);
- Involving the audience (pantomime style etc.);
- Local reference (relevant comments to the audience);
- Getting the message across.

○ Talk through the 'Dos and don'ts for street theatre drama' on page 78.
○ Warm up. (It may be awkward doing warm ups but the drama will be much better if you have a warm up first.) Try standing in a circle and making animal noises (for example, dog, cat, chicken, cow).
○ Then try acting out stereotype characters (for example, angry wife, drunk husband, beggar, mayor).
○ Decide with the participants the message to be promoted in the community. Then allocate titles to groups.
○ Explain that the plays should be 5 to 10 minutes long and will be done outside in the street or around water points etc.
○ Allow 1–2 hours to work out roles and for preparation of plays and making/gathering of props.

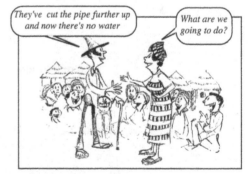

They've cut the pipe further up and now there's no water

What are we going to do?

○ Ask each group to perform its drama in turn.
○ After each play give feedback on what worked and what did not work. The performers themselves should be the first to feed back then other groups can feed back. Facilitators should feed back last.
○ The logistics and arrangements for the performance of the drama(s) in the community setting must be discussed and planned.
○ THEN PRACTICE AGAIN... and perform!

When preparing plays for public performance:

○ Organize people to help seat the crowd in readiness for the performance. Play music while the crowd gathers and is seated.
○ Announce the start and ask for applause. Wait for crowd laughter to die down before continuing speech. Don't rush the performance.
○ Ask questions of the crowd at the end of the show and repeat correct answers. Ask for applause for each correct response. At the end, thank the crowd and ask them to disperse.

Box A3.2. Example story (see page 65)

Long long ago, before you and I can remember, lived a proud and foolish young prince called Mujwashema. Prince Mujwashema liked hunting. One day he decided to ask his friend the fly to go hunting with him. You must remember that this was in the days when the fly was on the best terms with man. If only things had stayed that way!

On this occasion the fly was very pleased to accept and quickly gathered together his hunting spear and set off with the prince. They headed off towards the Forest of Sighs. On the way there they spotted a gazelle darting through the thicket. It was the fly who managed to spear it first and they both rushed to examine their prey. The prince said that they should build a fire straight away so that they might feast on the gazelle and then continue their hunt the next day.

The fly felt very proud of his skill in killing the animal and said that to make the meal even more delicious he would go into the woods to find some wild berries. He returned within a few hours imagining the sight of the gazelle roasting away on the spit and his taste buds began to water. He could not believe his eyes when he returned to see the prince and the embers of the fire. The prince ran up to his friend saying that a terrible thing had happened and that the roasting gazelle had been stolen by a wild cat who had the cheek to sit eating the animal in front of his very eyes and that was why the fly could now see the bones scattered around. The fly was most disappointed and had to content himself with the berries he had gathered. He was surprised that the prince refused to eat anything saying that he was too upset at the loss of their catch.

The next day they both arose very early and set off to hunt anew. It was not long before they saw a monkey and this time the prince took aim and managed to spear him. As they were very hungry they decided to build a fire and cook the monkey straight away. While it was roasting, the fly offered to go and collect some fruits of the forest that might make their meal even more enjoyable. On his return he found the prince sleeping by the fire but there was no monkey to be seen. The prince explained that a wild hyena had come along and stolen the roasting monkey. The prince had given chase but had not been able to catch up with the cunning old hyena. He was so tired on his return that he had collapsed and fallen asleep where the fly had now found him. The two of them decided to continue and to see if they could track down something else. It was not long before the prince spotted another monkey lurking in an acacia tree. He took aim and hurled his spear. The monkey dropped to the ground. The fly urged the prince to build another fire straight away, while he went off to look for some edible leaves.

Once again the fly returned to find that the monkey had disappeared. The prince tried to explain that a large pack of wild dogs had smelled the monkey cooking and had run off with it before he could stop them. The fly was very disappointed as by now he was getting very, very hungry. So he told the prince that they should set off again without delay before it got dark. After a short while the fly spotted the footprints of a wild boar and followed them until he saw the creature in a clearing in the middle of the forest. He took aim with his spear and there was no escape for the wretched creature. Now this time the fly had begun to get a little suspicious of the prince and waited until the boar was almost ready and then volunteered to collect some edible roots to eat with it. This time, instead of disappearing into the depths of the forest he circled the clearing and returned to hide behind a tree. And from there, just as he had expected, he saw the prince devouring the boar that was meant to be for the two of them. The fly was enraged and immediately flew off home to his family.

For days he fumed and raged and ranted and vented his anger against the prince. When he had calmed down a little his wife suggested a plan. Why did he not call together the whole tribe of flies and let them decide on what to do. As you will know, there are several billions of Mr Fly's friends and relatives, so he called them all together and told them what had happened and how he had been betrayed. What we must do he said is somehow to take advantage of man's stupidity. You know well the way that man excretes in the open without any regard for hygiene. What we could do is to walk all over this dirtiness and then when they are not looking we will walk all over their next meal and in this way we will force them to eat their own excreta. The billions of flies who were listening all laughed, cheered and applauded this cunning plan and to this day man has forfeited his friendship with the fly and he has suffered the consequences of his greed.

Source: Chiles, 1994, 'Samaritan's Purse, Rwanda', personal communication.

Making puppets

Simple puppets can be made from mounting cardboard cut-out figures on sticks or painting features on to wooden spoons, cardboard tubes or paper bags. (Glove puppets are easy to make and effective to perform with as they are able to pick things up.)

To make the body, fold a long piece of paper and put your second finger on the fold (see Figure A3.4). Draw round you hand and forearm as far down as your elbow, leaving a margin to make a template as shown in the picture. Cut the template along the drawn line, unfold it and pin it to a double layer of cloth. Cut out the cloth and sew it up, leaving the bottom and the neck open. Turn it right side out. The hands and the head can be attached to the body. The puppeteer's fingers must still be able to reach to the top of the puppet's hands.

To make a puppet head (see Figure A3.5), take thin foam, (0.5cm) and dye it in a solution of water and brown poster paint or strong black tea. Squeeze out the water and dry. Cut a head shape out of double thickness foam, sew these pieces together and stuff with kapok/wadding/cotton wool. Make a cardboard tube, wide enough for two fingers and insert it into the neck. Make sure that you sew through the card as well as the cloth when attaching the body to the head. Sew on foam ears and stick on a foam nose. Draw features with marker pens. Make hair by attaching strands of wool, or with marker pens.

To make a portable screen (see Figure A3.6), a length of cloth can be attached to two sticks and supported by people or roped to chairs.

Source: Howell, 1990.

Figure A3.4 Making puppet's body

How to make posters

○ Keep the details in the poster to a minimum and communicate one message at a time.

○ Make sure that the pictures are as accurate as possible and are familiar to the audience.

○ Do not distort the size of an object and try to avoid using sections of the body out of context as it may cause confusion.

○ Avoid using abstract symbols, especially if people are not literate, as they are unlikely to understand them. Similarly, trying to indicate movement in a picture may not be understood in the way intended.

○ Do not assume that a sequence of activities that makes sense to you will necessarily be understood by the viewer.

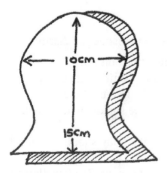

Figure A3.5 Making puppet's head

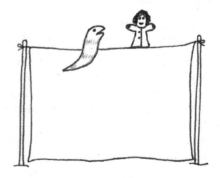

Figure A3.6 Puppet show

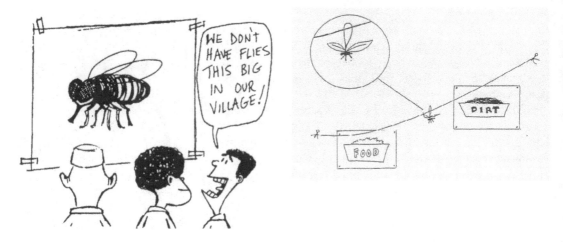

Figure A3.7 Vector on a string

○ Write words only if most of the target population can read. If words are to be included, use them sparingly and keep the message clear and simple. Try to convey positive messages whenever possible.
○ If using colours try to make sure that they resemble the real colour of the object they are depicting, to avoid confusion.
○ Insect vectors can be depicted with movement by using a cut-out vector attached to a piece of string with a paper clip (see Fig. A3.7). The string should then be attached with tape to the poster so that the string passes over the places where the vector might visit. The vector can then be moved along the string and over the different places represented in the poster. In this way flies can be depicted moving from food to faeces and back again.

Experiments

Wilted plant experiment
The purpose of this exercise is to show children that water is necessary for life. Plants, like people, suffer and die when they do not have sufficient water.

○ Cut two flowers or plants.
○ Put one flower in a container of water and leave the other without water for a few hours.
○ Discuss with the children why the plant without water is wilting.

Hollow gourd experiment
A hollow gourd or container can be used to show how fluid is lost through episodes of diarrhoea.

○ Make a hole in the top of a gourd and another small hole with a plug in the bottom.
○ Draw a mouth and eyes on the gourd. Fill it with water and cover the top opening with a small thin damp cloth. Pull out the plug and let the children see how the cloth sinks into the hole.
○ Discuss how this compares to the soft spot on the baby's head that will be sunken when the baby is dehydrated.
○ Mark a water level line on the gourd and explain that the fluid inside the body should never fall below this or the baby will become dehydrated and may die.
○ Show how each cup of water that is lost must be replaced by another that is poured in (swallowed) to prevent dehydration.

Coloured rice experiment

This experiment demonstrates how flies can spread dirt and contaminate food. It is most effective when the food used is white or when it is considered to be pure in the culture of the participants. Test it out first in your local setting before doing a public demonstration.

o Put cooked rice on one plate near the participants. Put some faeces on a leaf some 10 metres from the participants (a pit latrine nearby might also be effective).
o Cover the faeces in red powder (such as the red powder used by Hindu women for tikka and their hair partings).
o Leave the rice and the faeces for 30 minutes.
o Flies will move from the faeces to the food and gradually turn the white rice red.
o Discuss the implications of the results with the participants.

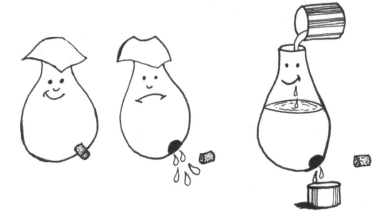

Figure A3.8 Three gourds

A4

Sample job descriptions

Job description for community facilitators

The role of the facilitator is to work directly with community groups or representatives to help them identify and seek solutions to problems and to take action to improve health.

Essential qualities

○ Confident communicator
○ Able to speak the local language
○ Available for full-time work
○ Willing to work in a collaborative way with the community
○ Has the trust of can easily build the trust of the community

Desirable qualities

○ Literacy and numeracy are less important than attitude and ability to communicate effectively with a range of different people
○ Good listening skills
○ Reasonable understanding of health and hygiene issues

Tasks

○ Enable the community to find solutions to water- and sanitation-related problems
○ Liaise with community leaders and other sectors and agencies working locally in order to promote the project
○ Take part in the monitoring and evaluation of the hygiene promotion project and ensure that feedback is given to the community
○ Plan and implement other communication strategies when appropriate, for example, the use of drama and campaigns
○ Assist with the planning and implementation of training for other community members, e.g. water committees, volunteers/animators
○ Assist volunteers/animators in their work
○ Supervise the activities of water-point attendants and latrine attendants
○ Develop and use appropriate education materials as required
○ Provide the project with regular work reports
○ Other duties as requested

Job description for children's facilitators

The role of the children's facilitator is to work directly with children and teachers to help them identify and seek solutions to problems and to take action to improve health.

Essential qualities

- Able to communicate easily with children
- Must be acceptable to the community

Desirable qualities

- Lively and imaginative personality
- Reasonable understanding of health and hygiene issues
- Reasonable understanding of child development

Tasks

- Identify groups of children in the community to work with
- Implement interactive education activities with them
- Help the children to evaluate their activities
- Provide regular oral reports on their work to the project

Job description for supervisors

The role of the hygiene promotion supervisor is to train, support and manage the community and children's facilitators in their work, by assisting them to identify and seek solutions to problems and to provide feedback on how they are performing. The supervisor also plays an important role in assessment, planning, monitoring the project and coordinating with other organizations and other sectors, and reporting progress to the line manager.

Essential qualities

- Commitment to capacity building and enhancing problem-solving skills in staff and communities
- Confident communicator, able to command respect from a wide range of people
- Available for full-time work
- Reasonable planning, negotiation and leadership skills; consultative management style
- Literate and numerate; able to analyse information, prepare plans and reports

Desirable qualities

- Practical experience of hygiene promotion with communities
- Previous experience of staff recruitment, support, supervision and training
- Reasonable understanding of health and hygiene issues

Tasks

- Responsible for the recruitment, supervision, support and training of six to eight community and children's facilitators and hygiene education campaign workers
- Undertake staff appraisals, observe staff at work with the community and provide feedback on a regular basis
- Liaise with community leaders and other sectors and agencies working locally in order to promote the project. Represent and promote the hygiene promotion project at coordination meetings
- Plan and organize needs assessment, implementation activities and monitoring and evaluation of the project; ensure that stakeholders are kept informed of progress
- Select and organize distribution of appropriate hygiene promotion materials

○ Prepare and distribute monthly reports to line manager
○ Other duties as requested

Job description for water-point attendants

The role of the water-point attendant is to ensure that water points are kept clean and are used appropriately at all times. Water-point attendants should also promote appropriate treatment of drinking water as required (for example, when there is an outbreak of diarrhoea).

Essential qualities

○ Must be able to command respect from, and be able to communicate effectively with, most community members and speak the local language
○ Must be prepared to undertake cleaning activities around the water point and other activities as necessary
○ Must maintain a high level of personal hygiene and cleanliness

Desirable qualities

○ Should live nearby to the water source
○ Preferably be a woman

Tasks

○ To ensure that water points are kept clean and free from contamination
○ To prevent people from washing in, or too close to, the water source
○ To prevent children and adults from defecating near the water point
○ To provide information to people on the problems associated with contaminated water and appropriate methods of water treatment

Job description for campaign workers

The role of the campaign worker is to spread specific hygiene messages quickly around the target community. Their role includes explaining the selected hygiene messages to groups of people in public places and to families in their homes.

Essential qualities

○ Must be able to command respect from the target community
○ Must be able to communicate effectively with most community members and speak the local language

Desirable qualities

○ Energetic and resourceful
○ Reasonable understanding of health and hygiene issues

Tasks

- To provide information to the population on ways of preventing the most significant water- and sanitation-related diseases
- To be deployed as necessary in a public place, for example, registration point, market, distribution areas
- To visit families at home to discuss the importance of using and constructing latrines, disposing of children's faeces, hand washing, and any other issues as determined by the project manager
- To provide feedback from information sessions through regular meetings with other team members and the project manager

Job description for latrine attendants

The role of the communal latrine attendant is to maintain the communal latrines in a clean and sanitary condition and to promote the use of latrines. (People will not use dirty, smelly latrines.) Latrine attendants should also encourage hand washing with soap or ash following use of latrines.

Essential qualities

- Must be able to command respect from, and be able to communicate effectively with, most community members and speak the local language
- Must be prepared to undertake cleaning activities in and around the latrine as necessary
- Must maintain a high level of personal hygiene and cleanliness

Desirable qualities

- Preferably a male latrine attendant for latrines assigned to males and a female latrine attendant for latrines assigned to females

Tasks

- To ensure that public latrines are kept clean following use (cleaning must be done frequently during the day)
- To encourage people to use the facilities provided to wash their hands following use of the latrine
- To ensure that water and soap are available at the facility
- To provide information to latrine users on the importance of disposing of all excreta in the camp in the latrine (including that of young children and babies), and on the necessity to dig family latrines
- To maintain a simple monitoring form on the condition and use of the latrines

A5

Sample training courses

Community facilitators' course: Objectives and sample timetable

To introduce participants to a variety of methods that can be used for carrying out data collection and hygiene education. By the end of the course, the participants should be able to:

- explain the relationship between hygiene and water- and sanitation-related diseases;
- demonstrate good listening and communication skills;
- facilitate a community group using participatory learning activities;
- initiate drama activities in the community.

Table A5.1 Community facilitator's course timetable

Time	Day 1	Day 2	Day 3	Day 4	Day 5	Day 6
09.00 to 10.00	**Introduction** to purpose of course, timetable housekeeping arrangements people introductions	**How People Learn** Discussion of own learning experiences, what makes learning new things easy/ difficult/fun	**Working with People** Case study on community participation. Setting objectives	**Communi-cation Skills** Oral and listening exercises followed by brainstorm and discussion of key points	**Using folk media** Discussion of local folk tradition (songs, story telling drama)	**Evaluation and feed back** Discussion on why to evaluate? Carry out course evaluation
10.00 to 11.00	Expectations and anxieties	Role play of health lecture Learning styles (learning styles pictures)	Group dynamics Individual in group (disrupter exercise) Coping with problems	Brainstorm and discussion about local beliefs and how to deal with them sensitively	Discuss ideas on street-theatre dramas (How to do street-theatre) Help participants prepare plots in small groups	Plans and practise giving feedback to the community
			Morning Break			
11.30 to 12.30	Prepare for local mapping exercise	**Simulate participatory exercise** (Time-line, flexiflans, Three-pile sorting cards)	**Simulate participatory exercise** (Comparative pictures, story with a gap)	**Simulate participatory exercise** (Unserialized pictures/ Serialized posters)	Participants prepare short (5-minute) street-theatre dramas, Present them to the other participants, Feedback to each group	**Plan afternoon session:** Community feedback using drama, songs or pictures

			Lunch Break		
13.30 to 16.00	Community activity Mapping	Community activity Timeline, Flexiflans, Three-pile sorting	Community activity Comparative pictures, Story with a gap	Community activity Unserialized posters, Sterialized pictures	Community activity Present the dramas to the community	Community activity Feeback – which activities have been most helpful/ enjoyable to the community
16.00 to 17.00	Debrief	Debrief	Debrief	Debrief	Debrief	Debrief
17.00 to 17.30	Evaluation	Evaluation	Evaluation	Evaluation	Evaluation	Where to we go from here? Plan work and follow up actions

Children's facilitators' course: Objectives and sample timetable

The objective of this training is to introduce participants to the child-to-child approach to working with children. By the end of the course, participants should be able to:

○ explain the relationship between hygiene activities and water- and sanitation-related diseases;
○ demonstrate a number of ways of engaging children in hygiene promotion activities.

Table A5.2 Children's facilitator's course timetable

Time	Day 1	Day 2	Day 3	Day 4	Day 5
09.00 to 10.00	**Introduction** to course, timetable arrangements, personal introductions Discussion on how children learn and different stage of child development based on participants' experience	**Learning about dehydration** Discussion of personal experiences and knowledge, Recognizing dehydration	**Learning how to prevent dehydration** Demonstration of making salt and sugar solution, How to give salt and sugar solution	**Thinking of ways to help children learn about hygiene** Brainstorm and discussion	**Learning about evaluation** Evaluating the course
10.00 to 11.00	Causes and prevention of diarrhoea using serialized pictures or other participatory activities	Use pictures and/ or hollow gourd or container to illustrate fluid loss Demonstrate need for water with two plants, one wilting	Discussion of what local fluids could be used, and Whether children should eat/breast-feed when they have diarrhoea	Ideas for using stories and games	How to help children review their activities? E.g. how often they help to make salt and sugar solution Drawing pictures of things they now do differently

Morning Break				
11.30 to 12.30	Talking with children about diarrhoea: Explore the use of games, stories, discussion, pictures	Preparing for afternoon activity How can children find out more?	Prepare song or rhyme about diarrhoea	Role play Presenting a story to children Explore ways of helping children to invent a story	Discuss ideas on drama and street-theatre, Small group work to consider how to organize children to prepare drama or street-theatre
Lunch Break				
13.30 to	Activities with children Using pictures and stories to find out more	Activities with children Fidning out about diarrhoea at home, How many children have had it? How to treat it? Can children identify causes in their homes?	Activities with children What have they found out What actions can they take? Help them draw a map of their compound or community	Activities with children Explore ways of helping children find out about dehydration – Help them replace words of a popular song with rehydration words, learn and sing them	Activities with children Assist participants to work with children to prepare short (5 minute) dramas, Practise the drama Present them to the other groups and feed back
16.00 to 17.00	Debrief	Debrief	Debrief	Debrief	Debrief Where to go from here? Plan work and follow up
17.00 to 17.30	Evaluation	Evaluation	Evaluation	Evaluation	Evaluation

Supervisors' course: Objectives and sample timetable

The course will provide the participants with opportunities to practice certain supervisory skills in a non-threatening context, and to plan a hygiene promotion project. By the end of the course the participants should be able to:

○ carry out preliminary needs assessment, planning implementation, monitoring and report writing activities;
○ recruit and select suitable facilitators for the project;
○ demonstrate reasonable negotiation skills.

This course assumes that the supervisors already have reasonable knowledge of water- and sanitation-related diseases and some experience in participatory hygiene promotion techniques.

Table A5.3 Supervisor's course timetable

Time	Day 1	Day 2	Day 3	Day 4	Day 5	Day 6
09.00 to 10.00	**Introduction** to purpose of course, timetable housekeeping arrangements people introductions	**Assessment** in small groups Prepare list of essential information needed for a rapid assessment	**Analyse information** matrix ranking of expected common risk practices in local community	**Recuitment and selection** discussion of job description, essential and desirable qualities	**Discussion** and preparation of sample contracts for facilitators	**Evaluation and feedback** Discussion on why to evaluate Small group work to develop indicators for monitoring
10.00 to 11.00	Expectations and anxieties	Rank in order of importance items on other groups' lists	Prepare charts and pictograms to present common risk practices expected	Preparation of list of essential and desirable qualities for each job in the team	**Negotiations** Discuss principles of good negoti-ations and win-win outcomes	Feedback ideas of groups on indicators in plenary
			Morning Break			
11.30 to 12.30	Role-play of health lecture Discuss learning style and how adults learn	**Simulated participatory exercise** (Time-line, three-pile sorting, explor-atory walk, mapping) using own local experiences	**Brainstorm** and discuss ideas on interventions necessary in expected local situation	**Simulation exercise** Role-play recruitment interviews – preparing interview questions	**Simulation exercise** Role-play negotiation – preparation of roles	Where do we go from here? Prepare plans and follow up actions
			Lunch Break			
13.30 to 15.30	**Attitudes of health workers** case study exercise and discussion	**Small group** discussions on how to obtain different type of essential information in a rapid assessment	**Planning** introduction to the log-frames	**Simulated exercise (continued)** Role-play recruitment intervies – role-play followed by discussion	**Simulated exercise (continued)** Role-play negotiation – role-play (for maximum of 30 minutes) followed by discussion of key points	Review plans, finalize and prepare action plans
15.30 to 17.00	Prepare list of important attitudes necessary for facilitators and supervisors	Finalize assessment list and ways to collect the information	Prepare aims, objectives and activities for assess-ment and implementation activities (in small groups)	**Debrief**	**Debrief**	**Report writing** Prepare report of the training and action plans
17.00 to 17.30	**Evaluation**	**Evaluation**	**Evaluation**	**Evaluation**	**Evaluation**	**Evaluation**

Campaign workers' course: Objectives and sample timetable

The objective of this training is to enable participants to communicate hygiene promotion information in an acute emergency. By the end of the training session the participants should be able to:

o explain the relationship between hygiene activities and water- and sanitation-related diseases;
o demonstrate the ability to communicate priority messages effectively to large crowds;
o understand the purpose of the campaign, and their roles and responsibilities within it.

Table A5.4 Campaign worker's course timetable

Time	
0.900 to 11.00	**Priority messages** o Introductions. o Divide participants into small groups, give each group a set of picture cards and ask them to carry out one of the participatory exercises as described in the appendices, e.g. three-pile sorting. o Encourage the participants to discuss their own knowledge and experience around this participatory exercise. Allow 30 minutes maximum for these discussions. o Ask the groups to give feedback to the plenary on the results of their discussions. Clarify and emphasize any points relating to safe defecation, water use and hand washing.
11.00 to 12.30	**Communication skills** o Organize a role-play of poor communication using a megaphone. The actor could mumble, use unclear and descriptive language and fail to give clear instructions as to water sites, chlorination practices. o Ask the whole group to brainstorm the problems they noticed with the communication. o Divide the large group into small groups of six to eight people and ask the small groups to practise communicating with the use of a megaphone. Participants should be asked to give each other feedback as part of this process. o Choose a participant who demonstrated the use of a megaphone message effectively. o Ask participants to discuss how to organize themselves to achieve maximum coverage of the target population.
12.30 to 13.00	o Clarify the purpose of the campaign. o Discuss roles and responsibilities of communicators in the campaign and their relationship with the community members, and with other organizers of the campaign. o Confirm logistical arrangements.

Latrine and water source attendants' course: Objectives and sample timetable

The objective of this training is to enable participants to understand the importance of using and maintaining clean water sources and latrine facilities and be able to communicate these messages to community members. By the end of the training session the participants should be able to:

o explain the relationship between hygiene activities and water- and sanitation-related diseases;
o demonstrate the ability to communicate priority messages effectively to users;
o understand the purpose of their roles in promoting hygiene and health in the community.

Table A5.5 Latrine and water source attendant's course timetable

Time	
0.900 to 11.00	**Priority messages** ○ Introductions. ○ Purpose of course, timetable, remuneration, etc. ○ Divide participants into small groups, give each group a set of picture cards and ask them to carry out one of the participatory exercises as described in the appendices, e.g. three-pile sorting. ○ Encourage the participants to discuss their own-knowledge and experience around this participatory exercise. Allow 30 minutes maximum for these discussions. ○ Ask the groups to give feedback to the plenary on the results of their discussions. Clarify and emphasize any points relating to safe defecation, water use and hand washing.
	Morning Break
11.30 to 12.30	**Communication skills** ○ Organize a role-play of a poor one-to-one communication message about dirty latrines or water sources. The actor could shout, point their fingers, use unclear and descriptive language and fail to give clear instructions about how to use the latrine or water-point etc. ○ Ask the whole group to brainstorm the problems they noticed with the communication. ○ Divide the large group into small groups of six to eight people and ask the small groups to practise communicating one-to-one more effectively. Participants should be asked to give each other feedback as part of this process. ○ Ask participants to demonstrate this who effectively demonstrated the use of one-to-one communication.
	Lunch Break
13.30 to 14.30	**Water and sanitation problems and solutions** ○ Brainstorm about water and sanitation problems in the camp ○ Discussion about possible solutions to the water and sanitation problems ○ **Role of latrine and water source attendant** ○ Discuss roles and responsibilities of attendants to fulfil those identified solutions. Identify the support required to enable them to perform their roles effectively (materials, logistics, etc.) ○ Discuss information requirements and demonstrate the filling in and compilation of information from the latrine and water source data collection sheets ○ Clarify and confirm job description of attendants
16.30 to 17.00	**Review and evaluation** ○ What will their roles be? ○ How can information help them and their families?

A6

Management tools

Expectations and ground rules

Where project goals and ways of working are not clarified, individuals work according to their own values and principles. Even the most well-intentioned individuals can have very different values and principles. This results in confusion and duplication of effort. The following training session has been used to develop ground rules or guiding principles for projects, training courses or sessions. This session will help participants to elaborate in detail what participants want and do not want from the project, training course or session. It provides a visible record of what people do and do not want, making it easier to determine just how much consensus exists beforehand, and to work towards a higher level of agreement.

For the session, you will need card or paper of two different colours. You will also need a number of dark marker pens (blue, black or green) for participants to use to write on the cards. You will also need drawing pins and a soft board, or tape or 'blu-tack' for sticking the cards or papers to a wall.

○ Give each participant three pieces of card or paper of each colour.
○ Decide which colour represents positive issues and which represents negative issues.
○ Prepare the question you wish to answer. Write it on a large piece of paper in large clear writing. For example 'What are your expectations of this team/project/training course?'.
○ On a coloured piece of paper matching the positive colour, write a positive statement summarizing positive answers to the question, and on a piece of paper the same colour as the negative papers write a negative statement summarizing the answers to the question. For example, for the question 'What are your expectations?', the positive statement would read 'Hopes' and the negative statement would read 'Fears'.
○ Distribute the coloured papers. Ask participants to write their answers to the question on the cards using one colour for positive answers, and the other colour for negative answers. For example, to the question, 'What are your expectations of this training course', participants may write their fears ('I will learn nothing new', 'late starts and late finishes'), and their hopes ('share experiences with new friends', 'what is said in the class will not be repeated outside'). For the question, 'What are your expectations of this project and team?', participants may write things like 'assist poor people first' and 'admit mistakes' as hopes, and 'favouritism', 'embezzlement', 'never delivering on promises' as fears.
○ As the papers are being written, take the papers and stick them on the soft board or wall. Cluster them together with other similar ideas under the positive or negative headings. When people are running out of ideas, sum up the answers and ask for clarification over any that are not obvious to read or understand. Papers can be rewritten to summarize a cluster of answers or to clarify an answer.
○ Discuss the answers among the group. Try to reach a consensus about which there are basic ground rules. This also provides an opportunity for you to respond to those expectations that are or are not likely to be met.

It is also helpful to refer back to these charts during the evaluation at the end of the session or course. If ground rules have been developed for a project, these can be written out to see the extent to which people's expectations have or have not been met.

○ Write all the different ideas on a new list. Ask two participants to select the most important principles from the list. Ask the group to review these principles and finally agree.
○ Prepare these as ground rules in the local language. Prepare a copy of the list for all staff members to sign. Keep the signed copies in their personnel files.
○ Share the ground rules with community members and other key stakeholders.

Source: Adapted from Pretty, et al, 1995.

Role play: Negotiation skills

Most people take part in negotiations every day. An ability to negotiate effectively is an important skill for managers and supervisors to develop. The purpose of this exercise is to help participants to understand the principles of effective negotiation and to practise negotiating win-win solutions in a non-threatening setting.

○ The course organizer should think of a situation that is likely to require negotiation in the context of hygiene promotion in emergencies. For example, this could be negotiations with community leaders about priority needs from the different perspectives of the community and project staff. The community might be concerned about lack of school facilities, while the project has identified lack of sanitation as a major health risk. Or perhaps the negotiation could focus on community contributions for the long term maintenance of facilities where the expectation of the leaders is that the project will take this responsibility. Write a brief explanation of the scenario on a flipchart and place it where the participants can see it. Provide the participants with a handout containing the points to bear in mind when negotiating (to be found on page 72).
○ Divide the participants into three groups: one for each side of the negotiation and one for observers. Each group should allocate roles to its members, i.e. the community groups could have a thoughtful elderly chairperson, an energetic youth leader, a school teacher, a business person, while the project group could have a community facilitator, a project supervisor and a project manager. Observers should select specific skills to look out for during the role play (using the handout for guidance). Roles could be distributed on pre-written cards if preferred.
○ Ask the participants to imagine themselves in their roles. Then ask each group to prepare their shopping lists of ideal and worst case scenarios (this might take 20 minutes). Then ask the group to consider the opposite group's role and imagine their shopping lists. Observers can also prepare the shopping lists for both sides of the negotiation.
○ Introduce the players and their roles. Ask them to role play the negotiation and ask the observers to take notes of what happens. Stop the negotiation if it is not complete at the end of 30 minutes.
○ Disengage the participants from their roles by asking them to get out of role and reintroduce themselves to the rest of the group with their real names and a quick summary of who they really are.
○ Ask the participants in turn how they behaved in the role play, why they behaved that way and what they learnt from it. How did they feel about the other people in the role play? Ask the observers to point out helpful and unhelpful aspects of the negotiation. How could it have been improved?

At the end of the discussion the issues can be summarized. If there is time, the groups could be asked to re-enact the scene with different negotiating styles. Remember, debriefing each participant individually from their roles is absolutely essential. If this is not done, uncomfortable feelings brought out by the roles and between the actors may cause problems later.

How to do a stakeholder analysis

The objective of a stakeholder analysis is to determine the influence and importance to the project of its stakeholders and the extent to which the interests must be satisfied in order to ensure the project's success.

Stakeholder analysis can be done in the following way:

○ Identify the community leaders and health workers in the community and discuss with them.
○ Ask them to identify all the stakeholders with responsibilities for, or influence on, hygiene.
○ Ask them to rank the stakeholders in terms of importance and influence using a scale of 0 for none to 10 for maximum. Mark these in a table. (*Influence* is the power that stakeholders have over a project to control what decisions are made, or to facilitate its implementation either positively or negatively. It is the extent to which stakeholders are able to persuade or coerce others into making decisions and following certain courses of action. *Importance* indicates the priority given by the project to satisfying those stakeholders' needs and interests through the delivery of the project. In general terms, they can be determined by examining the goal, purpose and outputs of the project.)
○ Discuss the possible interests (positive and negative) that the stakeholders may have in relation to hygiene promotion. Record these in the table.
○ Plot on a chart the rankings of influence and importance of the different stakeholders. Draw gridlines half way up the scale of both axes (i.e. for both influence and for importance). This divides the chart into four boxes of equal size. Note which groups fall into the different boxes. Note the findings in your report.

An example of a stakeholder analysis in an imaginary refugee camp can be found on page 225.

Source: Adapted from Reed and Skinner, 1998.

Example of a stakeholder analysis

The stakeholder analysis for hygiene promotion in an imaginary refugee camp has been prepared below:

In this example, the groups in the top right-hand box are of high importance and high influence. Stakeholders in these groups include the target community, donor agencies, camp administrators, health workers and facilitators, politicians, host government officials and teachers. Good relations with them, including meeting at least some of their needs, are essential for the success of the project. In this example, Group D has high influence and low importance. This group are the religious leaders and without their support the project could fail. Their opinions therefore need to be monitored.

Groups I, E and H have low influence and high importance. These groups include women and children with little formal education, community health workers, community-based organizations and the host community. Special initiatives are required to involve them in the project and to protect their interests. Groups G and F have low influence and low importance. These groups are the traditional healers and the traditional midwives. In this example they do not have to be considered specifically in project activities.

Source: Reed and Skinner, 1998.

Table A6.1 Example of stakeholder analysis

Stakeholders	Interest in hygiene improvement	Influence	Importance	Group
Male householder heads of target community	○ improved health ○ increased privancy ○ raised status	10	10	A
Uneducated women and children of target community	○ improved health of self and family ○ increased privacy ○ raised status ○ extra efforts and time required	4	10	I
Donor agencies	○ institutional learning ○ spending money ○ conserving staff inputs ○ sector objectives	10	10	A
Camp administrators	○ achievement of targets ○ salaries and allowances ○ control of funds and activities ○ need donors to fund the activities	9	8	B
Community facilitators	○ salaries and allowances ○ achievement of targets	9	7	C
Health workers	○ achievement of targets ○ may work only if receive allowance and transport	9	7	C
Politicians	○ political influence ○ control of activities ○ status ○ added responsibiliy	9	7	C
Host government officials	○ achievement targets and standards of service provision ○ more work	9	7	C
Teachers	○ improvement of school environment ○ achievement of targets	9	8	C
Religious leaders	○ social/religious influence ○ powerty reduction	9	4	D
Indigenous institutions	○ social influence	4	8	E
Community health workers	○ status ○ may want to work only if receive allowances or incentives	4	8	E
Community-based organisations	○ public image ○ improving local lives of people ○ improving local environment	4	8	E
Artisians	○ income generation ○ status	4	8	E
Traditional midwives	○ improve child survival ○ private incomes	4	4	E
Traditional healers	○ potential loss of income	4	2	G
Host population	○ employment opporunities ○ long-term development ○ resentment if not treated equally	3	6	G

Table A6.2 Stakeholder chart

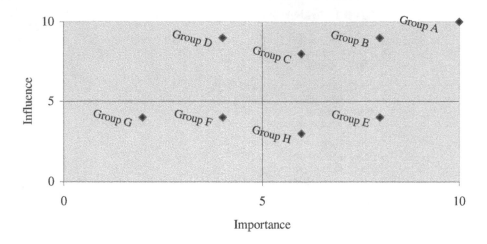

Example of a situation report (sitrep) outline

This guide has been developed for the person responsible for preparing written reports about the project. It is intended to give an idea of the sort of information that the agency is interested in, and the sort of information that you should be reporting to your manager, beyond the purely technical aspects of the project.

Box A6.1 Example of a situation report

Title of report...

Date of report...

Report intended for...

1 Main developments in emergency
   - Summary of main developments since last report including, where significant:
     - main changes in emergency needs, including security;
     - main developments in political situation and government activity towards agencies;
     - progress/problems in relevant operations of other organizations.

2 Progress of your project's response
   - Progress in implementing previous plans and difficulties or developments affecting progress; main issues occupying staff time.
   - How project is to change, or new projects to be added, to accommodate developments in the situation, and how problems facing the project are to be approached.
   - Priorities for action – plans for near and mid-term future, and assumptions on which these are based.

- Also report on deployment, movement and morale of staff, and proposed changes in staffing.

3 Visits
- Report on visits to local office or project by non-project staff, or by project staff to places relevant to the emergency.

4 Public profile
- Report on lobbying activity – main issues raised and with whom; priorities, aims and strategy to take these issues forward. Lobbying issues or changes of strategy that field would like HQ to take forward.
- Press line – should indicate which information is confidential and what might usefully be publicized and how.

5 Review of objectives
- Summary of main uncertainties in emergency situation or in overall relief effort and possible outcomes.
- What are the present priorities for your team?
- Have original project objectives, and activities designed to achieve them, been changed, or the emphasis within aims or strategies altered?

6 Reports produced
- List reports you have written (tours, meetings, projects) since last written a situation report, and their respective circulation lists.

Source: Davis and Lambert, 1995.

A7

Monitoring and evaluation tools

Example of facilitators' self-assessment tool

Self-assessment charts are a useful way to evaluate how you have performed as a facilitator. Charts can be kept over a long period and the facilitator can monitor how their performance has changed over time. This facilitators' assessment form is based on a radar chart.

After a training session or a training course, the facilitator can use a chart such as the one below to assess him or herself according to how they feel they have performed in each of the different categories. The better they feel they have performed, the further away from the middle they mark that line. Ideally, the facilitator will think that they have performed equally well in each of the areas. Where they have performed less well, they can use the form to identify areas for self-development.

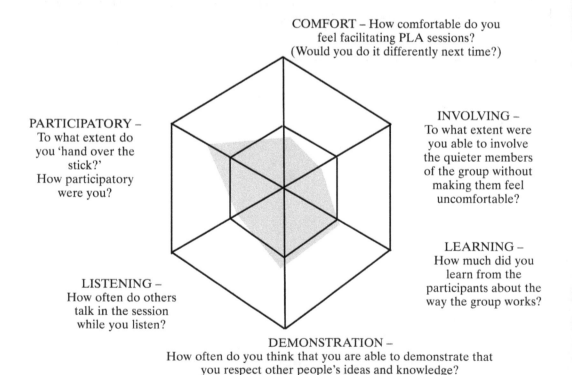

COMFORT – How comfortable do you feel facilitating PLA sessions? (Would you do it differently next time?)

INVOLVING – To what extent were you able to involve the quieter members of the group without making them feel uncomfortable?

PARTICIPATORY – To what extent do you 'hand over the stick?' How participatory were you?

LEARNING – How much did you learn from the participants about the way the group works?

LISTENING – How often do others talk in the session while you listen?

DEMONSTRATION – How often do you think that you are able to demonstrate that you respect other people's ideas and knowledge? (How much did you learn about people's own situations?)

Figure A7.1 Example facilitator's self assessment tool

Example of participants' course assessment flipchart

Flipcharts can be used as a way of allowing participants to give their ideas about a session or training course. They can be used to improve the training session or course for future occasions. This can be done without the individual's identity being revealed. In this example the facilitator writes a relevant title on the flipchart and places it in a convenient location. The facilitator then explains the purpose of the chart and what will happen to the comments collected. Participants are then given some time to post their comments on the flip chart, such as during a lunch or tea break. Discussion about the comments is not required unless some of them are unclear.

Box A7.1 Participants' comments about the course

Good things:
o   Enjoyed sharing ideas with other participants;
o   Surprised how much the community knew already;
o   More confident now about doing my job.

Bad things:
o   Too much packed into too short a time;
o   Session on how people learn was too long.

Example of the findings of a focus group discussion

Table A7.1 Summary of focus group discussion

Group details	Group characteristics	Group needs
General	Mostly farmers eight women and three men	1. Water 2. Income generating activities
Water	Collect water from public water points that are open once in four days. All use unprotected springs at other times. Mostly women and girls fetch water, sometimes men also. Big queues at springs, sometimes fighting. Laundry done at springs by women.	Would like existing public water points to operate each day for two hours. Prepared to manage the water points themselves and to pay more for a better water service. Think the problem is not a shortage of water but a problem with the water department.
Sanitation	Most use latrines, few defecate in open areas. Males and females use the same place, but at different times. Those in rented housing do not have latrines. Women clean latrines. Latrines collapse if pits not lined with stone or brick. Solid waste generally burned.	Those without latrines, mostly in rented housing, would like community latrines. Prepared to help with the construction. Would like water at the latrine but difficult to arrange. Require local authorities to allocate site for solid waste disposal.
Health	Health awareness was good, people were aware of the link between water, sanitation and diarrhoea. Health education carried out at the health centre, but need more in the community. Diseases include TB (from dust), malnutrition in children and diarrhoea.	More health education through health workers at community level, which is more appropriate to the needs of the local people and the culture than the methods that have been utilized before.

Source: JICA, 1994.

Example of community monitoring for latrine use

Self-monitoring forms can be provided to people in communities to monitor events in that community. For example, a hygiene promoter may encourage some mothers to complete self-monitoring forms for latrine use and maintenance or for mortality and morbidity over one month. Each selected mother would be given a form to fill in over the following five weeks. The words or symbols used on the form should preferably be selected by the people who are going to use the form. If this is not possible, agreement should be reached with the whole group about what the symbols represent and how the forms are to be completed.

	Week 1	Week 2	Week 3	Week 4	Week 5
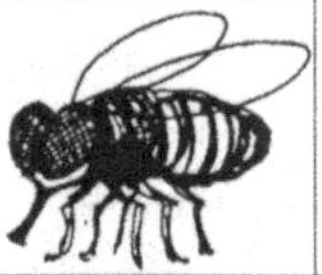					
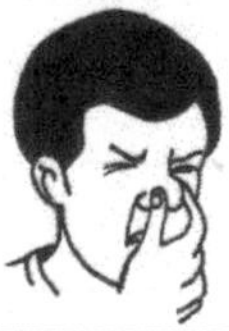					
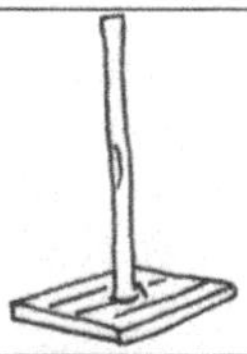					
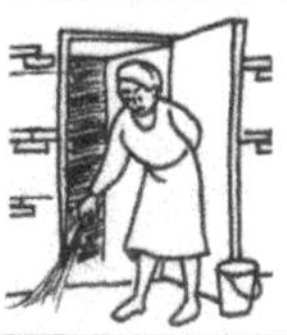					
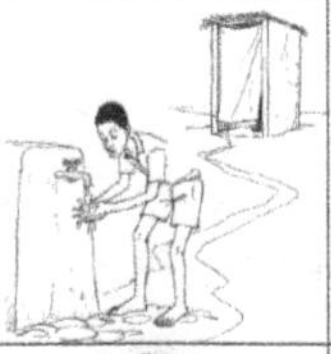					
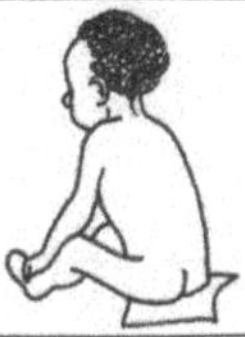					

Figure A7.2 Example of community monitoring for latrine use

231

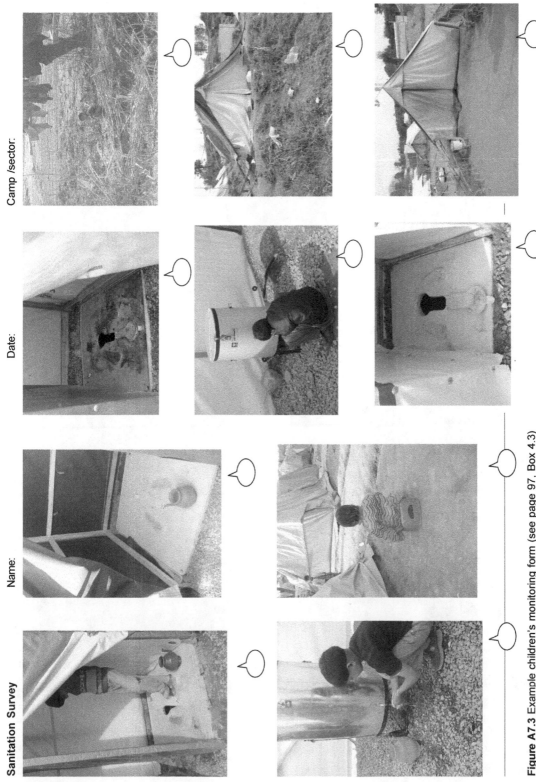

Figure A7.3 Example children's monitoring form (see page 97, Box 4.3)

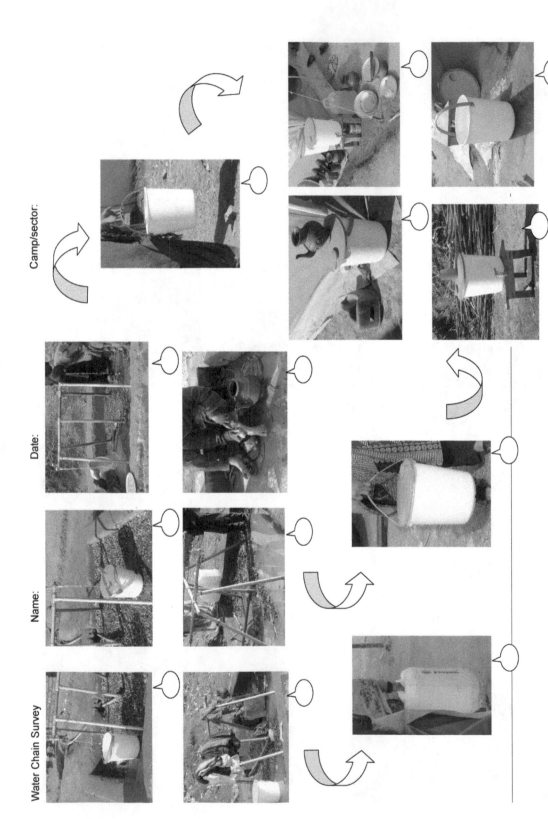

Figure A7.4 Example children's monitoring form 2

A8

Common water- and sanitation-related diseases in emergencies

This section provides a brief outline of the water- and sanitation-related diseases which are common in emergencies. It includes an estimate of the general global morbidity and mortality associated with the diseases, their transmission patterns and ways to prevent them. There is a detailed section on each of the diseases with special reference to prevention in emergencies.

Increased vulnerability of people affected by emergencies

Refugees, displaced people or returnees may be particularly vulnerable to disease.
  For the following reasons:
○ They will often be living in cramped and overcrowded conditions where maintaining hygiene is very difficult.
○ They will probably have suffered severe stress from the fear and ordeal of their journey and from the loss of loved ones; this may make them more prone to illness.
○ Trauma may have caused blood loss and anaemia, making them more likely to become ill.
○ Malnutrition or under-nutrition may make them less able to fight off infections.
○ They may move into an area where there are new diseases that they are not used to.

Transmission patterns and preventive measures for water- and sanitation-related diseases common in emergency situations

Faecal–oral diseases
The diseases in this category are caused by faeces from a person infected with the disease entering the mouth of another person. Faecal–oral diseases include simple diarrhoea and various diarrhoeal diseases (dysentery, cholera, giardia), typhoid and intestinal worms.

Symptoms of diarrhoea
Diarrhoea is defined as the passing of three or more watery stools in 24 hours and there are many different types. It is a major cause of morbidity and mortality in populations affected by emergencies. It is responsible for a significant proportion of the burden of disease in non-emergency situations. Diarrhoea can be caused by bacteria, protozoa or viruses, and can be accompanied by other symptoms such as fever and vomiting. Diarrhoea may result from swallowing relatively few organisms which can quickly multiply in the intestines.

  Babies excrete disease-causing organisms in their faeces; in fact, infants' faeces contain more disease-causing organisms per gram than do adults' faeces. As babies and young children are more susceptible to these diseases, their faeces should be considered more dangerous than adults' faeces.

Table A8.1 Transmission patterns and preventive measures for water- and sanitation-related diseases common in emergency situations

Infection	Transmission pattern	Human excreta disposal	Solid waste disposal	Waste water disposal	Safe water chain	Hand wash-ing	Food hygi-ene	Washing clothes and body
Various types of diarrhoea, dysentery, poliomselitis, typhoid and paratyphoid, hepatitis A	From human faeces to mouth (faceal-oral) via multiple routes of faceal contaminated water, fingers and hands, food, soil and surfaces. Animal faces may also contain diarrhoeal disease organisms.	✓	✓		✓	✓	✓	
Roundworm (Ascariasis), Whipworm (Trichuriasis)	From faeces to mouth. Worm eggs in human faeces develop in soil before being ingested through raw food, dirty hands and playing with things that have been in contact with infected soil. Soil on feet and shoes can transport the eggs long distances. Animals eating human faeces pass on the eggs in their own faeces.	✓	✓			✓	✓	
Hookworm	From faeces to skin (especially feet): Worm eggs in the faeces deposited in moist soil, hatch into larvae which enter the skin of people's feet	✓						
Schistosomiasis (Bilharzia)	From faeces to urine to skin: Worm eggs in human faeces or urine have to reach water where they hatch and enter the snails. In the snails they develop and are passed on as free swimming 'cercariae' which penetrate the skin when people come into contact with infested waters.	✓			✓			
Scabies, Ringworm, yaws	From skin to skin: both through direct skin contact and through sharing of clothes, bedclothes and towels							✓
Trachoma, Conjunctivitis	From eyes to eyes: both direct contact with the discharge from an infected eye and through contact with articles soiled by a discharge, such as towels, bedding, clothing, wash basins, washing water. Flies may also act as transmission agents.							✓
Louse-borne typhus, Louse-born relapsing fever	From person to person: Through bites of body lice which travel from person-to-person, through sharing clothes and bedclothes, particularly when underwear is not washed regularly.							✓
Malaria, Dengue fever, Yellow fever	From person to person through the bite of infected mosquitoes. The mosquito breeds in standing water			✓				
Leishmaniasis	From person to person through the bite of infected phlebotomine sandflies. The sandflies breed in damp organic debris, including excreta and solid waste.	✓	✓					

Source: Adapted from Boot and Cairncross, 1993; Ministry of Health Uganda, 1998a and 1998b.

There are a variety of organisms that cause diarrhoea: the following represent only some of them. With the majority of diarrhoeas it may not be possible to diagnose a particular cause.

Dysentery

Dysentery is a form of bloody diarrhoea transmitted through the faecal–oral route. When people become infected, they excrete large numbers of the infective organisms in their stools. If the bacteria from these stools come into contact with food, water or hands the infection can be passed to other people.

A person with dysentery passes faeces containing blood and often mucus. This is accompanied by fever, vomiting and stomach pains. It is usually caused by an organism known as *Shigella*, which has a variety of different forms. *Shigella* dysentery is endemic in many countries in the tropics, reaching its highest incidence in the rainy seasons. The disease usually occurs in two phases – an initial phase with fever and watery stools that can be very serious and cause dehydration and delirium, especially in children. The latter phase is accompanied with loose, frequent stools containing blood and mucus and may cause severe discomfort and pain. The only proven way of preventing infection and transmission of all types of *Shigella* dysentery is hand washing with soap (and breastfeeding for infants). Methods for preventing other forms of diarrhoea are also likely to reduce the transmission of dysentery.

Amoebic dysentery is the type of diarrhoea or dysentery (diarrhoea with blood) caused by the protozoa called *amoeba*. Amoebae may also cause abscesses in the liver, which can result in extreme pain in the right upper belly. Usually the diarrhoea comes and goes and there may even be constipation. There are cramps in the belly and the person experiences an urgent need to pass stools even when there is very little stool there. With amoebae there is usually no fever.

Cholera

Cholera is caused by one particular type of bacterium called *Vibrio cholerae*. Symptoms are usually mild but in a minority of cases there is a rapid onset of severe watery diarrhoea and vomiting, and sometimes cramps in the stomach, arms or legs. So much water and salts may be lost from the body of a person with cholera that the person becomes thirsty, stops urinating, and quickly becomes weak and dehydrated. Dehydration can lead to circulatory collapse and death. To prevent dehydration, the person must drink at least the volume of fluid the body is losing. Drinking ORS will replace salts and sugars which have also been lost from the body. Oral cholera vaccination is said by the WHO to be safe and to offer 70 per cent protection from infection. It is recommended by the WHO for helping to prevent and control cholera outbreaks in displaced populations. See www.who.int/cholera

Special measures to prevent the spread of cholera during an outbreak

o   Try to identify the source of the cholera, and whether particular areas or people are affected.
o   Prevent use of contaminated water sources.
o   Intensify the information campaign to promote hand washing, use of latrines and prompt identification and treatment (it may be necessary to appoint/employ case finders who identify patients on home visits).
o   Establish emergency isolation centres for sick patients (special precautions for disinfection should be in operation here).
o   Establish ORS centres to provide rehydration of less severe cases.

Management of cholera patients in an outbreak

o   Help them to drink plenty of fluid (preferably ORS) to prevent the dehydration that kills.
o   Help them get medical attention immediately.

Box A8.1 Making oral rehydration solution

Drinking plenty of any drink available in the home will help to prevent dehydration.

ORS is a special mixture of salts and sugars. When ORS solution is given to someone with dehydration, it will assist rehydration very quickly. ORS sachets are available for mixing with water. They can be obtained at health units, pharmacies and at other retail outlets.

To make ORS, follow the instructions on the packet. Usually these are the instructions:

1. Add one sachet of ORS salts to 1 litre of drinking water,
2. Mix thoroughly,
3. Taste the drink to make sure it is no more salty than tears.
4. Give a dehydrated person as much as they seem to want and if severely dehydrated, give sips to drink every five minutes, day or night, until they begin to urinate normally. This may take 3–5 days.
5. If a child vomits up the solution, wait ten minutes and continue to give small sips of the solution from a teaspoon (the child will absorb more of the solution than she or he vomits).
6. If the diarrhoea continues, seek medical help.

The person should also drink plenty of other fluids such as water, porridge drinks, soups, coconut milk and continue to eat solid food. Breastfeeding should be continued. If no ORS is available, a home made solution can be prepared using eight level teaspoons of sugar and one level teaspoon of salt in one litre of water. If available, some squeezed orange juice or mashed banana can be added to provide potassium. It is very important to ensure that the solution does not contain too much salt as this can be very dangerous, especially for a baby. *Always* taste the mixture to make sure that it is not more salty than tears.[3]

A useful website on ORS is: www.rehydrate.org/dehydration/treatment_plans.htm

---

○ Dispose of faeces in a latrine.
○ Wash hands frequently and thoroughly with soap and water.

Typhoid

Typhoid is a faecal–oral disease causing loose stools and a gradually increasing fever often accompanied by a relatively slow pulse. People with typhoid fever usually feel very unwell with generalized aches and pains and loss of appetite. Delirium (not being able to think clearly or make sense) may also be present as the illness progresses. The organism that causes typhoid is known as *Salmonella typhi*. The illness may cause death if not treated.

Giardia

Giardia is a faecal–oral disease. The symptoms are foul-smelling yellow diarrhoea that has bubbles in it. If blood or mucus is present it is probably not Giardia. In addition, the belly is swollen and uncomfortable and produces lots of gas. Giardia can clear up without medical treatment but if the diarrhoea goes on for more than 10 days it is best to seek medical advice. Long-term infection with Giardia can cause significant weight loss.

Hepatitis A

Hepatitis A is another faecal–oral disease. The disease causes acute inflammation of the liver. It usually starts with fever, chills, headaches and fatigue. A few days later there is often loss of appetite, vomiting, dark urine and light-coloured faeces, and jaundice of the skin or the outer coating of the eyeballs. In young children there may be few symptoms but in older people the jaundice may be severe

---

[3]The amount of salt and sugar and container for measuring the amount of water (for example, beer bottle, fizzy drink bottle) recommended in different countries may vary. Always check with the ministry of health in the country you are working in and follow their guidelines.

and prolonged; complete liver failure may occur and the patient may lapse into a coma. There are other forms of hepatitis, hepatitis B and C, with similar symptoms but that are not transmitted through the faecal–oral route but through blood and sexual contact.

Hepatitis E
Hepatitis E is also transmitted via the faecal–oral route. Contaminated water or food supplies have been implicated in major outbreaks. Epidemics have been reported in central and South East Asia, North and West Africa and Mexico. Death rates range between 0.5 and 4 per cent, and during pregnancy death rates can be as high as 20 per cent in the last three months of pregnancy. The disease is most common in young adults between 15 and 40 years of age. It occurs frequently in children but is usually mild or without symptoms. The typical signs include jaundice, loss of appetite, nausea, vomiting and fever – similar to Hepatitis A and the distinction is usually made on laboratory examination.

Roundworm
As their name suggests, these worms are round and can be up to 30 cm in length. They live in the intestines and feed off whatever food is ingested. This may make the person feel very weak as he or she is not getting enough food to eat. The worms may also block the intestine and cause problems with defecation.

The roundworm eggs follow the faecal–oral route of transmission usually through unclean fingers or unwashed fruit and raw vegetables. Raw fruit and vegetables may become contaminated when people with roundworm defecate on the ground near to where vegetables or fruit are growing. Because children often put their fingers and other objects in their mouths they are more at risk.

Whipworm
Whipworms are small thin worms and look like sewing threads. Infection occurs in a similar way to roundworm, but infection is less likely to be from eating contaminated fruit and raw vegetables as the eggs are more easily killed by drying or by direct sunlight.

Pinworm
Pinworms are very small, thin worms. The worms live in the intestines and at night they emerge from the anus to lay eggs around the opening. Pinworms cause severe itching around the anus. Whenever the person scratches, the eggs will contaminate the fingers and they may re-infect the person if they then put their fingers in their mouth.

Transmission and prevention of all faecal–oral diseases
The 5'Fs' diagram below illustrates the main ways in which diarrhoea may be transmitted and the ways it can be prevented. It summarizes the main ways in which faecal–oral diseases are spread – by faecal germs contaminating fields, fluids, fingers, flies or food, then eventually being swallowed. Most latrines will stop the 'fluids' and 'fields' transmission routes. Some of the more sophisticated latrines, such as the ventilated improved pit (VIP) latrine and pour-flush latrine, may also break the 'flies' route. Using a latrine does not prevent the contamination of hands and fingers. Good hygiene practices are needed for this, particularly the washing of hands with soap after contact with faeces (i.e. after defecation or after cleaning a child).

Hookworm
Hookworms are not strictly a faecal–oral disease, instead they are a faecal–soil-related disease. It can be one of the most damaging diseases of childhood and thrives in overcrowded unsanitary conditions. Hookworms are small and red in colour. They live in the intestines and feed on the blood by

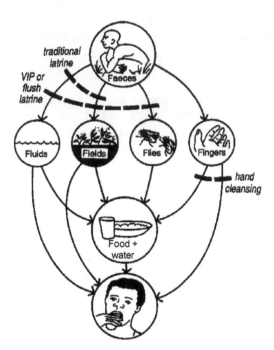

Figure A8.1 5 'F's diagram of transmission of faecal oral disease.
Source: Winblad, 1994.

hooking on to the wall of the gut. If there are many worms, the person may become anaemic and feel very weak and tired. Hookworm eggs are excreted in the stools. Once outside the body they develop into tiny worms (larvae). If someone walks on contaminated ground without any shoes, the worms will pierce the skin of the feet, enter the bloodstream and eventually find their way to the lungs where they develop and feed on blood. When they are mature, the worms are coughed up from the lungs and if the person swallows them in the sputum, they enter the intestine, lay their eggs and the new host then excretes their eggs and the life-cycle starts again.

Prevention of hookworm

○ Build and use latrines;
○ Children should not walk around barefoot.

Hygiene practices that prevent all faecal–oral diseases

The magnitude of risk varies with different hygiene practices. Three practices are considered to be the most significant and cost-effective in preventing faecal–oral diseases. These are:

○ Dispose of faeces safely. Use a latrine or bury faeces, including young children's and babies';
○ Clean hands frequently with soap or ashes, especially after defecation and after clearing up babies' faeces;
○ Maintain drinking water free from faecal contamination.

Other less significant prevention methods related to food hygiene are:

○ Wash hands with soap before preparing or eating food;
○ Protect food from flies;
○ Cook meals thoroughly;
○ Wash raw vegetables and fruit in clean water before eating.

Vector-borne diseases

Certain diseases are spread by insect vectors that live in, or breed near, water. This group includes such diseases as malaria, filariasis, dengue fever, yellow fever, river blindness, leishmaniasis, sleeping sickness and Guinea worm infections. Displaced people may be at particular risk because there may be diseases that they are not used to in the new area of settlement. They will therefore not have built up protection or immunity against these diseases.

Malaria

Malaria is the single most important vector-borne disease. The malaria-spreading mosquitoes are known as *Anopheles* mosquitoes and can be distinguished from other mosquitoes because they rest at an angle with their 'head' down.

There are several species of *Anopheles* mosquitoes; most can breed in still, unpolluted water including swamps and containers. Until recently mosquitoes could not breed above 3,000m altitude but have now started to breed at higher altitudes. *Anopheles* feed on people at night. It is only the females that bite because they need a

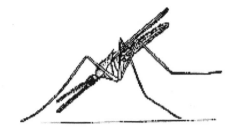

Figure A8.2 Enlarged picture of malarial mosquito (actual length 0.5 cm)

blood meal every 2–3 days to develop each batch of 100–200 eggs. When a mosquito bites its victim to suck blood, it first injects saliva to prevent the blood from clotting and blocking its mouth-parts. In malaria infected mosquitoes, the saliva contains infective forms of the parasite that actually cause malaria known as *Plasmodium*. There are four main types of *Plasmodium* and the most serious is the one that causes cerebral malaria known as *Pl. falciparum*. Most *Anopheles* can fly up to 2km from their breeding site to feed. The adults live for about 30 days. Different types of *Anopheles* mosquitoes live in different habitats, for example *Anopheles gambiae* larvae prefer the sun or partial shade and do not like thick bush. *Anopheles funestus* and *Anopheles mucheti* may infest shaded waters such as lakes and swamps. *Anopheles bwambae* lives in hot salt springs in some places. In emergencies, people may become more at risk of malaria when they have been displaced from an area of low transmission to an area of high transmission as they will have failed to develop sufficient immunity to the disease. For example, malaria and deaths from malaria increased significantly when Rwandans from malaria-free highland areas were forced to flee into lowland areas in Zaire and Tanzania during 1994.

Control of malaria

Control of malaria and other mosquito-borne infections is difficult and requires multiple measures. One of the most important measures may be the choice of settlement. Other measures that can be taken locally include:

o Ensuring adequate drainage around shelters or houses and water collection points using ditches and soak-aways;
o Covering water storage jars, rainwater tanks;
o Draining or filling in places where rain and washing water collects, including ponds or small puddles;
o Distributing and promoting the correct use of insecticide treated bed nets (malaria only);
o Planting of neem trees (*Azadriachta indica*) that repel mosquitoes;
o Removing anything that might collect stagnant water, such as tin cans, broken bottles (mainly effective against dengue);
o Spraying the walls and ceilings of shelters with insecticide may be an option (indoor residual spraying) but care must be taken to use trained personnel who are properly protected.

Dengue fever

Dengue is transmitted mainly by the *Aedes aegypti* mosquito that bites during the day. This mosquito breeds predominantly in containers such as old tins, coconut husks and discarded tyres. Prevention focuses on destroying these habitats or using chemicals to destroy the larvae that breed there.

Dengue causes a high fever, headache and aching joints. Severe bleeding can also occur and death rates can be as high as 40–50 per cent. Subsequently it can cause prolonged tiredness and depression.

Schistosomiasis (bilharzia)

Bilharzia or schistosomiasis is an infection caused by a kind of worm or fluke that gets into the bloodstream. It is becoming an increasingly common disease. In addition to being painful, causing weakness and fever, the kidneys or liver may be badly damaged, which can eventually cause death. There are several types of blood flukes, including:

o *Schistosoma haematobium* that can cause blood in urine and is spread through infected urine;
o *Schistosoma mansoni* that causes bloody diarrhoea and is spread through faeces.

Blood flukes are not spread directly from person to person. Part of their life must be spent inside a certain small water snail (*Bulinus* or *Biophalaria* species). An infected person urinates or defecates in water, passing the worm eggs into the water too. Worm eggs hatch and pass into the snails. Young stages of the worm leave the snail and then bury into the skin of a person who enters the water. In this way, someone who washes or swims in water where an infected person has urinated or defecated also becomes infected.

Prevention of schistosomiasis

Control and prevention of schistosomiasis is difficult, but measures include:

o Safe disposal of faeces and urine by all members of the community. (Even if one infected person urinates in snail-infested water, those snails will continue to produce worms for a long period of time.);
o Avoid skin contact with contaminated water. This means avoiding swimming, washing, clothes washing, walking or playing in contaminated water;
o If contaminated water is collected, all the worms will die within 48 hours providing all the snails are removed, and the water will then be safe for washing in.

Hygiene-related skin and eye infections

These diseases are not caught by drinking or bathing in infected water but, like the diarrhoeas and some of the worm infections, they can be prevented by the use of an increased quantity of water for personal and household hygiene.

Scabies

Scabies is a disease causing very itchy little bumps on the skin. The bumps can appear anywhere on the body but are most common between the fingers, on the wrists, around the waist, on the genitals and between the toes. The bumps are small mites living just under the skin, which make it itch. Scratching the infected skin can help to spread the disease and may also lead to skin lesions that in turn can become infected with bacteria. Scabies is spread by touching the infected skin, clothes or bedclothes of a person with scabies. The disease is very common in children and spreads most rapidly in overcrowded conditions.

Increasing the amount of water available and providing soap can help to reduce the spread of scabies. Treatment is with a solution of Benzyl Benzoate, which is applied to the skin. All bedding and clothes should be washed and hung in the sun to dry.

Prevention of scabies

○ Bathe and change clothes regularly.
○ Wash all clothes and bedding regularly and hang them in the sun.
○ If possible, do not let untreated infected children have contact with uninfected children.

Ringworm

Ringworm is caused by a fungal infection. It appears as small rings on the skin usually on the head, between the legs, between the toes, and under the nails. If it appears on the head it often causes scaly patches or rings on the scalp and the hair around these may fall out. Finger and toe nails infected with ringworm become rough and thick. The disease is very common in children and spreads most rapidly in overcrowded conditions.

Prevention of ringworm

○ Bathe and wash clothes regularly.
○ Do not let a child with ringworm sleep with others.

Trachoma

Trachoma is a chronic eye infection that gets slowly worse. It may last for months or years and can cause blindness if not treated. Trachoma begins with red, watery eyes like conjunctivitis but after a month or more, small lumps begin to develop inside the upper eyelids. These small lumps begin to disappear in a few years to leave scars that make the eyelids thick and may keep them from opening and closing all the way. The scarring may pull the eyelashes down into the eye, scratching the eye and causing blindness. Trachoma produces a discharge from the eyes and is usually spread when the discharge from an infected person comes into contact with another person by flies, contaminated fingers, cloths, towels or bedclothes. It is very common in dry, dusty areas where water is in short supply, and particularly among young children.

Prevention of trachoma

○ Wash the face every day with soap and water.
○ Keep flies away from the face.

Conjunctivitis

Conjunctivitis is another eye disease. It causes the eyes to become red and watery. The eye becomes sore. The eyelids often stick together after sleep. It is especially common in children. It is easily spread from one person to another by flies, fingers, cloths, towels or bedclothes that have been contaminated by the eyes of an infected person.

Prevention of conjunctivitis

○ Wash the face every day with soap and water.
○ Keep flies away from the face.

Typhus and plague

Rats carry fleas which can spread diseases such as typhus. Typhus can also be spread by lice or ticks carried by other animals. Typhus begins like a bad cold and leads to fever and aches and pains in the head and muscles. A rash appears after a few days, first in the armpits and then on the body, then the arms and legs. The rash looks like small bruises. The plague is also spread by rodents. The symptoms include high fever, headache, muscular pains, shaking chills, and often pain in the groin or armpit. The fatality rate for people with plague is 60–65 per cent.

Prevention of typhus and plague

○ Bathe and wash clothes regularly. Delouse the whole family regularly.
○ Hang clothes and bedding out in the sun frequently.
○ Keep animals such as dogs out of dwellings.
○ Discourage rats by burning or burying rubbish and protecting food supplies.
○ Kill rats. Set traps and destroy the rats that are caught.

Poison should be used only if strict controls are possible, as some rodents may be a source of human food, or poison may be allowed to contaminate other food for human consumption.

A9

Excreta disposal technologies for emergency situations

The following excreta disposal technologies have been used effectively in emergency situations.

Defecation trench

Defecation trenches confine excreta to one designated area and may be useful as a first measure in refugee camp situations. Two areas (one for males, one for females) are divided into 1.5m wide strips with poles and tape (or fences). Shallow trenches about 150mm deep are dug along one side of the strip. Defecation is allowed within each opened strip. Several strips can be opened if large numbers of people are using the trenches at the same time. After use, excreta should be covered with loose soil to prevent fly breeding and reduce smells. Hand washing facilities should be available near to the exit of the defecation trenches. Each site requires at least one full-time caretaker, and the system requires strict supervision and management to be effective.

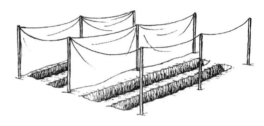

Figure A9.1 Trench latrine

Table A9.1 Advantages and disadvantages of trench latrines

Advantages	Disadvantages
○ Cheap ○ Quick to set up, even for large populations ○ Suitable for initial stages of an emergency	○ Difficult to maintain in a hygienic condition ○ In wet conditions, larvae of hookworms can develop if in contaminated soil ○ Lack of privacy ○ Problems with fly infestation

Pit latrine

This consists of a timber and mud slab or concrete slab over a pit that may be 2m or more in depth. The slab should be firmly supported on all sides and raised above the surrounding ground so that surface water cannot enter the pit. If the sides of the pit are liable to collapse they should be lined with brick, stone or, for short-term use, timber or bamboo. They can also be made in a trapezoidal shape. A squat hole in the slab or a seat is provided so that the excreta falls directly into the pit. A tight-fitting wooden cover over the squat hole when the latrine is not in use will reduce the access of flies into the pit. A small concrete slab or 'sanplat' (0.5m × 0.5m) can be placed over the squat hole for ease of cleaning.

Table A9.2 Advantages and disadvantages of pit latrines

Advantages	Disadvantages
○ Low cost ○ Can be built by householder ○ Needs no water for operation ○ Can be built with a number of squat holes over a larger pit and used communally by a number of users (30 maximum per squat hole)	○ Considerable fly nuisance (and mosquito nuisance if the pit is wet), unless lid is placed over squat hole when not in use ○ Smell problems ○ Wooden slabs may rot within three years ○ Life of latrine limited by size of pit and number of users or the strength of slab

The smell and fly nuisance can be reduced by throwing handfuls of ash or lime into the pit each week, or by smoking the pit. Solutions to common problems with pit latrines can be found below.

Place a tight-fitting wooden or concrete lid over the squat hole. A mud floor can be moulded to fit the lid exactly.

Family latrines take time to construct but are usually a better used and maintained option. Families may be able to build one latrine each or share with a few other families. Large communal latrines are usually unsuitable because there is no sense of ownership and therefore people are rarely motivated to keep them clean; where space is limited there may be no alternative. Recruiting latrine attendants to clean and organize the use of the latrines may help. Squatting holes should be covered with a lid to prevent access by flies.

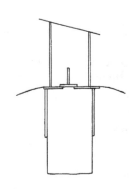

Figure A9.2 Pit latrine

Solutions for common problems with pit latrines

Cost

○ Construct a shallower pit (each person produces only 0.05m dry sludge over one year).

Figure A9.3 Cross section of pit latrine

○ Use local materials for slab and superstructure (banana leaf, papyrus for walls/roof).

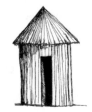

Figure A9.4 Pit latrine hut

○ Use scrap materials for superstructure (For example, scrap metal for doors or walls).

Figure A9.5 Pit latrine curtain

Bad smells

○ Throw handfuls of ash or lime into the pit over the excreta.

Figure A9.6 Hand sprinkling ash

○ Smoke the pit by throwing burning grass, papers or fire embers into the latrine pit.

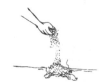

Figure A9.7 Flaming stick

○ Provide the latrine with a vent pipe (see VIP latrine option, below).

○ Use a timber and mud slab and keep it clean by smearing frequently with fresh mud and cow dung.

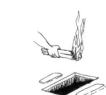

Figure A9.8 Cross section of pit latrine with vent pipe

Problems with flies

Place a tight-fitting wooden or concrete lid over the squat hole. A mud floor can be moulded to fit the lid exactly.

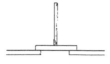

Figure A9.9 Lid over squat hole

Difficult for children, elderly, pregnant and disabled to use

○ Keep the squat hole small. A rectangular hole 25cm × 12cm or a keyhole shaped hole will be easy to use and small enough to prevent children falling through.

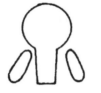

Figure A9.10 Keyhole shape

○ Children's latrines can be built for small children. These can be shallower, with hand-rails for support and less screening. Encourage the child to use a potty, then throw the contents of the potty into the pit latrine. Improve access by making a gently inclining path, and where steep install steps with handrails.

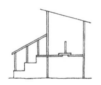

Figure A9.11 Cross section of steps and latrine

○ Provide a squatting seat. High seats are easier for the person to sit on, but aiming into the squat hole is more difficult.

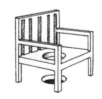

Figure A9.12 Chair over hole

○ Provide hand-rails to support the person while using the latrine.

Termite damage

Use local termite-resistant timbers such as fence-post palm. Paint the timber with old engine oil prior to use.

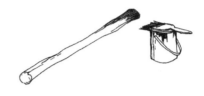

Figure A9.13 Painting timber

Collapsing soils

○ Make round pits and line them with stone, bricks, concrete blocks or concrete rings.

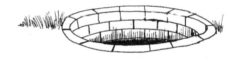

Figure A9.14 Block-lined hole

○ Use narrow pits and line with perforated clay pots or oil drums.

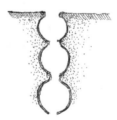

Figure A9.15 Cross section of hole lined with jars

○ Dig shallow pits that are wider at the top than at the base (most stable with a 45° angle or less).

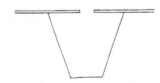

Figure A9.16 Cross section of trapezoidal hole

Hard rock

○ Use pickaxes or crowbars to break through the rock, crack the rock by heating with fire and quenching with water.

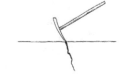

Figure A9.17 Pick and crack

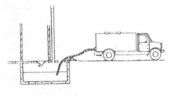

Figure A9.22 Vacuum tanker

○ Full pits can be emptied with a vacuum tanker if the contents of the pit are wet.

High watertable

Do not use groundwater for drinking within 200m radius of the latrine if the soils are made of coarse gravel of fissured rock. In areas with fine soils and clays a shorter distance may be acceptable. Construct pit above the ground with the latrine above it.

○ Build pit over natural crack or crevice (but do not use groundwater for drinking).

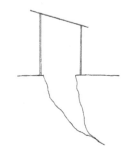

Figure A9.18 Profile of latrine over crack

○ Construct pit above the rock. Slab may be above ground level.

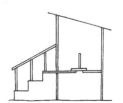

Figure A9.19 Cross section of steps beside latrine

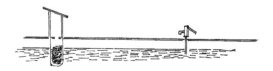

Figure A9.23 Cross section of latrine and water pump with aquifer

Latrine already full

○ Dig a new pit for a new latrine in another location.

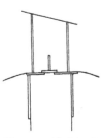

Figure A9.20 Cross section of simple latrine

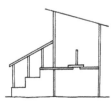

Figure A9.24 Cross section of steps beside latrine

○ Empty the full latrine pit. Handle sludge with care and bury it. The old latrine superstructure may need to be demolished.

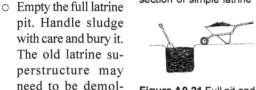

Figure A9.21 Full pit and wheelbarrow

Alternating pit latrine

This 'ecosan' variation on the simple pit latrine can use a timber and mud slab or a concrete slab over two pits, which may each be 2m or more in depth. The slab should be firmly supported on all sides and raised above the surrounding ground so that surface water cannot enter the pit. The pits must be lined with brick or stone, and be large enough to take an accumulation of faecal solids over a period of two years or more. A squat hole in the slab is provided over each pit so that excreta falls directly into the pit. Using a tight-fitting wooden cover over the squat hole when the latrine is not in use will reduce the access of flies into the pit. A second, larger hole is required over each pit so that a person with a bucket or the pipe of a vacuum truck can remove the contents of the pit. One pit is used until it is full. It is then closed and the second pit is used until that too is full, by which time (one year or more) the contents of the first pit will have completely decomposed and even the most persistent pathogens will have

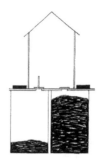

Figure A9.25 Cross section of latrine with two pits

been destroyed. The contents of the first pit are then dug out (it is easier to dig out than undisturbed soil). The first pit can then be used again.

These latrines can be built on a larger scale as communal latrines. However, communal latrines are often poorly maintained; a possible solution is the recruitment of communal latrine attendants.

Table A9.3 Advnatages and disadvantages of alternating pit latrines

Advantages	Disadvantages
○ Low cost, can be built by householder ○ Needs no water for operation ○ Once constructed, pits are more or less permanent ○ Easy removal of solids ○ Pit contents safe to use as a soil conditioner after one year if ash or lime are added to the pit weekly ○ Can be constructed as communal facilities with additional stances and larger pit volumes	○ Considerable fly nuisance (and mosquitoes if the pit is wet), unless there is a tight fitting cover over the squat hole when the latrine is not in use ○ Bad smell ○ Vacuum tankers are expensive to hire and people may not be willing to dig out the pit contents

Source: Adapted from Franceys et al, 1992.

Ventilated improved pit latrine

Variations of the traditional pit latrine include the ventilated improved pit (VIP) latrine. Fly and odour nuisance may be substantially reduced if the pit is ventilated by a pipe extending at least 0.5m above the latrine roof, with fly-proof netting (preferably with 1.5mm mesh) across the top of the pipe. Wind blowing across the top of the vent pipe causes air in the vent pipe to move upwards. When there is no wind, air in the vent pipe moves upwards if it is heated by the sun. Smells from the pit are carried up the pipe and escape from the top. Flies from outside are attracted to the pipe by smell but cannot get through the netting. Flies hatching in the pit are attracted by light at the top of the vent and fly upwards, but cannot get out through the fly

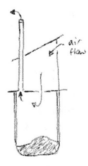

Figure A9.26 Cross section of latrine with vent pipe and air flow

screen. It is essential that the superstructure shades the squatting hole to prevent flies from exiting. It is also essential that the vent pipe extends above the superstructure, nearby trees and other buildings by at least 0.5m. While in theory VIP latrines are simple to build and should provide effective fly control, they are often poorly constructed, badly sealed or incorrectly ventilated and do not live up to their reputation.

It is difficult to construct VIP latrines as communal facilities; increasing the number of squat holes and the number and size of vent pipes can prevent the effective circulation of air and cause the smells to rise into the latrine house. Check the ventilation by performing the smoke test (see below).

Table A9.4 Advantages and disadvantages of VIP latrines

Advantages	Disadvantages
○ Medium cost	○ Does not control mosquitoes if pit is wet
○ Needs no water for operation	○ Need to replace the vent fly-screen every three months or before
○ Can be built by householder	it becomes rotten
	○ Difficult or expensive to empty pit once it is full
	○ Difficult to keep the airflow patterns as intended when constructed as communal facilities

Source: Adapted from Franceys et al, 1992.

Alternating ventilated pit latrine

This 'ecosan' variation on the VIP latrine can have either a timber and mud slab or a concrete slab over twin pits, which may each be 2m or more in depth. The slab should be firmly supported on all sides and raised above the surrounding ground so that surface water cannot enter the pit. The pits must be lined with brick or stone and be large enough to take an accumulation of faecal solids over a period of two years or more. A squat hole in the slab or a seat is provided over each pit so that the excreta falls directly into the pit. Again, a tight fitting wooden cover over the squat hole when the latrine is not in use will reduce the access of flies into the pit. A second, larger, hole is required over each pit so that a person or the pipe of a vacuum truck can remove the contents of the pit. A third hole is required in each slab for the vent pipe. The operation is the same as that of the alternating pit latrine. One pit is used until it is full, and then the second pit is used until that too is full, by which time the contents of the first pit can be dug out (it is easier to dig out than undisturbed soil) and the first pit can then be used again.

These latrines can be constructed as communal facilities but caution must be taken to ensure that the circulation of air within the latrine structure is maintained as intended. Ventilation can be tested by performing the smoke test (see below).

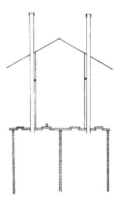

Figure A9.27 Latrine with two vaults and two vent pipes

Smoke test

The air movement in VIP latrines can be tested before using the latrine. When the latrine construction is complete, drop a smouldering bundle of dry grass or crumpled paper down the squat hole. Smoke should flow out of the top of the vent pipe and not out of the squat hole. If smoke does come up through the squat hole, the ventilation is not working correctly. Try to seal the gaps between the slab and the ground and perform the smoke test again. If ventilation is still not working correctly, place a well-fitting lid over the squat hole.

Table A9.5 Advantages and disadvantages of alternating VIP latrines

Advantages	Disadvantages
○ Medium cost, can be built by householder ○ Needs no water for operation ○ Once constructed the pits are more or less permanent ○ Easy removal of solids from the pits as they are shallow ○ Pit contents can be safely used as a soil conditioner after one year without treatment if ash/lime are added to the pit weekly	○ Does not control mosquitoes if pit is wet ○ Cost of providing a vent pipe may be more than the rest of the latrine ○ Need to replace the vent fly-screen every three months or before it becomes rotten ○ Vacuum tankers are expensive and people may not be willing to dig out the pit contents ○ Difficult to keep the airflow patterns as intended when constructed as communal facilities

Source: Adapted from Franceys et al, 1992.

Dry-box latrine

The dry-box 'ecosan' latrine is usually built above ground. Its receptacle consists of two sealed boxes or vaults, each with a hatch on the outside. On top of the vaults there is a squat hole with a urine collector from which the urine flows via a pipe into a soakpit or is collected in a jar and diluted to be used as liquid fertilizer. After using the latrine the user sprinkles ashes, soil or a soil/lime mixture over the faeces. Every week the contents of the box need to be stirred with a long stick and more ashes added. On the same principle as alternating pit latrines, when the first box is nearly filled up it should be closed off and then the second box is used. A year later and before the second box is full, the first box can be emptied and the contents safely used as a soil conditioner. The dry-box latrine can be attached to a house and is suitable for high-density areas. It is important to keep all liquids out of the box because they slow down the decomposition and result in foul smells and fly infestations. If the urine collector is considered too difficult, a pipe can be installed at the base of the box to drain the liquids into a soak-away pit.

Table A9.6 Advantages and disadvantages of dry-box latrines

Advantages	Disadvantages
○ Medium cost ○ Low smell ○ Once constructed the system is more or less permanent ○ Easy removal of solids from the pits as they are shallow ○ Pit contents can be safely used as a soil conditioner after one year ○ System can be used in rural or urban areas	○ Requires much more attention than other latrine types ○ Contents of the pit must be kept dry to avoid smell and fly problems ○ Faeces require covering with a thin layer of crushed lime/soil mixture or ashes after use in order to reduce fly problems and encourage composting process ○ Contents of pit require stirring every week to encourage composting ○ System less appropriate for people who use water for anal cleansing

Water-borne excreta disposal facilities

In some situations with high water tables, or very high population densities and good piped water supply, water-borne facilities may be appropriate. Details of these and other sanitation facilities can be found in other sanitation text books, such as Franceys et al (1992).

Hand washing facilities without piped water

Proper hand washing is one of the most effective ways of preventing the spread of diarrhoeal diseases, including cholera and dysentery. Disease-causing organisms cannot be seen on hands. Water alone is not sufficient to remove them. Soap or wood ash are both cleansing and disinfecting agents when used with water. They actually kill disease-causing organisms and sterilize hands and utensils. The most important times that hands should be washed with soap or ash are:

○ After going to the toilet;
○ After cleaning a child who has gone to the toilet.

Hand washing before handling food and before eating should also be encouraged. Promoting hand washing may require mobilization and education activities. However, to make hand washing part of the daily routine, hand washing facilities, water and soap/ash must be located near to the places where they should be used (i.e. kitchens and latrines). This section contains some suggestions for hand washing facilities, where running water is not available and convenient.

Container with tap
A container, such as an oil-can or bucket fitted with a tap or even pierced with a large nail, is the simplest way of providing hand washing facilities where they are needed. Some are available mounted on stands with a ledge on which to place soap. The larger the container, the less frequently water needs to be topped up.

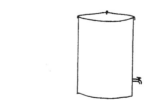

Figure A9.28 Container with tap

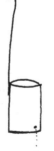

Leaking container
A container, such as an oil barrel, can easily be contaminated when people with unwashed hands collect water from it. A leaking jug, such as a tin can with holes in its base and fitted with a long handle with a hooked end, can be used to scoop water from the large container. By hooking it over the rim of the large container it provides a measured stream of running water for hand washing.

Figure A9.29 Leaky container

Tippy tap

A tippy tap is a suspended container which, when tipped, pours water on to the hands of the person using it. They can easily be made out of the plastic cooking oil containers or drinking water bottles and use a minimal amount of water.

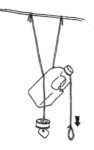

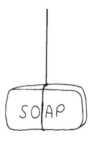

Figure A9.30 Tippy tap

Soap on a rope

Soap can be kept clean by suspending it off the ground. Tying string round the centre of the soap, or through a hole made in the middle of the soap can help to keep the soap off the ground and near the place of use.

Figure A9.31 Soap on a rope

A10

Community management and sustainability

As discussed previously, the long-term maintenance of water and sanitation installations should always be taken into account, even in emergency situations. This is especially important where permanent water supplies are being constructed or renovated. People will not automatically assume responsibility for keeping the system functional in the longer term, and may think that this will be taken care of by the agency concerned. The community may well have 'participated' in construction work but this does not automatically mean that they feel a sense of ownership for the completed project. Beneficiaries need to be involved in the decision-making process from inception to completion – from selection of water sources to be used, locations for installations, actions to be taken to improve health, to the financial arrangements for the longer term. However, it is also important not to expect that community management can work without outside support and a thorough assessment of the situation is important as soon as feasible.

To ensure community management is optimized in any emergency water, sanitation and hygiene project, the following points should be considered:

○ Do people in the community consider that the project responds to a priority felt need?
○ Have all sections of the community been consulted? A thorough assessment is necessary which identifies different groups in the community, their views about water, sanitation, health and their perceptions of the proposed project. Consensus will need to be reached on the siting of installations.
○ Have women been involved as far as possible in the initial discussions on the proposed project? (Women are often the main water carriers and users. This may involve work on building up self-esteem and confidence among women and ensuring that men are aware of the necessity for involving women.).
○ Are the disabled involved and will they have access? Will other disadvantaged groups such as minority groups or the very poorest have access?
○ Does the project have the support of the local government and community leaders? If respected community leaders are available they, rather than the agency involved, should lead the discussions.
○ Ensure that you have consulted and involved the water authorities as far as possible and that issues of long-term management have been discussed.
○ Have those involved in the community management and hygiene promotion aspects, and those involved in the engineering components, met to discuss how they can work together to achieve the goal of community management? If not, organize a short workshop to discuss the importance of this, and to formulate strategies for its inclusion.
○ Initiate training of committees/user groups as early as possible.
○ Try to ensure open and ongoing dialogue about the project. It is important to remain flexible and to encourage suggestions from community members on how the project should proceed.
○ If people do not attend meetings, try to find out why as soon as possible by discussing with people at places where they naturally meet, for example, at the water source. Find out if alternative arrangements can be made.

o Ensure that the issue of long-term maintenance is raised as soon as possible with community groups. Ask them how they intend to repair the system if it breaks down or what provision they have made for this in the past. This might involve discussion of the need for user fees or other payments, who will administer and collect these fees, financial accountability and the need for further training in such things as accounts and financial management. They will also need to identify who will actually do the maintenance and whether they need to be trained. Water committees may be set up.
o Maintenance issues should then be discussed in an open forum in order to arrive at some consensus from all users.
o Different groups may have alternative plans for the same water points. Visits by community members to other successful or unsuccessful projects in the vicinity may be considered.
o Formal agreements and contracts should be drafted when discussions have been finalized.
o Formulate objectives, indicators and means of verification to evaluate the capacity for community management, level of participation, and degree of integration of software and hardware components to the satisfaction of the intended project beneficiaries.

How to measure/evaluate community management?

Community management can be evaluated using the indicators suggested by Narayan (1993) in her capacity-building framework, focusing particularly on sustainability and replicability (also see page 91):

Framework of capacity-building indicators

Sustainability

o reliability of systems – quality of water at source, number of facilities in working order, maintenance arrangements;
o human capacity development – management abilities, knowledge and skills, confidence/self-esteem;
o local institutional capacity – autonomy, supportive leadership, systems for ongoing learning and problem-solving;
o cost sharing and unit costs – community contribution, agency contribution, unit costs;
o collaboration among organizations – planning, activities, level of coordination.

Replicability

o community ability to expand services – additional water/latrine facilities built, upgraded facilities, new development activities initiated;
o transferability of agency strategies – proportion and role of specialized personnel, established institutional framework, budget size, documented administrative and implementation procedures;
o other special unique conditions.

Source: Adapted from Narayan, 1993.

Measuring participation

The spider gram matrix given overleaf can be used to help measure the concept of participation which is vital to effective community management and sustainability. How to use a spider gram is explained on page 94.

Table A10.1 Participation spider gram matrix

Indicator	1 (bad)	2 (poor)	3 (fair)	4 (good)	5 (excellent)
Assessment	Assessed by agency	Assessed by agency but with community involvement	Leaders and agency assessed needs	Leaders assessed needs but without consulting the community	Leaders in consultation with community assessed needs and informed agency
Planning	Planning done by agency staff in office	Planning done in consultation with community leaders	Planning done in consultation with community leaders, men and women but fixed agenda	Planning decisions made following discussions with variety of community members including marginalized groups	Community members able to request agency to organise work differently and make suggestions about what they want
Implementation	Agency requests community to participate - community sees project as belonging to agency	Community leaders are consulted about ongoing work	Community leaders and others are consulted about ongoing work	Problems arising in course of work are taken to community meetings for resolution	Representative group monitors implementation and is able to easily access agency staff for discussions
Monitoring and Evaluation	Indicators are set by agency staff only	Community members asked to carry out monitoring tasks	Community members take part in monitoring activities and providing feedback	Community helps to define own indicators for programme	Community members take an active part in both monitoring and evaluating programme
Involvement of women	No women involved in decision making	Women on committees but in a minority and do not talk	Women represented equally but talk occasionally	Women talk as much as men	Decisions taken equally by men and women

Example of a community contract

The example on the next page of a community contract could be adapted to suit the agreements made between the development partners that you are dealing with. Details of the facilities to be constructed, services to be provided, contributions to be made, etc., by whom and in what time-frame, should all be clearly specified so that all parties understand and no confusion remains.

Box A10.1 Example of a community contract

This contract outlines the agreement between ...x... (Name of community) and ...y... (Name of Organization/s) regarding the provision of ...z... (details of facilities and services).

...y... organization undertakes to work in partnership with ...x... community in order to facilitate the provision of ...z... number and location of facilities in ...x... location within the community area. ...y... organization will facilitate only the provision of ...z... facilities or services. ...y... organization will NOT be responsible for providing manual labour, locally available materials, payment for community members or for long-term maintenance of ...z... facilities. ...y... organization's involvement in this project is reliant on the commitment of ...x... community. Each party is bound by the terms of this agreement. Both parties reserve the right to sever relations if either side does not comply with the terms of the agreement or if materials supplied by either party are misappropriated.

Under the terms of the agreement the community will have the following obligations:
...x... community will settle all rights of ownership and rights of way prior to commencement of any other activities.

Labour:
...x... community will provide the necessary labour for the construction of ...z... facilities, including extraction and removal of soil, provision of masons and carpenters, labour to assist the masons or carpenters, and any other assistance that may be required.

Materials:
...x... community will provide the necessary locally available materials such as sand, sticks, clay, soil blocks and clean water for the construction work. The community will be responsible for project materials and will secure them as necessary.

Accommodation and food:

...x... community will provide accommodation for the project staff if required. A contribution for food will be sought from ...y.. organization for the labourers only but ...x... community will prepare this food.

Maintenance:
On completion of the work the community will immediately become responsible for the longterm maintenance of the ...z... facilities. In order to minimize damage to the facilities and to minimize the risk of disease, all community members will be responsible for day-to-day use, care and maintenance. The community will be required to finance the cost of spare parts where and when necessary. (Where latrines are provided, those responsible for organizing a system to providing handwashing facilities including water and soap, and cleaning and maintaining the latrines should be specified.)

The community will establish and support a water, latrine or community development committee. If such a committee does not already exist, the community should elect at least four male and four female representatives. Members of the committee will be assigned roles, including that of chairperson, secretary and treasurer. The community will identify two suitable people (one man and one woman) to be trained in basic maintenance of each facility. These two people should also be included on the committee.

Under the terms of the agreement ...y... organization has the following obligations:

Labour:
...y... organization will be responsible for the supervision of construction of facilities. ...y... organization will provide training in basic maintenance of the facilities for two caretakers chosen by the community. In addition ...y... organization will work with members of the community to ensure that people are aware of how they can best prevent contamination of water supplies.

Materials:
...y... organization will be responsible for providing all materials that are not available locally, as specified in the community obligations above. ...y... organization will provide advanced notice of two days prior to any construction work. In case of a deteriorated security situation or during the period of heaviest rains, ...y... organization reserves the right to cease all the agreed work. This work will be resumed as soon as conditions allow.

Signatories of the agreement

Parish Chief:

Village Chief:

Elders:

Women's Leader:

Representative of ...y... organization:

DATE:

Assessment tool for sustainable water supplies

Below is a list of key questions that need to be answered in order to support the design and implementation of a sustainable water system. Useful methods that can be used to collect this data and help the community to explore the issue of maintenance are also suggested but there may be other methods that are more suitable for a particular context. (These could be adapted for sanitation and for hygiene.)

Social dynamics and livelihoods

Venn diagram

- How is the community organized – who are the leaders and opinion makers (male and female), what groups exist (youth, women, NGOs, CBOs, co-ops), what committees/management groups exist?
- Are there differences in terms of access and use for different tribes, religions, clans or castes?
- How influential is current leadership and/or administration?
- Who are the stakeholders in any proposed project (consider above groups, local government – including different ministries, local enterprises, NGOs etc.)?
- What potential do they have to support sustainability (experience and skills in sector, management systems and accountability, mobility, community mobilization and conflict resolution skills)?

Gender role analysis/pocket voting

O Gender differences: who collects water, who controls decision making, who controls finances? Attitude to women technicians etc.

Mapping

O What are the livelihood groups and what are the water requirements?
O Who are vulnerable groups and where do they live (older people, disabled, chronic illness, single parent headed household)?
O Educational level of men and women.
O Do men and women understand the importance of management of water system?

Government policy and legal considerations

O What is the government policy and strategy for water supply systems?
O Does the government support community management?
O What hand pumps does the government approve?
O What government level arrangements for maintenance are in place (village-level operation and maintenance, public-private operation and maintenance etc.)?
O Who owns the water supply systems?
O Who owns the land on which systems are built or could be built?
O What legal frameworks are accepted by the government with regard to water supply?

Choice of technology

Mapping

O What systems have been used previously (in this and surrounding areas) and why did they fail/succeed? (Consider ownership, control, government policy and support.)
O Groundwater levels and seasonal variation.
O What are the maintenance requirements for different systems (skills required, spare parts, cost, ease of repair, expected frequency of repair/maintenance for each type of technology)?

Training requirements

Mapping (some questions can be combined with the above)

O Were committees identified – are they functioning? If not, why not?
O What sort of water and sanitation related training was carried out?
O What systems exist for providing ongoing training and support?
O What are people's expectations in terms of access and quantity of water required? (Consider all water needs including those needed to sustain livelihoods and extra requirements for people with special needs.)
O What are people prepared/able to pay for water? Consider current situation and more stable situation (look at different livelihood/income groups).
O When are people best able to pay water charges (seasonal income etc.)?
O Who needs support in paying?
O What are the water requirements of community institutions (clinic, school, mosque etc.)?

A11
Glossary

AIMS: the final long-term goal of the project. In a health promotion project this can be seen as an improvement in the quality of life.

BASELINE DATA: the information gathered at the beginning of the project cycle that will subsequently be compared with information from the evaluation in order to determine the effect of the project. Ideally it should inform the project plan.

CLUSTER SAMPLING: a type of sampling used to obtain a random selection of people/households. This approach overcomes the constraints associated with working with a very dispersed population. The area is divided into 'clusters' of villages or towns and can be sub-divided into smaller groups of households. When all the units of the selected cluster are interviewed, this is referred to as 'one-stage cluster sampling'. If the subjects to be interviewed are selected randomly within the selected clusters, it is called 'two-stage cluster sampling'.

COMMUNITY PARTICIPATION: a catchall phrase currently popular in development circles. It is often supported as a means to promote community ownership and the sustainability of a project. It may be used simply as a way of obtaining cheap labour, which is unlikely to generate commitment to the project. Different levels of participation are, however, possible and people must be able to choose whether they want to participate or not. It is a term best avoided unless it is defined adequately and attempts are made to measure if it is happening or not.

COMPLEX EMERGENCIES: these are emergency situations that are caused by a complex web of political, social, economic and environmental factors, which are compounded by conflict.

DIDACTIC TEACHING: or 'empty vessel' teaching tries to pour knowledge into people (as if they were empty vessels) and assumes that lecturing people is sufficient for learning to take place.

FIELDWORKER: anyone who works at the grassroots level with communities, be this in an emergency or in a developmental situation.

FORMATIVE EVALUATION: an evaluation carried out when the project is in progress to assess whether it is on track and likely to meet its goals and objectives. Mid-term evaluations are formative evaluations. Formative evaluation tries to analyse project processes and assess their effectiveness.

INDICATORS: these will serve to indicate if objectives have been achieved. They may involve numbers such as percentages or descriptions of processes.

LOGICAL FRAMEWORK (LOGFRAME): a tool for project planning that employs a four square matrix detailing different levels of objectives and what is necessary for achieving these. A logical sequence can be traced between each square of the matrix and the next square, such that without fulfilling one condition another condition cannot be met.

MEANS OF VERIFICATION: these are the tools used to measure the indicators. They may include the use of PLA/participatory evaluation techniques or questionnaire surveys or monitoring forms.

MONITORING: an ongoing process of data collection. Monitoring examines individual aspects of the project by maintaining project records and assessing whether aspects of the project are working as planned.

OBJECTIVES: the successive steps that are necessary in order to achieve the final goal. Objectives may be broken down into intermediate goals and outputs.

OUTCOMES: the results of the project activities and outputs, for example, people drinking clean water or using latrines to dispose of excreta. If this happens then it is assumed that the project will achieve its impact on health and the reduction of diarrhoea.

OUTPUTS: the results of undertaking the project activities such as constructing wells and latrines or training outreach workers. The outputs will be in the form of systems for improved drinking water or excreta disposal. However, the fact that these systems have been provided does not necessarily mean that people will be using them to optimal effect and every project should strive to ensure that the outcomes are also achieved.

PARTICIPATORY EVALUATION: a process of actively involving community members in the process of data collection and evaluation so that they have access to information that is necessary for future planning and action.

PARTICIPATORY LEARNING AND ACTION: a philosophy of learning that respects the existing knowledge that people have. New learning is generated through the analysis of existing conditions and this often leads to action. PLA often uses techniques derived from anthropology which allow people to visualize particular problems or situations through the use of pictures or symbols. These techniques also stimulate dialogue and discussion. In pure PLA, power and control lie with the participants and they direct the process. PLA has evolved from PRA and RRA.

PARTICIPATORY METHODS OF LEARNING: these should involve the learner in interaction with the teacher or facilitator. They may include such things as the use of drama, songs and visual aids which are used to encourage discussion and enhance the capacity for problem-solving. It differs from PLA in that the teacher or facilitator usually sets the agenda and controls the process.

PARTICIPATORY RESEARCH: this is similar to PLA and draws on many of the same techniques. It is an approach that is more closely associated with health promotion than PLA but which is less political.

PARTICIPATORY RURAL APPRAISAL: an approach to project assessment and appraisal using anthropological techniques. The emphasis is on people's participation in the process of data collection and how the results of the assessment can be used by them. This has now come to be known as PLA.

PROXY INDICATOR: an indicator that substitutes for the measurement of impact, for example, use of latrines can substitute for health indicators that are difficult to obtain and measure accurately. Proxy indicators often measure outcomes rather than impact.

PURPOSIVE SAMPLING: a non-random sampling method which selectively identifies people in order to ascertain data from specific groups.

RAPID RURAL APPRAISAL: an approach originally used in agricultural projects to bypass more detailed ethnographic studies. RRA provided a rapid and effective alternative.

SAMPLING: a way of finding out about the whole population by studying just a small part of it.

THE SPHERE PROJECT: a project aiming to improve accountability of agencies working in emergencies. A set of standards and indicators have been produced as well as training on the use of these.

SUMMATIVE (OR FINAL) EVALUATION: an evaluation conducted at the end of the project cycle to ascertain if project aims and objectives have been met. It attempts to sum up the effectiveness of the project.

SUSTAINABILITY: another popular development term. It refers to the important concept of ensuring that the project has long-term feasibility. This means not only that the outputs of the project will continue functioning once the agency has left, but that the effects of the project do not compromise the feasibility of other development goals.

TRIANGULATION: a way of cross checking assessment or baseline data by using at least three other methods/tools to collect similar information

A12

Annotated bibliography

Boot, M. T. (1991) *Just Stir Gently: The Way to Mix Hygiene Education with Water Supply and Sanitation*, IRC, The Netherlands.
This book provides options and methods for integrating hygiene education with water supply and sanitation projects. Aspects covered include the process of behavioural change, hygiene education planning, implementation and evaluation, programme organization, manpower and costs. It is primarily intended for those involved with the planning and implementation of hygiene education.

Boot, M. T. and Cairncross, A. (1993) *ACTIONS Speak: The Study of Hygiene Behaviour in Water and Sanitation Projects*, IRC, The Netherlands.
This book is the outcome of a workshop on the measurement of hygiene behaviour, held in Oxford in 1991. The papers and discussions from this workshop form the basis of a comprehensive analysis of the ways that hygiene behaviour can best be studied and interpreted so as to provide the information needed to get the best out of water supply, sanitation and hygiene education projects.

Curtis, V. and Cairncross, S. (2003) 'Effect of washing hands with soap on diarrhoea risk in the community: A systematic review', *The Lancet Infectious Diseases*, **3** (5), pp 275–81.
The authors showed that, on current evidence, washing hands with soap can reduce the risk of diarrhoeal diseases by 42–47 per cent.

Curtis, V. and Kanki, B. (1998) *Hygienic, Happy and Healthy: How to Set Up a Hygiene Promotion Programme* (Volumes 1, 2, 3, and 4), UNICEF, WHO, LSHTM, MoH Burkino Faso.
This useful series of four short manuals, using the techniques of social mobilization, show the reader how to use formative research to encourage people to adopt safer hygiene practices in a development context. No. 1 in the series covers how to plan a hygiene promotion programme, No. 2 covers setting up a hygiene promotion programme, No. 3 covers motivating behaviour change and No. 4 covers designing a hygiene communication programme.

Davis, J. and Lambert, R. (1995) *Engineering in Emergencies: A Practical Guide for Relief Workers*, Intermediate Technology Publications, London.
This comprehensive book draws on the experience of a wide range of relief workers who have worked in numerous emergencies around the world. It covers the very practical issues of how to improve water supplies and sanitation, and the options available. It also includes sections on refugee needs, personal effectiveness and the international relief system.

Esrey, S. A., Potash J. B., Roberts, L. and Shiff, C. (1991) 'Effects of improved water supply on ascariasis, diarrhoea, dracunculiasis, hookworm infection, schistosomiasis and trachoma', *Bulletin of the World Health Organization*, **69** (5), pp 609–21.
This academic paper compares 144 epidemiological studies to examine the impact of improved water supply and sanitation facilities on six water- and sanitation-related diseases. It concludes that 65 per cent of child diarrhoea mortality was reduced by the provision of water and sanitation facilities. The research also separated the effects of different interventions on diarrhoeal disease morbidity; sanitation alone was associated with a 36 per cent reduction, improved hygiene was associated with a 33 per cent reduction, water quantity was associated with a 20 per cent

reduction, and water quality with a 15 per cent reduction.

Feuerstein, M. (1986) *Partners in Evaluation: Evaluating Development and Community Programmes with Participants*, Macmillan, London.
This book paved the way for development in participatory evaluation. It gives details of how to plan and conduct an evaluation and how to provide useful feedback to the community. It has a large section on how to carry out questionnaire surveys, sampling and report writing. The illustrations provide useful examples of how to represent information in a pictorial way so that non-literate people can understand it.

Fewtrell, L. Kaufmann, R. B., Kay, D., Enanoria, W., Haller, L., Colford, J. M. (2005) *Lancet Infectious Diseases*, **5** (1), pp 42–52.
This meta-analysis of recent health impact studies of water, sanitation and hygiene interventions provides percentage reduction figures for the reduction of diarrhoea: sanitation 31 per cent (was 37 per cent) reduction, water availability 25 per cent (was 20 per cent) reduction, water quality giving a 31 per cent (was 15 per cent) reduction, hygiene promotion 38 per cent (was 33 per cent) reduction and handwashing a 44 per cent (was 41 per cent) reduction. (Former meta-review figures (mostly Esrey et al, 1986) in brackets.)

Freire, P. (1972) *Pedagogy of the Oppressed*, Penguin Books, London.
This seminal text details Freire's ideas on 'conscientisation' and education for freedom. In it he explains how the so-called 'helping professions' can often undermine people's quest for self-determination by their patronizing approach to teaching. He outlines the approach of conscientisation, which involves the stimulation of dialogue to produce group-generated learning that will lead to group-determined actions.

Gordon, G. (1986) *Puppets for Better Health*, Macmillan, London.
This book describes the contribution that puppets can make to health promotion, with examples from the author's experience in northern Ghana. The importance of community participation is stressed, particularly in developing stories with local people so that they reflect local problems, options and values. Detailed instructions are given for making different types of puppets, props and theatres using local materials and skills. The book includes suggestions of follow-up activities after the show, and how it can be evaluated so that puppet shows are not 'just entertainment'.

Hanbury, C. (Ed) (1993) *Child-to-Child and Children Living in Camps*, Child-to-Child Trust, London.
This book provides numerous different activities that can be used with children. It has sections on clean water, how to prevent diarrhoea and other illnesses, and caring for children with diarrhoea. It also has a chapter on how to work with the special needs of traumatized children.

Hartford, N. and Baird, N. (1997) *How to Make and Use Visual Aids*, Heinemann, London.
The book offers many practical, low-cost suggestions for visual aids. It is both a starting point for those with little experience and a rich source of new ideas for those who already use a variety of visual aids. It shows how visual aids can be used to support both teaching and development work, covers a wide range of visual aids – from chalkboards to card games, from posters to puppets – is easy to use with clear illustrations and step-by-step instructions.

Hope, A. and Timmel, S. (1984) *Training for Transformation*, Intermediate Technology Publications, London and Mambo Press, Zimbabwe.
Three separate manuals comprise this training handbook. They provide an excellent introduction to participatory development and are full of practical ideas, suggestions, case studies and training exercises. They have been widely used by many organizations.

Hubley, J. (1993) *Communicating Health: An Action Guide to Health Education and Health Promotion*, Macmillan, London.
This book explores the role of communication in improving people's health and discusses strategies for health education, health promotion and

the empowerment of individuals and communities to take action on health issues. Practical guidelines are given on how to carry out effective communication in a wide range of settings including family, community, schools and health services employing different media of communication.

IT Publications (1988) *The Copy Book – Copyright-free Illustrations for Development*, IT Publications, London.
This useful book contains lots of pictures with clear instructions on how to copy the pictures and make pictures and posters of your own.

Jones, H. and Reed, B. (2005) *Water and Sanitation for Disabled People and Other Vulnerable Groups: Designing Services to Improve Accessibility*, WEDC, Loughborough.
This publication shares ideas on how water and sanitation facilities have been adapted by and for disabled people in developing countries, including Bangladesh, Uganda and Cambodia. Available in CD and book formats.

Linney, B. (1995) *Pictures, People and Power*, Macmillan, Hong Kong.
This book provides an in-depth analysis of how pictures can be used in a more empowering way to support learning by drawing on indigenous knowledge. It covers such issues as visual literacy, people producing their own visual representations and how pictures can support multi-channel communication rather than the single-channel communication of message-based posters. Linney argues that visual literacy is a skill that can be easily learned and he suggests that this can either be done in a dominating way by people with 'superior knowledge' or as a means of empowering people.

Narayan, D. (1993) *Participatory Evaluation: Tools for Managing Change in Water and Sanitation*, World Bank, Washington DC.
This excellent introduction to participatory evaluation in the water and sanitation sector provides a framework for setting targets and indicators with the community and subsequently evaluating the effectiveness of specific interventions. It gives numerous examples of projects that have successfully managed to incorporate participatory techniques into planning and evaluation.

Pretty, J., Guijt, I., Thompson, J. and Scoones, I. (1995) *Participatory Learning and Action: A Trainer's Guide*, IIED, London.
This book provides a very comprehensive description of the theory and practice of PLA. It gives detailed explanations of how to conduct PLA exercises and what the pitfalls are. The style is easy to read and the illustrations provide additional explanation of some of the methods. This is an excellent resource for trainers, as over 100 different exercises are described.

Röhr-Rouendaal, P. (1997 and 2007) *Where There Is No Artist: Development Drawings and How to Use Them*, Intermediate Technology Publications, London.
A very useful copyright-free collection of over 1200 drawings for anyone wanting to prepare visual aids and materials. Clear instructions on making up your own pictures, comics, flexiflans and puppets. Also plenty of copy pictures of people doing various activities, including some related to hygiene. The example flexiflans are included in this manual. Now available on CD.

Rowntree, D. (1981) *Statistics Without Tears: A Primer for Non-Mathematicians*, Penguin Mathematics, UK.
A statistics book written in simple clear terminology. Provides help for those interested in using project data to evaluate project progress and outcomes. Even so, it requires the reader to have some understanding of or aptitude for statistics.

Smith, A. (2002) *HIV/AIDS and Emergencies: Analysis and Recommendations for Pratice*, HPN Network Paper 38, ODI, London.
This paper considers the way in which emergencies increase the susceptibility of affected populations to HIV transmission and the potential impact of emergencies on the lives and livelihoods HIV infected and affected individuals and communities.

Srinivasan, L. (1990) *Tools for Community Participation: A Manual for Training Trainers in*

Participatory Techniques, PROWESS/UNDP Technical Series Involving Women in Water and Sanitation, Lessons Strategies Tools, Washington DC.
Tools for Community Participation tries to address the problem of integrating both hardware and software elements of a water and sanitation programme. It provides example activities that can be carried out with different stakeholders in the project, from community groups to engineers, programme managers and other project staff. It also details how to run a training workshop and provides very useful theoretical information on the use of participatory techniques.

Sphere Project (2004) Sphere Humanitarian Charter and Minimum Standards in Disaster Relief, Sphere Poject, www.sphereproject.org/handbook
The internationally agreed standards for disaster response; including eight core common standards on processes and people and technical standards for sectors such as hygiene promotion/sanitation/water supply. Each has minimum standards, indicators and guidelines on how to apply the standards and indicators.

Walden V. M., O'Reilly, M. and Yetter, M. (2006) *Mainstreaming HIV in Humanitarian Programmes: A Practical Approach*, Oxfam, in press.
Developed as a manual for field practitioners, this book contain case examples and guidance on mainstreaming HIV in water, sanitation and hygiene promotion programmes.

WEDC (1998) *DFID Guidance Manual on Water Supply and Sanitation Programmes*, WEDC for DFID, London.
A comprehensive manual on all aspects of water supply and sanitation in development contexts. It includes information on the social and health aspects of water and sanitation programmes as well as chapters on social marketing and the programme and project cycle.

Werner, D. (1993) *Where There Is No Doctor: A Village Health Care Handbook*, Macmillan Education, London.
This book covers a wide range of illnesses that might affect communities, from water and sanitation-related diseases to AIDS and drug addiction. It gives details of signs and symptoms and common treatment regimes. It also devotes much attention to prevention and emphasizes the importance of hygiene, a healthy diet and immunization.

Werner, D. and Bower B. (1982) *Helping Health Workers Learn*, Hesperian Foundation, USA.
This book has lots of ideas on how to train health workers and how to work more effectively with communities. The focus of the book is educational rather than medical. Rather than try to change people's attitudes and behaviour, this community-based approach tries to help people analyse and change the situation despite the constraints.

WHO (1997) *Participatory Hygiene and Sanitation Transformation: PHAST*, WHO, Geneva.
This book comes in two parts – an introductory report providing the underlying principles of PHAST and case studies from four pilot countries and a step by step guide for extension workers comprising various tools and methodologies to use when promoting improved sanitation

Wilson, J., Chandler, G. N., Mushlihatun and Jamiluddin (1991) 'Hand washing reduces diarrhoea episodes: A study in Lombok, Indonesia', *Transactions of the Royal Society of Tropical Medicine and Hygiene*, **85**, pp 819–21.
This paper describes research work carried out in Indonesia on hand washing. Hand washing with soap (particularly after defecation and after cleaning a child) was found to have a significant effect on diarrhoeal disease transmission.

Useful websites

CORE group – coalition of NGOs working in health for mothers, children and communities: http://www.coregroup.org/start.cfm

EpiInfo on www.cdc.gov

LQAS – (trainer's guide): www.coregroup.org/working_groups/ lqas_train.html

Teaching aids at Low Cost – www.talcuk.org

World Bank Empowerment Activities Database: http://web.worldbank.org

Oral Rehydration website: http://www.rehydrate.org/dehydration/ treatment_plans.htm

International Water and Sanitation Centre (IRC): http://www.irc.nl/page/115 and e-mail source weekly http://www.irc.nl/source

A training guide based on this manual is available on the web. It is called *Environmental health promotion capacity building: A training guide based on CARE's hygiene promotion manual* by Joy Morgan (2001), WELL task 0515. http:/www.lboro.ac.uk/orgs/well/resources/well-studies/full-reports-pdf

malaria control in complex emergencies e-mail: info@malariaconsortium.org

http://www.tearfund.org

http://www.healthlink.org.uk

http://www.unaids.org

http://hapinternational.org

References

Abbatt, F. and McMahon, R. (1985) *Teaching Health Care Workers – A Practical Guide*, Macmillan, London.

Almedom, A., Blumenthal, U. and Manderson, L. (1997) *Hygiene Evaluation Procedures: Approaches and Methods for Assessing Water- and Sanitation-Related Hygiene Practices*, International Nutrition Foundation for Developing Countries, London.

Bastable, A. (1998) Bucket (Nearly) Scoops Award, *RedR Newsletter*, **45**, Spring.

Bateman, M., Jahan, R. A., Brahman, S., Zeitlyn, S. and Laston, S. L. (1995) *Prevention of Diarrhoea Through Improving Hygiene Behaviours – The Sanitation and Family Education (SAFE) Pilot Project Experience*, CARE Bangladesh and ICDDR-B, Dhaka.

Boot, M. T. and Cairncross, A. (1993) *Actions Speak: The Study of Hygiene Behaviour in Water and Sanitation Projects*, IRC, The Netherlands.

CARE (1997) Dadaab Refugee Programme, internal project report, CARE Kenya, Nairobi.

CARE (1998) Siaya Health Education, Water and Sanitation Project, CARE Kenya, Nairobi.

Chambers, R. (1992) *Rural Appraisal: Rapid, Relaxed and Participatory, Discussion Paper*, Institute of Development Studies, Sussex University.

Clasen, T., Brown, J., Suntura, O. and Collin, S. (2004) 'Safe household water treatment and storage using ceramic drip filters: A randomised controlled trial in Bolivia', *Water Science and Technology*, **50** (1), pp 111–15.

Crisp, J. (1997) Complex Emergencies and Humanitarian Relief, *RedR Newsletter*, **43**, Summer.

Curtis, V. and Kanki, B. (1998) *Hygienic, Happy and Healthy, How to Set up a Hygiene Promotion Programme* (Volumes 1, 2, 3, and 4), UNICEF, WHO, LSHTM, MoH, Burkino Faso.

Curtis, V. and Cairncross, S. (2003) 'Effect of washing hands with soap on diarrhoea risk in the community: A systematic review', *Lancet Infectious Diseases*, **3**, pp 275–81.

Dale, R. (1998) *Evaluation Frameworks for Development Programmes and Projects*, Sage, New Delhi.

Darcy, J. and Hofmann, C. (2003) *ODA Briefing Paper No. 13*, ODI, London.

Davis, J. and Lambert, R. (1995) *Engineering in Emergencies: A Practical Guide for Relief Workers*, IT Publications, London.

Dawood, R. (1992) *Traveller's Health, How to Stay Healthy Abroad*, OUP, Oxford.

De Koning, K. and Martin, M. (1996) *Participatory Research in Health, Issues and Experiences*, Zed Books, London.

DFID (1997a) *Evaluation Synthesis of Rural Water and Sanitation Projects*, Evaluation Report EV 596, Department for International Development, London.

DFID (1997b) *Office Instructions Vol II, D5 Annex 3*, Department for International Development, London.

DFID (2004) *Water Action Plan, A DFID Policy Paper*, Department for International Development, London.

Duffield, M. (1994) 'Complex emergencies and the crisis of developmentalism', *IDS Bulletin*, **25** (4), pp 37–45.

Esrey, S. A. (1995) *Sustaining Health from Water and Sanitation Systems*, Proceedings of 21st WEDC Conference, Kampala, Uganda.

Esrey, S. and Habicht, J. (1986) 'Epidemiological evidence for health benefits from improved water and sanitation in developing countries', *Epidemiological Reviews*, **1**, pp 117–28.

Esrey, S. A., Potash, J. B., Roberts, L. and Shiff, C. (1991) 'Effects of improved water supply on ascariasis, diarrhoea, dracunculiasis, hookworm infection, schistosomiasis and trachoma', *Bulletin of the World Health Organization*, **69** (5), pp 609–21.

Ferron, S. (2003) *Oxfam Guidelines for Hygiene Promotion in Emergencies*, Oxfam, Oxford.

Feuerstein, M. (1986) *Partners In Evaluation, Evaluating Development and Community Programmes with Participants*, Macmillan, London.

Fewtrell, L., Kaufmann, R. B., Kay, D., Enanoria, W., Haller, L. and Colford, J. M. (2005) 'Water, sanitation and hygiene interventions to reduce diarrhoea in less developed countries: A systematic review and meta-analysis', *Lancet Infectious Diseases*, **5** (1), pp 42–52.

Franceys, R., Pickford, J. and Reed, R. (1992) *A Guide to the Development of On-site Sanitation*, WHO, Geneva.

Goma Epidemiology Group (1995) 'Public health impact of Rwandan refugee crisis: What happed in Goma, Zaire in July 1994?', *Lancet*, **11** 345 (8946), pp 339–44.

Gosling, L. and Edwards, M. (1995) *Toolkits: A Practical Guide to Assessment, Monitoring, Review and Evaluation*, SCF Development Manual 5, Save the Children, London.

Green, L. and Kreuter, M. (1991) *Health Promotion Planning, An Educational and Environmental Approach*, Mayfield Publishing Co., California.

Hanbury, C. (ed) (1993) *Child-to-Child and Children Living in Refugee Camps*, A Child-to-Child Publication, TALC, Child-to-Child, London.

Herson, M. and Mears, C. (1992) *Evaluation of Rohinga Refugee Programme*, internal report, Oxfam, Oxford.

Hubley, J. (1993) *Communicating Health: An Action Guide to Health Education and Health Promotion*, TALC Macmillan Press, London.

Howell, L. (1990) BNMT (Britain Nepal Medical Trust), Nepal

International Union for Health Promotion and Education (2000) The evidence of health promotion effectiveness – Shaping Public Health in a New Europe Parts 1 & 2, International Union for Health Promotion and Education.

JICA (1994) *Ethiopia*, internal report, JICA, Tokyo.

Khaw, A. J., Salama, P., Burkholder, B. and Dondero, T. J. (2000) 'HIV risk and prevention in emergency-affected populations: A review', *Disasters*, **24** (3), pp 181–97.

Kleinmann, A., Eisenberg, L. and Good, B. (1978) 'Culture, illness and care: Clinical lessons from anthropologic and cross-cultural research', *Annals of Internal Medicine*, **88** (2), pp 251–58.

Knowles, M. (1990) *The Adult Learner: A Neglected Species*, Gulf Publishing Company, Houston.

Linney, B. (1995) *Pictures, People and Power*, Macmillan, Hong Kong.

LWF (1997) *Seven Guiding Principles, In Conversation, Karamoja Agro-pastoral Development Project (KADP)*, LWF, Uganda

Ministry of Health Uganda (1998a) *Participatory Toolkit for Cholera Prevention*, Ministry of Health, Kampala.

Ministry of Health Uganda (1998b) *Documented experience from 1997/8 cholera epidemic (Draft)*, Ministry of Health, Kampala.

Morgan, J. (1994a) 'Sudanese refugees in Koboko', *Focus on Gender*, 2 (1), pp 41–44.

Morgan, J. (1994b) *Health Education Review*, internal document, Oxfam, Oxford.

Mulenga, D. (1994) *Participatory Research in Africa: A Critical Appraisal*, Proceedings of the International Symposium on Participatory Research in Health Promotion, Liverpool School of Tropical Medicine, Liverpool.

Naidoo, S. and Wills, J. (1994) *Health Promotion, Foundations for Practice*, Baillière Tindall, London.

Narayan-Parker, D. (1989) *Indonesia: Evaluating Community Management*, PROWESS/UNDP Technical Series, New York.

Narayan, D. (1993) *Participatory Evaluation: Tools For Managing Change In Water and Sanitation*, World Bank, Washington DC.

Narayan D. and Srinivasan L. (1994) *Participatory Development Tool Kit*, International Bank for Reconstruction and Development/World Bank, Washington DC.

Norwood, T. and Mears, C. (1993) *Evaluation of Tajik Refugee and Afghan Internally Displaced Emergency Programmes*, internal report, Oxfam, Oxford.

Oxfam (1994) *Azeri Displaced Programme Situation Reports*, internal reports, Oxfam, Oxford.

Oxfam (1995) *Goma Interim Evaluation*, internal report, Oxfam, Oxford.

Oxfam (1996) *Water Supply and Sanitation in Emergencies, Practical Guide – First Draft*, Oxfam Publications, Oxford.

Oxfam (2003) *Malawi HIV/AIDS and Orphans Home Based Care Programme*, Oxfam, Oxford.

Pretty, J., Guijt, I., Thompson, J. and Scoones, I. (1995) *Participatory Learning and Action, A Trainer's Guide*, IIED, London.

Reed, B. and Skinner, B. (1998) *Stakeholder Analysis, WEDC Uganda Training Course*, unpublished notes.

Rifkin, S. (1988) 'Primary health care: On measuring participation', *Social Science and Medicine*, **26** (9), pp 931–40.

Roche, C. (1999) *Impact Assessment for Development Agencies: Learning to Value Change*, Oxfam, Oxford.

Röhr-Rouendaal, P. (1997) *Where There Is No Artist: Development Drawings and How to Use Them*, Intermediate Technology Publications, London.

Ryan, M. A. K., Christian, R., Wohlrabe, J. (2001) *American Journal of Preventive Medicine*, 21 (2), pp 79–83.

Schouten, T. and Moriarty, P. (2003) *Community Water, Community Management from System to Service in Rural Areas*, ITDG, London.

Schroeder, G. (1997) *Refugee Relief in Somalia and Tanzania, Quick Impact, Sustainability, and Dependence Reduction*, MSc Thesis Humbolt State University, Humbolt.

Sphere Project (2004) *Humanitarian Charter and Minimum Standards in Disaster Response*, Geneva.

Srinivasan, L. (1990) *Tools for Community Participation: A Manual for Training Trainers in Participatory Techniques*, Prowess/UNDP, Washington DC.

Toole, K. (2001) DFID Logframe Training, Wolverhampton University.

Toole, M. J. and Waldman, R. J. (1990) 'Prevention of excess mortality in refugee and displaced populations in developing countries', *JAMA*, **263** (24), pp 3296–302 .

UNICEF (1999) *Towards Better Programming, A Manual on Communication for Water Supply and Environmental Sanitation Programmes*, Technical Guidelines Series, Number 7, UNICEF, New York.

UNFPA, Woman Studies Centre, Oxfam (2005) *Gender and Changes in Tsunami-affected Villages in NanggroeAceh Darussalam Province*, UNFPA, Woman Studies Centre, Oxfam, New York and Oxford.

Van Wijk, C. and Murre, T. (revised Esrey, S.) (1995) *Motivating Better Hygiene Behaviour: Importance for Public Health Mechanisms of Change*, UNICEF, New York.

Wallace, T. (1990) *Refugee Women: Their Perspectives and Our Responses*, internal document, Oxfam, Oxford.

White, S. C. (1996) 'Depoliticising development: The uses and abuses of participation', *Development in Practice*, **6** (1), pp 6–15.

Williams, S. (ed.) (1995) *Oxfam Handbook of Development and Relief*, Oxfam Publications, Oxford.

Winblad, U. (1994) 'Interrupting transmission', *Dialogue on Diarrhoea*, **57** p 2.

World Bank (1991) *A Common Vocabulary: Popular Participation Learning Group*, World Bank, Washington DC.

Index

Printed in the USA
CPSIA information can be obtained
at www.ICGtesting.com
JSHW051458221024
72172JS00011B/98

9 781853 396410

HYGIENE PROMOTION